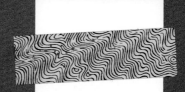

Glioblastoma

STEVEN BREM, MD
Hospital of the University of Pennsylvania
Philadelphia, PA, USA

KALIL G. ABDULLAH, MD
Hospital of the University of Pennsylvania
Philadelphia, PA, USA

ELSEVIER

ELSEVIER

1600 John F. Kennedy Blvd.
Ste 1800
Philadelphia, PA 19103-2899

Glioblastoma   ISBN: 978-0-323-47660-7

Notices

Knowledge and best practice in this field are constantly changing. As new research and experience broaden our understanding, changes in research methods, professional practices, or medical treatment may become necessary.

Practitioners and researchers must always rely on their own experience and knowledge in evaluating and using any information, methods, compounds, or experiments described herein. In using such information or methods they should be mindful of their own safety and the safety of others, including parties for whom they have a professional responsibility.

With respect to any drug or pharmaceutical products identified, readers are advised to check the most current information provided (i) on procedures featured or (ii) by the manufacturer of each product to be administered, to verify the recommended dose or formula, the method and duration of administration, and contraindications. It is the responsibility of practitioners, relying on their own experience and knowledge of their patients, to make diagnoses, to determine dosages and the best treatment for each individual patient, and to take all appropriate safety precautions.

To the fullest extent of the law, neither the Publisher nor the authors, contributors, or editors, assume any liability for any injury and/or damage to persons or property as a matter of products liability, negligence or otherwise, or from any use or operation of any methods, products, instructions, or ideas contained in the material herein.

Library of Congress Cataloging-in-Publication Data

A catalog record for this book is available from the Library of Congress

Content Strategist: Charlotta Kryhl
Content Development Specialist: Alison Swety
Design Direction: Renee Duenow

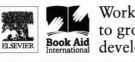

Working together
to grow libraries in
developing countries

www.elsevier.com • www.bookaid.org

Contributors

KALIL G. ABDULLAH, MD
Department of Neurosurgery
Perelman School of Medicine
Hospital of the University of Pennsylvania
Department of Bioengineering
University of Pennsylvania
Philadelphia, PA, USA

COREY ADAMSON, MD, PhD, MPH
Department of Neurosurgery
Emory University Hospital
Atlanta, GA, USA

MANISH K. AGHI, MD, PhD
Professor, Department of Neurologic Surgery
University of California
San Francisco, CA, USA

MAYA A. BABU, MD, MBA
Department of Neurological Surgery
Mayo Clinic
Rochester, MN, USA

RABAA BAITALMAL, MBBS
Microvascular and Molecular Neuro-Oncology
  Laboratory
Department of Pathology
NYU Langone Medical Center
New York, NY, USA;
Department of Pathology
King Abdulaziz University
Jeddah, Saudi Arabia

GENE H. BARNETT, MD, MBA
Department of Neurosurgery
Rose Ella Burkhardt Brain Tumor &
  Neuro-Oncology Center
Neurological Institute, Cleveland Clinic
Cleveland, OH, USA

JILL S. BARNHOLTZ-SLOAN, PhD
Professor, Case Comprehensive Cancer Center
Case Western Reserve University School
  of Medicine
Cleveland, OH, USA

TELMO BELSUZARRI, MD
Department of Neurosurgery
Hospital Celso Pierro, PUC-Campinas
Campinas, Sao Paulo, Brazil

MITCHEL S. BERGER, MD
Professor, Department of Neurological
  Surgery
University of California
San Francisco, CA, USA

RODICA BERNATOWICZ, MD
Resident, Neurological Institute Cleveland
  Clinic Foundation
Cleveland, OH, USA

FLORIEN W. BOELE, PhD
Edinburgh Centre for Neuro-Oncology
Western General Hospital
Edinburgh, United Kingdom

STEVEN BREM, MD
Co-Director, Brain Tumor Center Director
  of Neurosurgical Oncology
Professor of Neurosurgery, Hospital of the
  University of Pennsylvania
Philadelphia, PA, USA

JASON A. BURDICK, PhD
Department of Bioengineering
University of Pennsylvania
Philadelphia, PA, USA

BOB S. CARTER, MD, PhD
Department of Neurosurgery
University of California
La Jolla, CA, USA

SAMUEL T. CHAO, MD
Department of Radiation Oncology
Rose Ella Burkhardt Brain Tumor &
  Neuro-Oncology Center
Cleveland Clinic
Cleveland, OH, USA

STEPHANIE CHEN, MD
University of Miami Miller School
  of Medicine
University of Miami Hospital
Miami, FL, USA

ANDREW S. CHI, MD, PhD
Department of Neurosurgery
NYU Langone Medical Center
Departments of Neurology and Medicine
NYU School of Medicine
Laura and Isaac Perlmutter Cancer Center
NYU Langone Medical Center
NYU School of Medicine
New York, NY, USA

JOHN CHOI, MEd
Johns Hopkins University School of Medicine
Baltimore, MD, USA

ROBERTO JOSE DIAZ, MD, PhD, FRCS(C)
University of Miami Miller School of Medicine
University of Miami Hospital
Miami, FL, USA

LINDA DIRVEN, PhD
Department of Neurology
Leiden University Medical Center
Leiden, The Netherlands

HUGUES DUFFAU, MD, PhD
Professor, Department of Neurosurgery
Gui de Chauliac Hospital
National Institute for Health and Medical
   Research (INSERM)
Team "Brain Plasticity, Stem Cells and Glial
   Tumors"
Institute for Neurosciences of Montpellier
Montpellier University Medical Center
Montpellier, France

YI FAN, MD, PhD
Assistant Professor, Departments of Radiation
   Oncology and Neurosurgery
University of Pennsylvania
Perelman School of Medicine
Philadelphia, PA, USA

JAVIER M. FIGUEROA, MD, PhD
Department of Neurosurgery
University of California
La Jolla, CA, USA

PATRICK FLANIGAN, BS
Department of Neurologic Surgery
University of California
San Francisco, CA, USA

JEAN-PIERRE GAGNER, MD, PhD
Microvascular and Molecular Neuro-Oncology
Laboratory
Department of Pathology
NYU Langone Medical Center
New York, NY, USA

**CONSTANTINOS G. HADJIPANAYIS,
MD, PhD**
Department of Neurosurgery
Mount Sinai Health System
New York, NY, USA

ZHENQIANG HE, MD
Department of Radiation Oncology
University of Pennsylvania
Perelman School of Medicine
Philadelphia, PA, USA;
Department of Neurosurgery
Sun Yat-sen University Cancer Center
State Key Laboratory of Oncology in South China
Collaborative Innovation Center for
   Cancer Medicine
Guangzhou, China

SHAWN L. HERVEY-JUMPER, MD
Assistant Professor
Department of Neurosurgery
University of Michigan
Ann Arbor, MI, USA

ANDREAS F. HOTTINGER, MD, PhD
Departments of Clinical Neurosciences
   and Oncology
Lausanne University Hospital
Lausanne, Switzerland

MICHAEL E. IVAN, MD, MBS
University of Miami Miller School of Medicine
University of Miami Hospital
Miami, FL, USA

ARMAN JAHANGIRI, BS
Department of Neurologic Surgery
University of California
San Francisco, CA, USA

EDWARD W. JUNG, MD
Therapeutic Radiology Associates
Hagerstown, MD, USA

ANELIA KASSI, BSc
University of Miami Miller School of Medicine
University of Miami Hospital
Miami, FL, USA

JOHAN A.F. KOEKKOEK, MD, PhD
Department of Neurology
Leiden University Medical Center
Leiden, The Netherlands;
Department of Neurology
Medical Center Haaglanden
The Hague, The Netherlands

RICARDO J. KOMOTAR, MD, FACS
University of Miami Miller School of Medicine
University of Miami Hospital
Miami, FL, USA

PETER LIAO, BS, MD, PhD Student
Case Comprehensive Cancer Center
Case Western Reserve University School
  of Medicine
Cleveland, OH, USA

EDWIN LOK, MS
Brain Tumor Center & Neuro-Oncology Unit
Department of Neurology
Beth Israel Deaconess Medical Center
Harvard Medical School
Boston, MA, USA

MARCELA V. MAUS, MD, PhD
Cancer Center
Massachusetts General Hospital
Harvard Medical School
Boston, MA, USA

JACOB A. MILLER, BS
Lerner College of Medicine
Cleveland Clinic
Cleveland, OH, USA

RICHARD ALAN MITTEER Jr, MS
Department of Radiation Oncology
University of Pennsylvania
Perelman School of Medicine
Philadelphia, PA, USA

YONGGAO MOU, MD
Professor, Department of Neurosurgery
Sun Yat-sen University Cancer Center
State Key Laboratory of Oncology in South China
Collaborative Innovation Center for
  Cancer Medicine
Guangzhou, China

ERIN S. MURPHY, MD
Department of Radiation Oncology
Rose Ella Burkhardt Brain Tumor &
  Neuro-Oncology Center
Cleveland Clinic
Cleveland, OH, USA

DONALD M. O'ROURKE, MD
Department of Neurosurgery
Perelman School of Medicine
University of Pennsylvania
Philadelphia, PA, USA

QUINN T. OSTROM, MPH, MA
Research Coordinator
Case Comprehensive Cancer Center
Case Western Reserve University School
  of Medicine
Cleveland, OH, USA

DAVID PEEREBOOM, MD, FACP
Professor of Medicine
Lerner College of Medicine
Director, Clinical Research
Rose Ella Burkhardt Brain Tumor &
  Neuro-Oncology Center
Solid Tumor Oncology
Cleveland Clinic
Cleveland, OH, USA

H. WESTLEY PHILLIPS, MD
Department of Neurosurgery
NYU Langone Medical Center
NYU School of Medicine
New York, NY, USA

JONATHAN J. RASOULI, MD
Department of Neurosurgery
Mount Sinai Health System
New York, NY, USA

CHRISTOPHER A. SARKISS, MD
Department of Neurosurgery
Mount Sinai Health System
New York, NY, USA

JAMES ERIC SCHMITT, MD, PhD
Assistant Professor of Radiology
Division of Neuroradiology
Department of Radiology
Hospital of the University of Pennsylvania
Philadelphia, PA, USA

MAYUR SHARMA, MD
Department of Neurosurgery
Rose Ella Burkhardt Brain Tumor &
  Neuro-Oncology Center
Cleveland Clinic
Cleveland, OH, USA

DANILO SILVA, MD
Department of Neurosurgery
Rose Ella Burkhardt Brain Tumor &
  Neuro-Oncology Center
Cleveland Clinic
Cleveland, OH, USA

JOEL M. STEIN, MD, PhD
Assistant Professor of Radiology
Division of Neuroradiology
Department of Radiology
Hospital of the University of Pennsylvania
Philadelphia, PA, USA

LINDSAY C. STETSON, PhD
Post-Doctoral Scholar
Case Comprehensive Cancer Center
Case Western Reserve University School
   of Medicine
Cleveland, OH, USA

ROGER STUPP, MD
Professor, Department of Oncology
Zurich University Hospital
Zurich, Switzerland

YOURONG SOPHIE SU, MD
Department of Neurosurgery
University of Pennsylvania
Philadelphia, PA, USA

JOHN H. SUH, MD
Department of Radiation Oncology
Rose Ella Burkhardt Brain Tumor &
   Neuro-Oncology Center
Cleveland Clinic
Cleveland, OH, USA

KENNETH D. SWANSON, PhD
Brain Tumor Center & Neuro-Oncology Unit
Department of Neurology
Beth Israel Deaconess Medical Center
Harvard Medical School
Boston, MA, USA

MARTIN J.B. TAPHOORN, MD, PhD
Department of Neurology
Medical Center Haaglanden
The Hague, The Netherlands;
Department of Neurology
Leiden University Medical Center
Leiden, The Netherlands

JAYESH P. THAWANI, MD
Department of Neurosurgery
Hospital of the University of Pennsylvania
Philadelphia, PA, USA

CHEDDHI J. THOMAS, MD
Division of Neuropathology
Department of Pathology
NYU Langone Medical Center
New York, NY, USA

ERIC T. WONG, MD
Brain Tumor Center & Neuro-Oncology Unit
Department of Neurology
Beth Israel Deaconess Medical Center
Harvard Medical School
Boston, Massachusetts;
Department of Physics
University of Massachusetts
Lowell, Massachusetts

ANDREW I. YANG, MD, MS
Department of Neurosurgery
Perelman School of Medicine
University of Pennsylvania
Philadelphia, PA, USA

DAVID ZAGZAG, MD, PhD
Division of Neuropathology
Microvascular and Molecular Neuro-Oncology
   Laboratory
Department of Pathology
Department of Neurosurgery
Laura and Isaac Perlmutter Cancer Center
NYU Langone Medical Center
New York, NY, USA

PREFACE

Glioblastoma: Translating Scientific Advances to Innovative Therapy

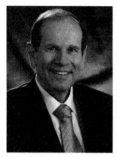
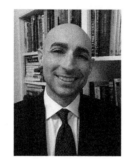

Steven Brem, MD, *Editor*   Kalil G. Abdullah, MD, *Editor*

Our main business is not to see what lies dimly at a distance, but to do what clearly lies at hand

—*Thomas Carlyle*

In your hands you will find in this unique volume a current and comprehensive look at glioblastoma, and emerge with an enhanced understanding that reflects an explosion of information and innovation. There has been an unmet need for a single, systematic treatise on glioblastoma. With the enthusiastic participation of luminaries in neuro-oncology, we redefine the numerous facets of glioblastoma, from its history, epidemiology, and pathogenesis to principles of surgery, radiation therapy, and chemotherapy. The early detection of glioblastoma through biomarkers and response to therapy promises to inform future clinical trials and accelerate the pace of discovery to continuously increase survival. We include novel approaches such as antiangiogenic therapy, T-cell immunotherapy, laser interstitial thermocoagulation, electric field therapy, and local therapies.

Glioblastoma has long been refractory to treatment because of its molecular, cellular, and spatial heterogeneity, depicted by its original surname *multiforme*. Accordingly, the book distills the multiple dimensions of glioblastoma in a rare collection of brief, but informative, summaries of classic and emerging modalities to tackle glioblastoma. The pieces of the puzzle are here for the reader to digest and discover. This robust, dynamic, interdisciplinary approach paves the way for further breakthroughs to enhance survival and quality of life.

For those entering the field, or for seasoned clinicians and researchers, there is a sense of genuine excitement this year. President Barack Obama declared a "cancer moonshot" to harness advances in genomics, informatics, and immunotherapy towards the ultimate cure of cancer. Vice-President Joe Biden has traveled across the United States to speak with leaders in the war against cancer. There is a feeling of increasing optimism that this war is winnable. Data presented on epidemiology and survival demonstrate the basis for optimism and the progress made to tame glioblastoma. Included in this text are chapters on socioeconomics that highlight the challenges we face in providing the most advanced care in the context of a shifting healthcare landscape. Dr. Duffau's chapter on neuroplasticity provides insight and hope as we move from scientific discovery to functional recovery. Taken together, the reader will develop a profound understanding of glioblastoma from multiple vantage points. We believe the reader will find the best work of the most established thinkers, scientists, and surgeons in our field. We hope you enjoy these gems as as much as we have.

We thank all the authors who so kindly contributed these erudite and well-researched chapters. We are ever grateful to Charlotta Kryhl and Alison Swety at Elsevier for their professionalism and timely publication of this book.

We thank our families and loved ones; Dr. Brem especially thanks his wife, Hana, an angel throughout his career, including during the time to prepare this book. We also thank our patients and their families, who have been touched by glioblastoma. As with all cancer, glioblastoma disrupts not only the life of the patient, but the lives of the family, loved ones, and community. Each and every day our patients provide us with the inspiration, strength, and purpose to treat this disease. They are our heroes, and we dedicate this book to them.

Most sincerely,

Steven Brem, MD
Department of Neurosurgery
Hospital of the University of Pennsylvania
Philadelphia, PA, USA

Kalil G. Abdullah, MD
Department of Neurosurgery
Hospital of the University of Pennsylvania
Philadelphia, PA, USA

Contents

Part I: Disease Origins and Context

1 The Story of Glioblastoma: History and Modern Correlates, 1
Jayesh P. Thawani and Steven Brem

2 Epidemiology of Glioblastoma and Trends in Glioblastoma Survivorship, 11
Quinn T. Ostrom, Peter Liao, Lindsay C. Stetson, and Jill S. Barnholtz-Sloan

3 The Molecular Pathogenesis of Glioblastoma, 21
Kalil G. Abdullah, Corey Adamson, and Steven Brem

4 Translating Molecular Biomarkers of Gliomas to Clinical Practice, 33
Cheddhi J. Thomas, Jean-Pierre Gagner, Rabaa Baitalmal, and David Zagzag

5 Multimodality Targeting of Glioma Cells, 55
Zhenqiang He, Richard Alan Mitteer, Yonggao Mou, and Yi Fan

Part II: Standards of Medical and Surgical Treatment

6 Current Standards of Care in Glioblastoma Therapy, 73
Andreas F. Hottinger, Kalil G. Abdullah, and Roger Stupp

7 Radiographic Detection and Advanced Imaging of Glioblastoma, 81
James Eric Schmitt and Joel M. Stein

8 Principles and Tenets of Radiation Treatment in Glioblastoma, 105
Edward W. Jung, John Choi, Samuel T. Chao, Erin S. Murphy, and John H. Suh

9 Chemotherapeutics and Their Efficacy, 133
H. Westley Phillips and Andrew S. Chi

10 Antiangiogenic Therapy for Glioblastoma, 143
Arman Jahangiri, Patrick Flanigan, and Manish K. Aghi

11 Recurrent Glioblastoma, 151
Kalil G. Abdullah, Jacob A. Miller, Corey Adamson, and Steven Brem

12 Principles of Surgical Treatment, 167
Shawn L. Hervey-Jumper and Mitchel S. Berger

13 Awake Craniotomy for Glioblastoma, 177
Roberto Jose Diaz, Stephanie Chen, Anelia Kassi, Ricardo J. Komotar, and Michael E. Ivan

14 Intraoperative Imaging of Glioblastoma, 187
Christopher A. Sarkiss, Jonathan J. Rasouli, and Constantinos G. Hadjipanayis

15 Minimally Invasive Targeted Therapy for Glioblastoma Laser Interstitial Thermal Therapy (LITT), 197
Danilo Silva, Mayur Sharma, Telmo Belsuzarri, and Gene H. Barnett

16 Local Drug Delivery in the Treatment of Glioblastoma, 207
Kalil G. Abdullah and Jason A. Burdick

17 Tumor-Treating Electric Fields for Glioblastoma, 213
Kenneth D. Swanson, Edwin Lok, and Eric T. Wong

Part III: Scientific Advances, Future Directions, and Socioeconomic Considerations

18 Brain Plasticity and Reorganization Before, During, and After Glioma Reseaction, 225
Hugues Duffau

19 General Principles of Immunotherapy for Glioblastoma, 237
Andrew I. Yang, Marcela V. Maus, and Donald M. O'Rourke

20 Early Detection of Glioblastoma, 247
Javier M. Figueroa and Bob S. Carter

21 Health-Related Quality of Life and Neurocognitive Functioning After Glioblastoma Treatment, 253
Florien W. Boele, Linda Dirven, Johan A.F. Koekkoek, and Martin J.B. Taphoorn

22 Socioeconomics and Survival, 265
Maya A. Babu

23 National and Global Economic Impact of Glioblastoma, 271
YouRong Sophie Su and Kalil G. Abdullah

24 Lessons Learned: Clinical Trials and Other Interventions for Glioblastoma, 279
Rodica Bernatowicz and David Peereboom

INDEX, 291

Glioblastoma

CHAPTER 1

The Story of Glioblastoma: History and Modern Correlates

Jayesh P. Thawani, MD[a],*, Steven Brem, MD[b]

Glioblastoma remains a formidable pathologic entity. Without the tools necessary to make a neurologic diagnosis, early medical and surgical clinicians were likely not only puzzled but also appalled by the downward trajectory of patients affected by this tumor. The development of neurosurgery and neuropathology served as the first necessary steps in understanding glioblastoma. Despite major diagnostic and therapeutic advances, clinicians continue to struggle in providing favorable outcomes for patients with glioblastoma. This chapter provides a historical context for glioblastoma and outlines the evolution of the diagnosis and management of this tumor.

HISTORY OF GLIOBLASTOMA: FROM TREPHINATION TO WORLD HEALTH ORGANIZATION CLASSIFICATION

Although evidence of trephination or trepanation has been found from ancient cultures dating back to the late Paleolithic period from around the world,[1] the first medical description of the procedure was documented by Hippocrates.[2] Practitioners performed trephination for traumatic injuries (to elevate depressed skull fractures) and for a variety of other reasons, including to alleviate seizures, headaches, superficial growths, and psychiatric maladies (**Fig. 1.1**). The ancient physician and surgeon, Abu al-Qasim Al-Zahrawi (Latinized to Albucasis) of Andalusia, developed and described numerous surgical instruments and procedures in the volumes of *Kitab al-Tasrif* (The Method of Medicine), including operations to treat neurosurgical disorders. These disorders included tumors of the central nervous system.[3]

The acceptance and formalization of the scientific method, advancements in clinical and laboratory medicine, and the development of equipment like the light microscope brought forth new knowledge and opportunities to study human disorders. Between 1856 and 1865, Rudolph Ludwig Carl Virchow first described neuroglia,[4] defined the gliomas and separated them into what are now considered low-grade and high-grade disorders, and developed the foundation for pathologic study.[5,6] At the time, tumors found in the brain at autopsy were named according to the presumed (normal) cellular counterpart.[7] Given the available staining and visualization techniques, many of the cell types that are now considered glial cells were not clearly defined; they were thought of as elements of connective tissue without a cellular origin. Based on Camilo Golgi's[8] work in identifying foot processes along neurons (1873), and Michael von Lenhossék's[9] description of the astrocyte (1891), the idea that glial cells provided support for neurons was propagated. Santiago Ramón y Cajal and Pío del Río-Hortega contributed much to the understanding of glial cells and the cellular architecture of the brain using gold-based (labeling glial fibrillary acidic protein) and platinum-based (labeling oligodendrocytes) agents.[10–12]

In 1926, Percival Bailey and Harvey Cushing,[13] both American Midwesterners by birth and upbringing, collaborated to publish *A Classification of the Tumors of the Glioma Group on a Histogenetic Basis with a Correlated Study of Prognosis*. Bailey used histologic staining techniques to study 254 gliomas from Cushing's series.[13] These and an additional 160 gliomas were used in classifying

a Department of Neurosurgery, Hospital of the University of Pennsylvania, 3400 Spruce Street, 3 Silverstein, Philadelphia, PA 19103, USA; b Department of Neurosurgery, Brain Tumor Center, Hospital of the University of Pennsylvania, 3400 Spruce Street, 3 Silverstein, Philadelphia, PA 19103, USA
* Corresponding author.
E-mail address: jayesh.thawani@uphs.upenn.edu

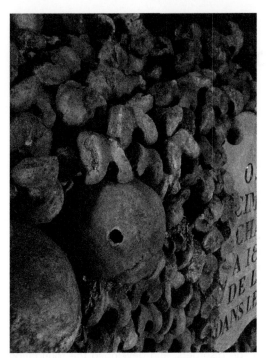

Fig. 1.1 The Catacombes of Paris, 2014. There is evidence of trephination dating back to the late Paleolithic time period. Although the first documented central nervous system tumor resection dates back to 900 to 1000 AD (*Kitab Al-Tasrif*, Albucasis of Cordoba), the first documented, controlled operation for a primary brain tumor was performed by Mr Rickman Godlee in 1884.

13 groups according to the cellular configuration. The classification scheme was later condensed.[14] In addition, tumors were grouped according to patient survival. Before this work, central nervous system tumors were generally considered gliomas; prognosis was not clearly linked to histopathologic diagnosis. Because of the important and practical implications of this work, it was received with great interest worldwide (**Figs. 1.2–1.4**).[13–15]

Cushing and Bailey identified spongioblastoma multiforme as a distinct tumor with a specific cell of origin based on its histologic appearance, which appeared different from the other gliomas (see **Fig. 1.2**). Despite heterogeneity (prompting the term multiforme) when visualized under the microscope, patients with these tumors uniformly experienced rapid declines in their clinical trajectories. By the 1940s, spongioblastoma multiforme became better known as glioblastoma multiforme.[16]

The German neuropathologist Hans Joachim Scherer[17] first hypothesized the concept of primary versus secondary glioblastoma in 1938 and published a series of articles substantiating this into the 1940s. His ideas were ahead of his time in both a theoretic and scientific sense. He noted that patients with secondary glioblastoma had long clinical courses compared with those with primary glioblastoma, emphasizing that they could be distinguished from biological and clinical perspectives.[17–20] Although this was noted by both Scherer and Cushing,[21] both were in disagreement over systems of classification. Penfield, Kernohan, Sayre, Schaffer, Bergstrand, Purdy, and Olivecrona proposed differing systems of classification based on novel clinical and histopathologic findings; these systems were introduced with considerable bias.[22]

A consensus system for classification was needed. From 1956 to 1979, the World Health Organization (WHO) recruited 23 centers worldwide consisting of approximately 300 pathologists to provide microscopic samples of brain tumors for classification. In 1979, the first edition of the *WHO Classification of Tumors of the Central Nervous System* was published.[23] Subsequent editions were published in 1982, 2000, and 2007.[24,25] At the time of this writing, a fifth edition is due for release (See Chapter 4 for details).

HISTORICAL PERSPECTIVES ON THE DIAGNOSIS OF GLIOBLASTOMA

Imaging technologies such as radiograph (Roentgen, 1895),[26] ventriculography (Dandy, 1919),[27] angiography (Lima and Moniz, 1927),[28] computed tomographic imaging (Hounsfield and Cormack, 1971),[29] and magnetic resonance (MR) imaging (Lauterbur, Mansfield, and Damadian, 1977)[30] significantly changed the diagnosis and subsequent management of glioblastoma. At the time of this writing, T1-weighted and T2-weighted imaging sequences on MR imaging, with and without gadolinium administration, serve as standard imaging sequences for newly diagnosed glioblastoma. Advanced imaging sequences developed in the last 15 to 20 years can be used to ascertain recurrence and differentiate this from radiation-related changes. The current contrast agent of choice (gadolinium) results in enhancement on T1-weighted imaging within the major cellular components of a tumor based on breakdown of the blood-brain barrier (BBB).

Even at present, many clinicians consider areas of contrast enhancement on MR imaging to equate to borders of neoplastic disease in the brain. It is now understood that the genetic and phenotypic heterogeneity of glioblastoma is spatial and may account for neoplastic cells identified in the brain outside of enhancing regions on

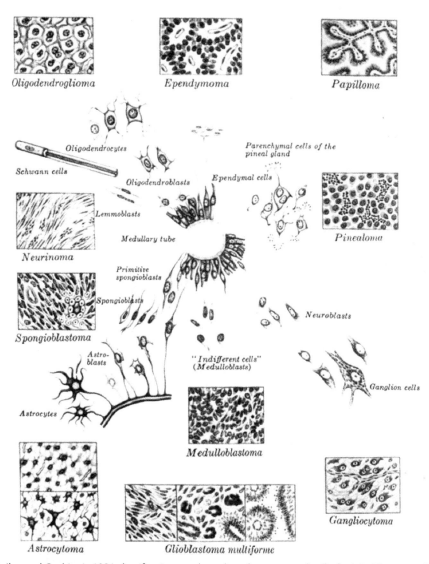

Fig. 1.2 Bailey and Cushing's 1926 classification was based on the presumed cell of origin. The term glioblastoma multiforme was in the literature by the 1940s. (*From* Zülch KJ. The historical development and present state of classification. In: Brain tumors. New York: Springer US; 1957. p. 9.)

MR imaging. When Walter Dandy[31,32] performed right hemispherectomy procedures on patients with this tumor in 1928, relapses were noted (**Fig. 1.5**). Several decades later, Patrick Kelly performed stereotactic biopsies outside of regions of contrast enhancement on imaging, showing neoplastic disease in nonenhancing tissue (**Fig. 1.6**).[33] Over time, through these and numerous other studies, clinicians developed an understanding that glioblastoma is a microscopic and not a macroscopic disease.

The many scientific and biomedical advancements made in the twentieth century contributed to the present understanding of the genetic and environmental basis for disease. In 1974, the p53 tumor suppressor gene was discovered.[34] Its role in the pathogenesis of glioblastoma was later shown through a large body of scientific evidence.[35–37] It is now understood that primary glioblastoma is hallmarked by epidermal growth factor (EGFR) overexpression and that p53 mutations characterize secondary tumors.[18,35,37] Collaboration among centers and data from integrated genomic profiling have identified subtypes of glioblastoma typified by genetic alterations and variability in expression. In the last 10 years, isocitrate dehydrogenase (IDH) mutations were found with a high frequency in secondary

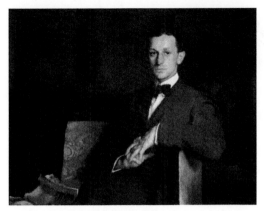

Fig. 1.3 Harvey Williams Cushing, father of neurosurgery in America. ("Dr. Harvey Cushing," oil on canvas, by the American artist Edmund Tarbell. *Courtesy of* the Dittrick Medical History Center.)

glioblastomas, and patients with these mutations have a longer survival than patients with wild-type IDH status.[38–40] In the early 2000s, The Cancer Genome Atlas group defined classic, proneural, neural, and mesenchymal subtypes. Earlier studies showed 3 dominant subtypes (mesenchymal, proneural, and proliferative.[41,42] The genetic and expression variation between these groups, along with common clinical manifestations between these groups, are discussed later because they are beyond the scope of this chapter, but their establishment is an example of the use of advanced computing and genomic sequencing to better understand a disease first recognized almost a century ago.

Clinicians continue to improve on their ability to diagnose glioblastoma. Developing methods

to detect circulating tumor cells or circulating elements of a glioblastoma (eg, vesicles or other cell membrane components) in the circulation may improve the ability to screen for this condition or monitor for recurrence. Advancements made in molecular imaging will, in the future, allow clinicians to more precisely visualize neoplastic cells or tissues radiologically and in the operating room.

HISTORICAL PERSPECTIVES ON THE MANAGEMENT OF GLIOBLASTOMA

Amid changes in diagnosis, the nonsurgical and surgical management of glioblastoma has improved with technology. In the 1970s and 1980s, Judah Folkman[43] and others helped establish the angiogenesis concept in tumors.[21,43] Antiangiogenesis-based therapies such as bevacizumab (a vascular endothelial growth factor–neutralizing antibody) remain in the armamentarium with specific indications (recurrence) at the time of this writing.[44,45] Other targeted pathway inhibitors (eg, *mTOR* (mechanistic target of rapamycin), *PDGF*) have been developed and are under investigation in the modern era. As mentioned previously, mutations of *EGFR* were identified in a subset of patients with glioblastoma. In the past 5 to 10 years, targeted therapeutic agents have come to light; genetic factors, such as coexpression of EGFRvIII, phosphatase and tensin homolog (*PTEN*), and others may alter host susceptibility to therapeutic agents. In the early 2000s, the methylguanine methyltransferase (*MGMT*) excision repair enzyme was linked to tumor resistance to alkylating agents; thus methylation/inactivation was shown to predict outcome/survival in patients with glioblastoma receiving temozolomide chemotherapy.[35,46] Genetic factors are no longer solely prognostic; they now guide therapeutic strategies. Although the concepts of immunotherapies directed at cancer are not novel, human glioblastoma research using immunotherapy is in its infancy and shows promise. Challenges in terms of the antigens used, humoral versus cytotoxic mechanisms, and delivery with respect to the BBB and tumor remain.

Neurosurgical treatment has changed with improvements in operative technology and visualization, especially with the introduction of the microscope and loupe magnification in the operating theater. M. Gazi Yaşargil is an important figure in neurosurgery because of his development of novel techniques and tools, his relentless devotion to surgical nuance, and his teaching (**Fig. 1.7**). Influenced by Hugo Krayenbühl and R.M. Peardon Donaghy, his work advanced the practice of

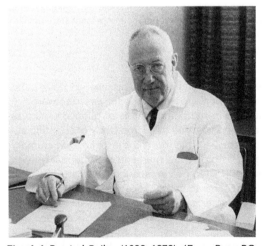

Fig. 1.4 Percival Bailey (1892–1973). (*From* Bucy PC. Percival Bailey, 1892–1973. J Neurosurg 1974;40(2): 281–8.)

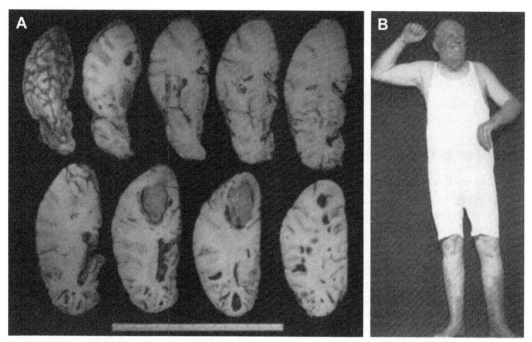

Fig. 1.5 (A) Coronal sections of a right hemisphere taken from a patient with a frontal/parietal glioma with cyst formation. (B) Patient with left hemiplegia following right hemispherectomy. Walter Dandy performed this procedure in patients with right hemispheric glioblastomas. However, recurrent disease following surgery was noted. (From Bell E, Karnosh LJ. Cerebral hemispherectomy; report of a case 10 years after operation. J Neurosurg 1949;6(4):285–93; with permission.)

neurosurgery not only in patients with cerebrovascular disorders but also in those with brain tumors.[47,48]

With advanced imaging techniques such as functional MR imaging or diffusion tensor imaging, clinicians are able to obtain approximations of functional regions of the brain. Awake functional mapping and preoperative language lateralization procedures serve as more accurate and precise means for ascertaining functional nodes or regions within the brain.[4,49–51] High-quality functional mapping techniques have improved the safety of neurosurgical resection for patients with gliomas. The utility of such techniques varies along with the spectrum of pathologic disease because patients with low-grade

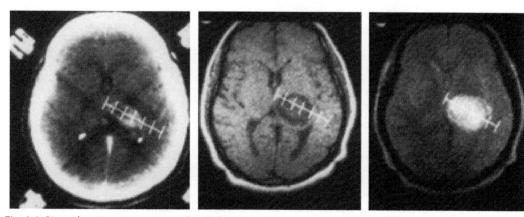

Fig. 1.6 Biopsy locations in a patient with a thalamic grade IV astrocytoma indicated by computer on the stereotaxic computed tomography slice (left) and on the T1-weighted (center) and T2-weighted (right) MR images. (From Kelly PJ, Daumas-Duport C, Kispert DB, et al. Imaging-based stereotaxic serial biopsies in untreated intracranial glial neoplasms. J Neurosurg 1987;66(6);865–74; with permission.)

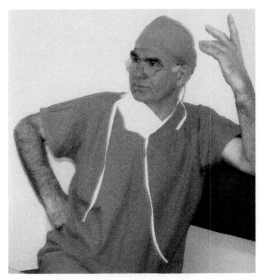

Fig. 1.7 M. Gazi Yasargil, who developed and popularized microsurgical techniques that, through further modifications, have improved the safety and efficacy of neurosurgical resection of brain tumors. (*From* Tew JM Jr, M Gazi Yaşargil: neurosurgery's man of the century. Neurosurgery 1999;45(5):1010–4; with permission.)

tumors and those making the transition from low-grade tumors have shown an increasing capacity for cerebral plasticity.[52] Penfield, Ojemann, Berger, Duffau, and others have built and substantiated the concept of a functional neuro-oncology; balancing (and optimizing) function while minimizing the oncologic burden of disease

remains the goal as clinicians learn more about the brain and develop novel technologies.[50,53–57]

In 1908, Victor Horsley and Robert Clarke developed the stereotactic method for use in animal experimentation.[58] Lars Leksell, Ernest Spiegel, and Henry Wycis developed technologies to perform stereotactic brain biopsies in humans.[59] Biopsy of tumors in deep-seated, vital regions where surgical resection was precluded because of safety is now possible through a variety of stereotactic technologies. Neurosurgeons were the first to deploy radiation therapies in treating gliomas. Hirsch and Gramegna used brachytherapy as early as 1912 to treat patients with acromegaly.[60] In North America, Charles Harrison Frazier implanted radium in a small series of patients undergoing craniotomies for tumors; several of these patients had gliomas.[61] In the 1930s, with some advancements in conformal dosing with brachytherapy, Cushing reported depositing radium in the resection cavities of gliomas (**Fig. 1.8**).[60] Over the next several decades, external beam radiation therapy and other modalities were refined and used in treating glioblastoma. Radiation therapy remains an important adjunct in treating glioblastoma. Throughout the world, groups continue to differ in terms of their operative and nonoperative strategies to treat glioblastoma. Surgical resection, biopsy, radiation therapies (radiosurgery, external beam radiation, proton beam radiation), and implantation of chemotherapeutic agents using platforms for controlled release are methods now in use. Based

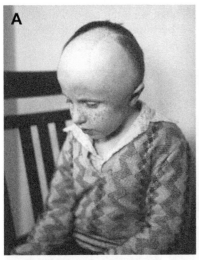
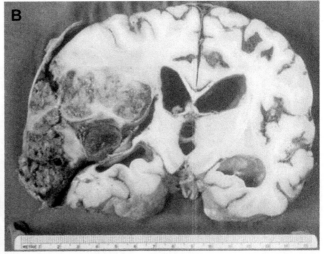

Fig. 1.8 (*A*) A 6-year-old boy with a diagnosis of astroblastoma underwent surgical resection and implantation of radium. The photograph was taken 2 months following the intervention with notable alopecia. (*B*) Autopsy specimen taken from the child shows gross invasion of central regions. (*From* Seymour ZA, Cohen-Gadol AA. Cushing's lost cases of "radium bomb" brachytherapy for gliomas. J Neurosurg 2010;113(1):141–8. Cushing/Whitney Medical Library/Yale University.)

on initial imaging studies suggestive of glioblastoma, no intervention might be recommended; this may be justifiable in special circumstances but, for most, it remains controversial given the many trajectories patients may have based on pathologic investigation.

Randomized clinical trial designs have changed the oncologic management of glioblastoma. About 10 years ago, concurrent chemoradiotherapy with temozolomide was established by Stupp and colleagues[45] as an effective means to treat patients with glioblastoma. Maintenance therapy with temozolomide has also been advocated. Various chemotherapies aimed at cell cycle targets and molecular pathway inhibitors, antibody-based therapies, and immunotherapy-based therapies are under investigation and are described in detail later.

Most studies from the current era advocate a maximal, safe resection when possible. This concept is vague to clinicians outside of neuro-oncology or neurosurgery. A maximal resection, based on multiple studies, has been established based on retrospective data and analyzing outcomes and extent of resection based on T1-weighted imaging with standard volumetric techniques. Given the infiltrative nature of glioblastoma, this concept of gross total resection may not be sufficient, because many tumor cells almost certainly exist outside of the contrast-enhancing regions of the tumor cavity. However, regardless of how it is measured, surgical resection provides for cytoreduction of glioblastoma and is associated with better outcomes for most patients when neurologic function is preserved. As discussed later in Chapters 12 - 15, neurosurgeons continue to improve on their ability to more effectively and safely manage this tumor through advances in operative guidance and technique.

SUMMARY

As neurosurgery and neuro-oncology have evolved, so has the classification system for central nervous system tumors, and glioblastoma multiforme has been chosen as the name for this vexing condition. As clinicians learn more about this entity, the word multiforme takes on a new meaning. In the past, the term referred to the histopathologic heterogeneity, but it now also represents the variety of genetic and phenotypic manifestations this tumor takes on. In the future, the name glioblastoma multiforme will likely become out of date as clinicians move to classify tumors based on personalized genotypic and advanced pathologic characteristics, but its origins still reflect its complexity and ability to evade and outmaneuver treatment and definitive cure.

REFERENCES

1. Gross CG. Trepanation: history, discovery, theory. Lisse (Netherlands): Swets and Zeitlinger; 2002.
2. Martin G. Craniotomy: the first case histories. J Clin Neurosci 1999;6:361–3.
3. Ghannaee Arani M, Fakharian E, Sarbandi F. Ancient legacy of cranial surgery. Arch Trauma Res 2012;1:72–4.
4. Duffau H, editor. Diffuse low-grade gliomas in adults. London: Springer London; 2013.
5. DeAngelis LM, Mellinghoff IK. Virchow 2011 or how to ID(H) human glioblastoma. J Clin Oncol 2011;29:4473–4.
6. Virchow R, Frankfurt M. Gesammelte Abhandlungen zyr wissenschaftlischen Medizin. Bayer, Staatsbibliothek: Verlag von Meidinger Sohn & Comp; 1856.
7. Parpura V, Verkhratsky A. Neuroglia at the crossroads of homoeostasis, metabolism and signalling: evolution of the concept. ASN Neuro 2012;4:201–5.
8. Golgi C. Suella struttura della sostanza grigia del cervello (comunicazione preventiva). Lombardia (Italy): Gazzetta Medica Italiana; 1873.
9. Lenhossék M. von: Zur Kenntnis der Neuroglia des menschlichen Rückenmarkes. Verh Anat Ges 1891;1:193–221.
10. Del Rio-Hortega P. Estudios sobre la neuroglia. La glia de escasas radiaciones oligodendroglia. Biol Soc Esp Biol 1921;21:64–92.
11. Iglesias-Rozas JR, Garrosa M. The discovery of oligodendroglia cells by Rio-Hortega: his original articles. 1921. Clin Neuropathol 2012;31:437–9.
12. Ramon y Cajal S. Contribution a la connaissance de la nevroglia cerebrale et cerebeleuse dans la paralyse generale progressive. Trab Lab Invest Biol Univ Madrid 1925;23:157–216.
13. Bailey P, Cushing H. A classification of the tumors of the glioma group on a histogenetic basis with a correlated study of prognosis. Philadelphia: Lippincott; 1926.
14. Ferguson S, Lesniak MS. Percival Bailey and the classification of brain tumors. Neurosurg Focus 2005;18:e7.
15. Bailey P. Histological atlas of gliomas. Arch Pathol Lab Med 1927;4:19–21.
16. Del Rio-Hortega P, Nomenclatura y. clasifieacion delos tumores del sistema nervioso. Buenos Aires (Argentina): López & Etchegoyen; 1945.
17. Scherer HJ. A critical review: the pathology of cerebral gliomas. J Neurol Psychiatry 1940;3:147–77.

18. Kleihues P, Ohgaki H. Primary and secondary glioblastomas: from concept to clinical diagnosis. World Health 1999;1(1):44–51.

19. Kubben PL, Ter Meulen KJ, Schijns OEMG, et al. Intraoperative MRI-guided resection of glioblastoma multiforme: a systematic review. Lancet Oncol 2011;12:1062–70.

20. Peiffer J, Kleihues P. Hans-Joachim Scherer (1906-1945), pioneer in glioma research. Brain Pathol 1999;9:241–5.

21. Agnihotri S, Burrell KE, Wolf A, et al. Glioblastoma, a brief review of history, molecular genetics, animal models and novel therapeutic strategies. Arch Immunol Ther Exp (Warsz) 2013;61:25–41.

22. Zülch KJ. Brain tumors. Berlin Heidelberg: Springer; 1986.

23. Scheithauer BW. Development of the WHO classification of tumors of the central nervous system: a historical perspective. Brain Pathol 2009;19: 551–64.

24. Kaye AH, Laws ER Jr. Brain Tumors - An Encyclopedic Approach. 3rd Edition. Elsevier; 2012.

25. Louis DN, Ohgaki H, Wiestler OD, et al. The 2007 WHO classification of tumours of the central nervous system. 4th edition. Geneva (Switzerland): WHO Press; 2007.

26. Morgan RH, Lewis I. The roentgen ray: its past and future. Dis Chest 1945;11:502–10.

27. White YS, Bell DS, Mellick R. Sequelae to pneumoencephalography. J Neurol Neurosurg Psychiatry 1973;36:146–51.

28. LIMA A. 25th anniversary of cerebral angiography. Med Contemp (Lisbon, Portugal) 1952;70: 439–44.

29. Hounsfield GN. Historical notes on computerized axial tomography. J Can Assoc Radiol 1976;27: 135–42.

30. Becker C. A sharper image. Father of the MRI honored for invention that forever changed diagnostics. Mod Healthc 2001;31(44):50.

31. Dandy WE. Removal of right cerebral hemisphere for certain tumors with hemiplegia. JAMA 1928;90–1.

32. Dandy W. Physiological studies following extirpation of the right cerebral hemisphere in man. Bull Johns Hopkins Hosp 1933;53:31–57.

33. Kelly PJ, Daumas-Duport C, Kispert DB, et al. Imaging-based stereotaxic serial biopsies in untreated intracranial glial neoplasms. J Neurosurg 1987;66:865–74.

34. Levine AJ. The road to the discovery of the p53 protein. The Steiner Cancer Prize Award Lecture. Int J Cancer 1994;56:775–6.

35. Ohgaki H, Kleihues P. Genetic pathways to primary and secondary glioblastoma. Am J Pathol 2007;170: 1445–53.

36. Shiraishi S, Tada K, Nakamura H, et al. Influence of p53 mutations on prognosis of patients with glioblastoma. Cancer 2002;95:249–57.

37. Watanabe K, Tachibana O, Sata K, et al. Overexpression of the EGF receptor and p53 mutations are mutually exclusive in the evolution of primary and secondary glioblastomas. Brain Pathol 1996;6:217–23.

38. Parsons DW, Jones S, Zhang X, et al. An integrated genomic analysis of human glioblastoma multiforme. Science 2008;321:1807–12.

39. Smith JS, Tachibana I, Passe SM, et al. PTEN mutation, EGFR amplification, and outcome in patients with anaplastic astrocytoma and glioblastoma multiforme. J Natl Cancer Inst 2001;93: 1246–56.

40. Yan H, Parsons DW, Jin G, et al. IDH1 and IDH2 mutations in gliomas. N Engl J Med 2009;360: 765–73.

41. Cancer Genome Atlas Research Network. Comprehensive genomic characterization defines human glioblastoma genes and core pathways. Nature 2008;455:1061–8.

42. Phillips HS, Kharbanda S, Chen R, et al. Molecular subclasses of high-grade glioma predict prognosis, delineate a pattern of disease progression, and resemble stages in neurogenesis. Cancer Cell 2006; 9:157–73.

43. Folkman J. Tumor angiogenesis: therapeutic implications. N Engl J Med 1971;285:1182–6.

44. Friedman HS, Prados MD, Wen PY, et al. Bevacizumab alone and in combination with irinotecan in recurrent glioblastoma. J Clin Oncol 2009;27: 4733–40.

45. Stupp R, Hegi ME, Mason WP, et al. Effects of radiotherapy with concomitant and adjuvant temozolomide versus radiotherapy alone on survival in glioblastoma in a randomised phase III study: 5-year analysis of the EORTC-NCIC trial. Lancet Oncol 2009;10:459–66.

46. Ohgaki H. Genetic pathways to glioblastomas. Neuropathology 2005;25:1–7.

47. Flamm ES, Professor M. Gazi Yaşargil: an appreciation by a former apprentice. Neurosurgery 1999;45: 1015–8.

48. Tew JM Jr. Gazi Yaşargil: neurosurgery's man of the century. Neurosurgery 1999;45:1010–4.

49. Duffau H. New concepts in surgery of WHO grade II gliomas: functional brain mapping, connectionism and plasticity–a review. J Neurooncol 2006;79:77–115.

50. Duffau H. Surgery of low-grade gliomas: towards a "functional neurooncology". Curr Opin Oncol 2009;21:543–9.

51. Tate MC, Herbet G, Moritz-Gasser S, et al. Probabilistic map of critical functional regions of the human cerebral cortex: Broca's area revisited. Brain 2014; 137:2773–82.

52. Duffau H. Is supratotal resection of glioblastoma in noneloquent areas possible? World Neurosurg 2014;82:e101–3.

53. Bloch O, Han SJ, Cha S, et al. Impact of extent of resection for recurrent glioblastoma on overall survival: clinical article. J Neurosurg 2012;117: 1032–8.

54. Feindel W. The contributions of Wilder Penfield to the functional anatomy of the human brain. Hum Neurobiol 1982;1:231–4.

55. Lucas TH, Drane DL, Dodrill CB, et al. Language reorganization in aphasics: an electrical stimulation mapping investigation. Neurosurgery 2008;63: 487–97 [discussion: 497].

56. Sanai N, Berger MS. Glioma extent of resection and its impact on patient outcome. Neurosurgery 2008; 62:753–64 [discussion: 264–6].

57. Sanai N, Mirzadeh Z, Berger MS. Functional outcome after language mapping for glioma resection. N Engl J Med 2008;358:18–27.

58. Rahman M, Murad GJA, Mocco J. Early history of the stereotactic apparatus in neurosurgery. Neurosurg Focus 2009;27:E12.

59. Gildenberg PL. Spiegel and Wycis - the early years. Stereotact Funct Neurosurg 2001;77:11–6.

60. Seymour ZA, Cohen-Gadol AA. Cushing's lost cases of "radium bomb" brachytherapy for gliomas. J Neurosurg 2010;113:141–8.

61. CH F. The effects of radium emanations upon brain tumors. Surg Gynecol Obstet 1920;31: 236–9.

CHAPTER 2

Epidemiology of Glioblastoma and Trends in Glioblastoma Survivorship

Quinn T. Ostrom, MPH, MA, Peter Liao, BS, MD,
Lindsay C. Stetson, PhD, Jill S. Barnholtz-Sloan, PhD*

INCIDENCE OF GLIOBLASTOMA

Gliomas are the most common type of malignant brain tumor in adults. Of the gliomas, glioblastoma (astrocytoma grade IV) is the most common, and represents approximately 27% of all primary brain tumors, and 80% of malignant primary brain tumors in the United States.[1] Incidence of glioblastoma in the United States varies significantly by sex, race, ethnicity, and age (**Fig. 2.1**). From 2006 to 2012, glioblastoma occurred at an overall average annual age-adjusted incidence rate (AAAIR) of 3.20 (95% confidence interval [95% CI], 3.17–3.22) per 100,000 population. Glioblastoma is 1.6 times more common in men than in women, with an AAAIR of 3.99 (95% CI, 3.94–4.03) per 100,000 in men, and 2.53 (95% CI, 2.50–2.56) per 100,000 in women. Incidence of glioblastoma is significantly higher in non-Hispanic people (AAAIR, 3.28, 95% CI, 3.25–3.31) compared with Hispanic people (AAAIR, 2.41; 95% CI, 2.33–2.50). Glioblastoma is most common in white people (AAAIR, 3.45; 95% CI, 3.42–3.48), compared with black people (AAAIR, 1.76; 95% CI, 1.69–1.82), American Indian/Alaska natives (AIAN) (AAAIR, 1.47; 95% CI, 1.25–1.70), and Asian/Pacific Islanders (API) (AAAIR, 1.60; 95% CI, 1.51–1.70). Incidence of glioblastoma increases with increasing age. Incidence is lowest among people 0 to 19 years old (AAAIR, 0.15; 95% CI, 0.13–0.16) and highest among those 75 years and older (AAAIR, 13.66; 95% CI, 13.42–13.91).

INCIDENCE TIME TRENDS

There was no significant increase in incidence of glioblastoma in the United States between 2000 and 2010.[2] This trend is similar to patterns of incidence in other countries, including Australia and the United Kingdom. Previous analyses showed an increasing incidence of malignant brain tumors during the 1980s and the 1990s, but this is thought to be the result of screening bias caused by increasing access to and use of medical imaging technologies such as computed tomography (CT) and MRI.

SURVIVAL AFTER DIAGNOSIS WITH GLIOBLASTOMA

Glioblastoma has one of the poorest survival rates of any malignant brain tumor,[1] and contributes disproportionately to cancer mortality and morbidity. Median survival after diagnosis with glioblastoma is approximately 12 months, and this survival period increases to approximately 14 months when patients are treated with current standard therapy, which consists of maximal safe surgical resection followed by concurrent radiation and temozolomide.[3] Between 2000 and 2012 in the United States, glioblastoma had a 1-year relative survival rate of 37.8% (95% CI, 37.3%–38.4%), with 5.1% (95% CI, 4.8%–5.7%) of persons surviving 5 years after diagnosis (**Fig. 2.2**). One-year survival rates have improved

---

Conflicts of Interest: The authors have any commercial or financial conflicts of interest to disclose related to this work.
Case Comprehensive Cancer Center, Case Western Reserve University School of Medicine, 1-200 Wolstein Research Building, 2103 Cornell Road, Cleveland, OH 44106-7295, USA
* Corresponding author. Case Comprehensive Cancer Center, Case Western Reserve University School of Medicine, 2-526 Wolstein Research Building, 2103 Cornell Road, Cleveland, OH 44106-7295.
E-mail address: jsb42@case.edu

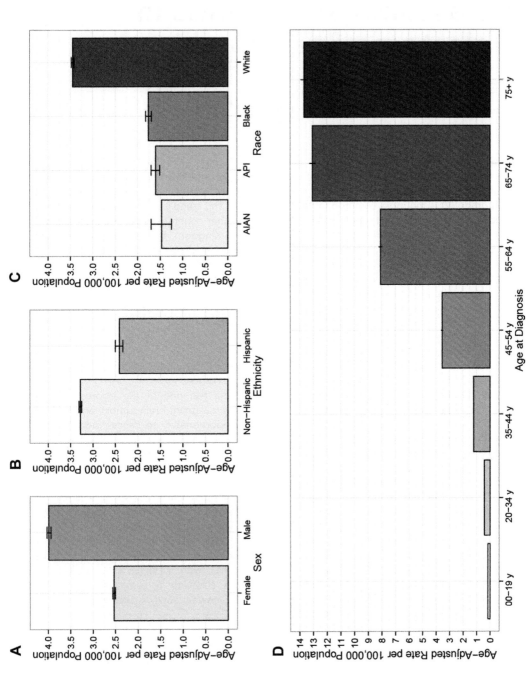

Fig. 2.1 Average annual age-adjusted incidence rates of glioblastoma by (A) sex, (B) Hispanic ethnicity, (C) race, and (D) age groups for diagnoses between 2008 and 2012. AIAN, American Indian/Alaska Native; API, Asian Pacific Islander. (*Data from* Central Brain Tumor Registry of the United States (CBTRUS). Available at: http://www.cbtrus. org/. Accessed April 27, 2016.)

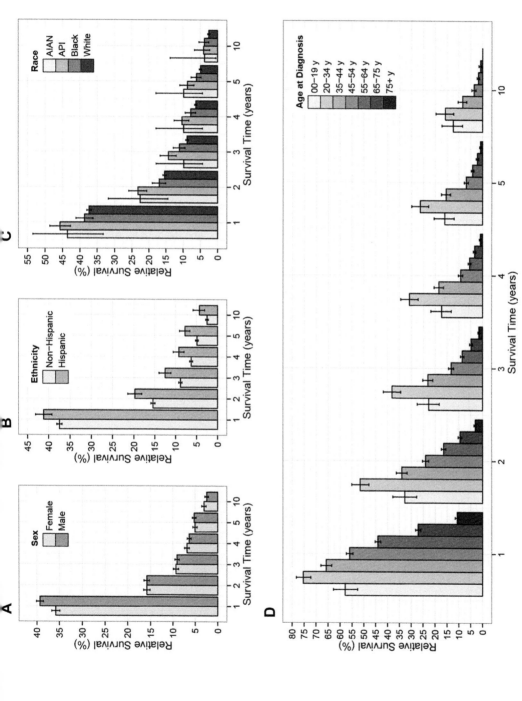

Fig. 2.2 One-year, 2-year, 3-year, 4-year, 5-year, and 10-year relative survival rates after diagnosis with glioblastoma by (A) sex, (B) Hispanic ethnicity, (C) race, and (D) age groups for diagnoses between 2000 and 2012. (*Data from* National Cancer Institute. Surveillance, Epidemiology and End Results Program. Available at: http://seer.cancer. gov/. Accessed April 27, 2016.)

since 2000, likely because of the current standard therapy being widely adopted. Survival rates over time vary significantly by age at diagnosis, with persons aged 20 to 34 years having the best overall survival. There are some small differences in 1-year survival by sex and ethnicity, but there are no significant differences by sex, ethnicity, and race in long-term survival with glioblastoma.

SURVIVAL TIME TRENDS

There have been significant increases in both 1-year and 5-year survival after diagnosis with glioblastoma since 1973 (**Fig. 2.3**). From 1997 to 2012, 1-year survival increased with an annual percentage change (APC) of 3.7% (95% CI, 3.1%–4.3%) from 24.3% (95% CI, 21.4%–27.2%) at the beginning of the time period, to 43.0% (95% CI, 37.6%–48.3%) at the end of the time period. Five-year survival also increased from 1997 to 2012, with an APC of 8.0% (95% CI, 5.1%–11.0%) from 2.1% (95% 1.3%–3.3%) at the beginning of the time period to 5.6% (95% CI, 4.7%–6.7%) at the end of the time period. This

trend may be caused by a wide variety of factors including increased screening and earlier detection caused by improvements in medical imaging technologies, as well as the introduction of new treatment modalities, such as the current standard therapy in the early to mid-2000s.

LONG-TERM SURVIVAL IN GLIOBLASTOMA

The National Cancer Institute's Surveillance, Epidemiology and End Results (SEER) has been collecting data on cancer diagnoses in population-based registries since 1973. This program initially started with 9 registries, but has since increased to 18 (comprising ~26% of the United States population). From 1973 to 2012, there were 51,152 persons diagnosed with a glioblastoma in the SEER data set; 1611 of these persons (3.1%) survived at least 5 years after diagnosis, and approximately 733 (54% of 1611) were still alive as of 2012. Compared with the population of persons who lived 18 months or less after their diagnoses, this population is significantly younger, with mean age at diagnosis of 48.3 years

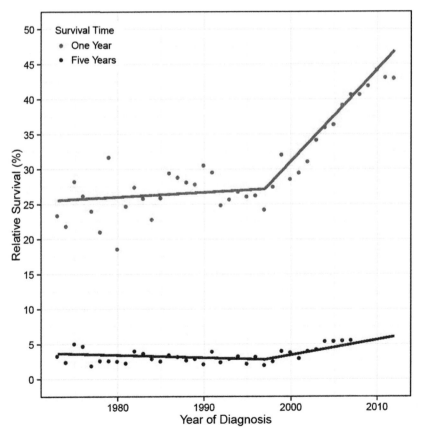

Fig. 2.3 Relative 1-year and 5-year overall survival after diagnosis with glioblastoma. (*Data from* National Cancer Institute. Surveillance, Epidemiology and End Results (SEER) 1973–2012. Available at: http://seer.cancer.gov/. Accessed April 27, 2016.)

compared with 63.4 years (P<.001). Slightly more long-term (> 5 years) and median-term (< 18 months) survivors were male, with no significant differences in gender distribution between the two groups. In addition, fewer in this population were white (88.4% compared with 91.4%; P<.001), with 5.9% and 4.9% of these long-term survivors being black and API, respectively. A larger proportion of these long-term survivors are Hispanic compared with those who lived 18 months or less (10.6% compared with 7.2%; P<.001).

RISK FACTORS FOR GLIOMA
Environmental Risk Factors
Many environmental and behavioral risk factors have been investigated as causative for glioma. The only well-validated factors are an increased risk associated with exposure to ionizing radiation[4] (the type of radiation generated by atomic bombs, therapeutic radiation treatment, CT scans, MRI scans, and x-rays) and a decreased risk in persons with history of allergy or other atopic disease[5] (including eczema, psoriasis, and asthma). Recent review articles have further elaborated on the current state of risk factor research in malignant brain tumors.[6]

Heritable Genetic Risk Factors
Several inherited, monogenic mendelian cancer syndromes are associated with increased incidence of glioblastoma, including Lynch syndrome (glioblastoma and other gliomas), Li-Fraumeni syndrome (glioblastoma and other gliomas), melanoma–neural system tumor syndrome (all gliomas), and Ollier disease/Maffucci syndrome (all gliomas).[6,7] However, these monogenic disorders account for only a small proportion of glioma cases (<5% overall). A small proportion (about 5%–10%) of gliomas occur in familial clusters, in which multiple members of a family have been diagnosed with a glioma. First-degree relatives of patients with glioma have a 2-fold increased risk of developing a brain tumor, and this effect is stronger with family members who are young at the time of diagnosis.[7] Linkage studies within families with multiple patients with glioma have not definitively identified risk variants that are strongly associated with diagnosis of glioma (highly penetrant). In the absence of a clear pattern of risk variants identifiable across many families, segregation analyses suggest that genetic risk factors for glioma are best explained with a multigene (polygenic) model.[8]

Five genome-wide association studies of patients with glioma have been conducted.[9–13]

Together, these studies identified 7 genomic variants that correlated with increased risk of developing a glioma. The variants and their respective genes are telomerase reverse transcriptase (TERT, rs2736100)[9–11,13,14]; epidermal growth factor receptor (EGFR, rs2252586[11,13,15,16] and rs11979158)[11,13,15,16]; coiled-coil domain containing 26 (CCDC26, rs55705857)[10,13,16–18]; cyclin-dependent kinase inhibitor 2B (CDKN2B, rs1412829)[9,10,13]; pleckstrin homologylike domain, family B, member 1 (PHLDB1, rs498872)[10,13,19]; tumor protein p53 (TP53, rs78378222)[12,20,21]; and regulator of telomere elongation helicase (RTEL1, rs6010620).[9,10,13,14] Four of these variants (TERT, RTEL1, EGFR, and TP53) increase risk of all types of glioma, whereas 3 of these only increase risk for specific grades and histologies of glioma (CDKN2B, PHLDB1, and CCDC26). Both CCDC26 and PHLDB1 are associated with tumors that have mutations in IDH1/IDH2 (most often World Health Organization [WHO] grade II and III gliomas), whereas CDKN2B is associated with astrocytic tumors in general (WHO grades II–IV).[6,22] Two variants in telomere-related genes increase risk for all glioma types (rs2736100 [TERT] and rs6010620 [RTEL1]). Telomere length has been associated with other types of cancer, but a recent case-control study did not find a significant overall association between this variant and risk of glioma.[23] A recent review article further elaborated on the current state of heritable genetic risk for glioma.[6]

GLIOBLASTOMA SUBTYPES AND SURVIVAL
Primary and Secondary Glioblastoma
Clinical presentation of glioblastoma follows 2 main paradigms: primary glioblastoma, which develops predominantly in elderly adults without previous evidence of a precursor malignancy, and secondary glioblastoma, which occurs mainly in younger patients as a progression from lower-grade glioma.[24] Secondary glioblastomas are rare; a population-based study showed that only 5% of all glioblastomas were secondary.[24] Although indistinguishable histologically, primary and secondary glioblastomas show key molecular differences. EGFR overexpression is observed in many primary glioblastomas, whereas TP53 mutations occur at high incidence in secondary glioblastomas; the mutual exclusivity of these features has suggested distinct pathways for primary and secondary glioblastoma development.[25] More recently, in 2008, mutations in IDH1/IDH2 mutations as a marker of secondary glioblastoma were reported and have subsequently been shown to be very frequent in secondary glioblastomas and rare in primary

glioblastomas (>80% and <5%, respectively).[26] A population-based study showed that only 3.4% of primary glioblastomas carried an *IDH1* mutation, and that these patients were younger than their counterparts with secondary glioblastoma, had frequent mutation of *TP53*, and lacked amplification of *EGFR*, suggesting that glioblastomas with isocitrate dehydrogenase 1/2 (*IDH1/IDH2*) mutations diagnosed as primary glioblastomas may be misclassified secondary gliomas (Table 2.1).[24,27] It has been proposed that *IDH1/ IDH2* mutation status rather than clinical history can be used as a more reliable marker of primary and secondary glioblastoma for the purposes of prognosis and treatment.[24] *IDH1/IDH2* mutations in glioblastoma are prognostically significant; patients with *IDH1/IDH2* mutations had a median overall survival of 94 weeks versus 31 weeks for those patients without mutations in *IDH1/ IDH2*.[28] In addition, lower-grade gliomas that lack mutations in *IDH1/IDH2* have significantly shorter survival times, and seem to be more glioblastomalike.[29]

Glioblastoma Somatic Mutations

The Cancer Genome Atlas (TCGA) initial analysis of genetic alterations in glioblastomas identified aberrations in 3 core pathways: *TP53*, retinoblastoma (*RB*), and receptor tyrosine kinase (*RTK*)/ Ras/phosphoinositide 3-kinase (*PI3K*) signaling. Seventy-four percent of the 206 analyzed glioblastomas in the study had genomic aberrations in *RB*, *TP53*, and receptor tyrosine kinase (*RTK*) pathways, and 87%, 78%, and 88% of samples showed somatic alterations in core components of each of the 3 pathways, respectively.[30] A statistical tendency toward mutual exclusivity of within-pathway alterations was also observed, suggesting that these genetic alterations are driver alterations that are important in glioblastoma pathogenesis. Within each pathway, common alterations to specific genes were identified. In the *RTK* pathway, in addition to *EGFR* mutation and amplification, *PDGFRA* amplification, *PI3K* mutation, and mutation and deletion of neurofibromatosis 1 (*NF1*) and *PTEN* were also observed. In the *TP53* pathway, homozygous deletions and mutations were observed in *CDKN2A* and *TP53*. In the RB pathway, homozygous deletion and mutations of *CDKN2A*, *CDKN2B*, and *RB1* were observed in conjunction with amplification in cyclin-dependent kinase 4 (*CDK4*). Expanded exome sequencing performed on 291 paired tumor and normal samples

---

TABLE 2.1
Prognostic and/or predictive molecular features of glioblastoma

Glioblastoma Subtype	Prognostic	Predictive	Note
DNA Methylation			
MGMT	Yes	Yes	Silencing of gene responsible for alkylated DNA repair; effect may be related to classic subtype
G-CIMP	Yes	No	Associated with proneural subtype, *IDH1* mutation status
Messenger RNA Expression			
Proneural	No	No	Proneural contains most secondary GBM, trends toward increased survival, younger age, enriched for *IDH1* mutation
Classic	No	No	Classic subtype may have role in *MGMT* survival benefit
Mesenchymal	No	No	Associated with increased expression of markers of necrosis and inflammation, endothelial markers. Moderately increased activation of MAPK pathway
Neural	No	No	Characterized by expression of neuronal markers
Somatic Alteration			
IDH1/IDH2 mutation	Yes	Yes	Potential marker of primary/secondary GBM status, with *IDH1/IDH2* mutation showing lower-grade gliomalike features with improved survival, attenuated response to aggressive treatment. *ATRX* mutation associated, *TERT* promoter mutation exclusive

Abbreviations: GBM, glioblastoma; G-CIMP, glioma CpG island (regions of DNA that are enriched for cytosine and guanine nucleotides) methylator phenotype; IDH1/2, isocitrate dehydrogenase 1/2; MAPK, mitogen-activated protein kinase; MGMT, O(6)-methylguanine-DNA-methyltransferase.

in a 2013 TCGA update identified novel somatic mutations in glioblastoma, including mutations in leucine zipper–like transcriptional regulator 1 (*LZTR1*), spectrin alpha 1 (*SPTA1*), Gamma-aminobutyric acid receptor subunit alpha-6 (*GABRA6*), Kell blood group, metallo-endopeptidase (*KEL*), and ATRX, chromatin remodeler (*ATRX*).[31] Of note, *ATRX* mutations most often coincided with *IDH1* mutation, consistent with secondary glioblastoma. In the same update, analysis of whole-genome sequencing data confirmed mutations of the *TERT* promoter region in 21 out of 25 glioblastoma cases with promoter mutation correlated with increased *TERT* expression levels. The 4 cases that did not harbor *TERT* promoter mutations and did not have increased *TERT* messenger RNA (mRNA) expression all harbored *ATRX* mutations concurrent with *IDH1*, which is suggestive of secondary glioblastoma. Taken as a whole, telomerase lengthening in glioblastoma pathogenesis seems to be accomplished via *TERT* mutation in most glioblastomas, whereas *IDH1/IDH2* mutant tumors exploit *ATRX* mutations to drive alternative lengthening of telomeres, as previously described in the literature.[31,32]

Gene Expression Subtypes

In 2010, 4 gene expression subtypes of glioblastoma were identified: proneural, neural, classic, and mesenchymal (see **Table 2.1**).[33] The classic subtype is characterized by higher levels of *EGFR* expression, relative lack of *TP53* mutations, deletion of *CDKN2A*, and high expression of Sonic hedgehog and Notch pathways and neural precursor and stem cell marker nestin relative to other subtypes. The mesenchymal subtype was characterized by deletion of *NF1* and lower *NF1* expression, as well as increased expression of genes in the tumor necrosis factor superfamily pathway and nuclear factor kappa-B pathway, suggesting increased necrosis and inflammation. The proneural subtype was characterized by alterations of *PDGFRA* leading to amplification and increased expression, as well as point mutations in *IDH1*. The neural subtype was identified by expression of neuron markers such as neurofilament, light polypeptide (*NEFL*), gamma-aminobutyric acid type A receptor alpha1 subunit (*GABRA1*), synaptotagmin 1 (*SYT1*), and solute carrier family 12 member 5 (*SLC12A5*). This initial analysis showed that the proneural subtype was associated with a younger age at diagnosis and a trend toward longer survival, whereas patients with the mesenchymal subtype had poorer survival. Most secondary glioblastomas in the data set were classified as proneural, leading to the

suggestion that it may be more accurate to understand the proneural subtype as a reflection of secondary glioblastoma status. In this interpretation, the survival benefit observed in the proneural subtype is reflective of the enrichment for secondary glioblastomas rather than existing as a true subtype. In an updated analysis using TCGA data from more than 500 glioblastomas, differences in survival between these 4 subtype groups was no longer shown, with the exception being the proneural tumors with *IDH1/IDH2* mutations and the hypermethylator phenotype.[31]

Epigenetic Alterations

Epigenetic alterations have been among the most clinically relevant findings in glioblastoma. Promoter methylation of the DNA-repair gene, O(6)-methylguanine-DNA-methyltransferase (*MGMT*), has been shown to be prognostically significant in glioblastoma (see **Table 2.1**).[34] *MGMT* activity confers resistance to DNA alkylation, blunting response to alkylating chemotherapeutic agents such as temozolomide, which in conjunction with radiation completes the current standard-of-care treatment of glioblastoma.[34] Methylation of the *MGMT* promoter has been shown to be a positive prognostic predictor of survival irrespective of treatment, with a hazard ratio of 0.45 (95%CI, 0.32–0.61) compared with glioblastomas with unmethylated *MGMT*.[34] *MGMT* methylation confers a stronger benefit to patients receiving both radiotherapy and temozolomide compared with radiotherapy alone (2-year survival rates of 46% and 23%, respectively).[34] Although promoter methylation of *MGMT* is an accepted glioblastoma prognostic biomarker, its clinical utility has been limited. Only 20% to 40% of patients with glioblastoma have methylation in the *MGMT* promoter, there is no consensus on how best to measure *MGMT* methylation, there exists no clear cutoff between methylated and unmethlyated *MGMT*, and there are no standard treatment alternatives for those patients with unmethylated *MGMT* promoters.[35,36]

DNA methylation changes have been observed to play biological roles in human cancers, most commonly in the context of global hypomethylation with CpG island (regions of DNA that are enriched for cytosine and guanine nucleotides) hypermethylation in promoter regions causing transcriptional silencing of associated genes.[37] Analysis of DNA methylation profiles of 272 TCGA glioblastoma samples identified a subset of samples with broad hypermethylation described as a glioma CpG island methylator phenotype (G-CIMP) (see **Table 2.1**).[37]

G-CIMP tumors were found to be highly overrepresented in the proneural expression subtype and tightly associated with *IDH1/IDH2* mutation status. Patients with these tumors have significantly improved outcome, median overall survival of 150 weeks for G-CIMP–positive patients, and median overall survival of 42 weeks for G-CIMP–negative patients.[37] Although this combination of biomarkers has been well validated, patients with proneural, G-CIMP–positive, *IDH1/IDH2*–mutated tumors represent ~6% of all glioblastomas, limiting clinical impact.[31] These findings were recently recapitulated in a TCGA analysis of more than 1000 diffuse gliomas.[38] This large study confirmed many previously observed epigenetic modifications in glioma and also identified new glioma subtypes; *IDH1/IDH2* mutant gliomas that were demethylated were shown to be associated with poor outcome, and a group of *IDH1/IDH2* wild-type gliomas was identified that were molecularly similar to pilocytic astrocytoma and had favorable survival.

REFERENCES

1. Ostrom QT, Gittleman H, Fulop J, et al. CBTRUS statistical report: primary brain and central nervous system tumors diagnosed in the United States in 2008-2012. Neuro Oncol 2015;17(Suppl 4):iv1–62.
2. Gittleman HR, Ostrom QT, Rouse CD, et al. Trends in central nervous system tumor incidence relative to other common cancers in adults, adolescents, and children in the United States, 2000 to 2010. Cancer 2015;121(1):102–12.
3. Stupp R, Mason WP, van den Bent MJ, et al. Radiotherapy plus concomitant and adjuvant temozolomide for glioblastoma. N Engl J Med 2005; 352(10):987–96.
4. Braganza MZ, Kitahara CM, Berrington de Gonzalez A, et al. Ionizing radiation and the risk of brain and central nervous system tumors: a systematic review. Neuro Oncol 2012;14(11):1316–24.
5. Turner MC. Epidemiology: allergy history, IgE, and cancer. Cancer Immunol Immunother 2012;61(9): 1493–510.
6. Ostrom QT, Bauchet L, Davis F, et al. The epidemiology of glioma in adults: a "state of the science" review. Neuro Oncol 2014;16(7):896–913.
7. Goodenberger ML, Jenkins RB. Genetics of adult glioma. Cancer Genet 2012;205(12):613–21.
8. de Andrade M, Barnholtz JS, Amos CI, et al. Segregation analysis of cancer in families of glioma patients. Genet Epidemiol 2001;20(2):258–70.
9. Wrensch M, Jenkins RB, Chang JS, et al. Variants in the CDKN2B and RTEL1 regions are associated with high-grade glioma susceptibility. Nat Genet 2009; 41(8):905–8.
10. Shete S, Hosking FJ, Robertson LB, et al. Genome-wide association study identifies five susceptibility loci for glioma. Nat Genet 2009;41(8):899–904.
11. Sanson M, Hosking FJ, Shete S, et al. Chromosome 7p11.2 (EGFR) variation influences glioma risk. Hum Mol Genet 2011;20(14):2897–904.
12. Stacey SN, Sulem P, Jonasdottir A, et al. A germline variant in the TP53 polyadenylation signal confers cancer susceptibility. Nat Genet 2011;43(11):1098–103.
13. Rajaraman P, Melin BS, Wang Z, et al. Genome-wide association study of glioma and meta-analysis. Hum Genet 2012;131(12):1877–88.
14. Chen H, Chen Y, Zhao Y, et al. Association of sequence variants on chromosomes 20, 11, and 5 (20q13.33, 11q23.3, and 5p15.33) with glioma susceptibility in a Chinese population. Am J Epidemiol 2011;173(8):915–22.
15. Walsh KM, Anderson E, Hansen HM, et al. Analysis of 60 reported glioma risk SNPs replicates published GWAS findings but fails to replicate associations from published candidate-gene studies. Genet Epidemiol 2013;37(2):222–8.
16. Jenkins RB, Wrensch MR, Johnson D, et al. Distinct germ line polymorphisms underlie glioma morphologic heterogeneity. Cancer Genet 2011;204(1):13–8.
17. Jenkins RB, Xiao Y, Sicotte H, et al. A low-frequency variant at 8q24.21 is strongly associated with risk of oligodendroglial tumors and astrocytomas with IDH1 or IDH2 mutation. Nat Genet 2012;44(10): 1122–5.
18. Enciso-Mora V, Hosking FJ, Kinnersley B, et al. Deciphering the 8q24.21 association for glioma. Hum Mol Genet 2013;22(11):2293–302.
19. Rice T, Zheng S, Decker PA, et al. Inherited variant on chromosome 11q23 increases susceptibility to IDH-mutated but not IDH-normal gliomas regardless of grade or histology. Neuro Oncol 2013; 15(5):535–41.
20. Egan KM, Nabors LB, Olson JJ, et al. Rare TP53 genetic variant associated with glioma risk and outcome. J Med Genet 2012;49(7):420–1.
21. Enciso-Mora V, Hosking FJ, Di Stefano AL, et al. Low penetrance susceptibility to glioma is caused by the TP53 variant rs78378222. Br J Cancer 2013; 108(10):2178–85.
22. Melin B, Jenkins R. Genetics in glioma: lessons learned from genome-wide association studies. Curr Opin Neurol 2013;26(6):688–92.
23. Walcott F, Rajaraman P, Gadalla SM, et al. Telomere length and risk of glioma. Cancer Epidemiol 2013;37(6):935–8.
24. Ohgaki H, Kleihues P. The definition of primary and secondary glioblastoma. Clin Cancer Res 2013; 19(4):764–72.
25. Watanabe K, Tachibana O, Sata K, et al. Overexpression of the EGF receptor and p53

mutations are mutually exclusive in the evolution of primary and secondary glioblastomas. Brain Pathol 1996;6(3):217–23 [discussion: 223–4].

26. Balss J, Meyer J, Mueller W, et al. Analysis of the IDH1 codon 132 mutation in brain tumors. Acta Neuropathol 2008;116(6):597–602.

27. Ohgaki H, Dessen P, Jourde B, et al. Genetic pathways to glioblastoma: a population-based study. Cancer Res 2004;64(19):6892–9.

28. Molenaar RJ, Verbaan D, Lamba S, et al. The combination of IDH1 mutations and MGMT methylation status predicts survival in glioblastoma better than either IDH1 or MGMT alone. Neuro Oncol 2014; 16(9):1263–73.

29. Cancer Genome Atlas Research Network, Brat DJ, Verhaak RG, et al. Comprehensive, integrative genomic analysis of diffuse lower-grade gliomas. N Engl J Med 2015;372(26):2481–98.

30. Cancer Genome Atlas Research Network. Comprehensive genomic characterization defines human glioblastoma genes and core pathways. Nature 2008;455(7216):1061–8.

31. Brennan CW, Verhaak RG, McKenna A, et al. The somatic genomic landscape of glioblastoma. Cell 2013;155(2):462–77.

32. Lovejoy CA, Li W, Reisenweber S, et al. Loss of ATRX, genome instability, and an altered DNA damage response are hallmarks of the alternative lengthening of telomeres pathway. PLoS Genet 2012;8(7):e1002772.

33. Verhaak RG, Hoadley KA, Purdom E, et al. Integrated genomic analysis identifies clinically relevant subtypes of glioblastoma characterized by abnormalities in PDGFRA, IDH1, EGFR, and NF1. Cancer Cell 2010;17(1):98–110.

34. Hegi ME, Diserens AC, Gorlia T, et al. MGMT gene silencing and benefit from temozolomide in glioblastoma. N Engl J Med 2005;352(10):997–1003.

35. Hegi ME, Liu L, Herman JG, et al. Correlation of O6-methylguanine methyltransferase (MGMT) promoter methylation with clinical outcomes in glioblastoma and clinical strategies to modulate MGMT activity. J Clin Oncol 2008;26(25):4189–99.

36. Suri V, Jha P, Sharma MC, et al. O6-methylguanine DNA methyltransferase gene promoter methylation in high-grade gliomas: a review of current status. Neurol India 2011;59(2):229–35.

37. Noushmehr H, Weisenberger DJ, Diefes K, et al. Identification of a CpG island methylator phenotype that defines a distinct subgroup of glioma. Cancer Cell 2010;17(5):510–22.

38. Ceccarelli M, Barthel FP, Malta TM, et al. Molecular profiling reveals biologically discrete subsets and pathways of progression in diffuse glioma. Cell 2016;164(3):550–63.

CHAPTER 3

The Molecular Pathogenesis of Glioblastoma

Kalil G. Abdullah, MD[a], Corey Adamson, MD, PhD, MPH[b], Steven Brem, MD[a,*]

The cellular origin of glioblastoma is complex. Despite decades of research, the understanding of the cellular, molecular, and pathogenetic architecture of this lethal disease is still evolving. Other chapters discuss the epidemiology, risk factors, associated clinical outcomes, and molecular targeting for glioblastoma. There are also chapters that describe the mechanisms of small molecule inhibitors, targets for therapeutics and their molecular basis, immune evasion, and mechanisms of angiogenesis and proliferation. This chapter provides a practical and concise overview for practicing clinicians of the well-understood and best-studied mechanisms that cause an innocuous glial cell to transform into glioblastoma.

CLASSIFICATION AND HISTOLOGY

The most commonly used and widely accepted classification schema for malignant gliomas is based on a consensus by the World Health Organization (WHO), first published in 1979, updated in 2007, which designated glioblastoma a WHO grade IV neoplasm. WHO grading was based on glioblastoma as a "cytologically malignant, mitotically active, necrosis-prone neoplasm typically associated with rapid pre- and postoperative disease evolution and fatal outcome."[1] Deficiencies with the use of the WHO schema include inability to account for molecular subtypes, therapeutic responses, or size and location of lesion. This shortcoming has led many scientists and clinicians to advocate for a molecular grading system that more accurately takes into account the evolving understanding of the molecular pathogenesis of glioblastoma. Some of which is outlined in the following chapter.

On histology, gliomas show several characteristic findings.[2] These findings include anaplasia, high levels of mitotic activity, cellular pleomorphism, nuclear atypia, and coagulation necrosis that accompanies microvascular proliferation. Necrosis is the result of ischemia caused by endothelial cell hyperplasia and hypertrophy. There is a hypercellularity present throughout the tumor, with atypical mitotic figures, bizarre nuclei, and multinucleated cells. Commonly referred to is the concept of pseudopalisading necrosis, which consists of tumor cells that appear to surround centralized necrotic zones. The presence of both necrosis and endothelial proliferation is necessary for the histologic diagnosis to be complete, to differentiate glioblastoma from anaplastic astrocytoma (**Fig. 3.1**).

These histologic findings have been in use for decades, and remain important in the initial classification after biopsy or resection of a tumor. Advances in modern molecular and genetic techniques, including large-scale profiling of data sets both at the national level (The Cancer Genome Atlas) and the international level (International Cancer Genome Consortium), have resulted in a more expansive and complex understanding of the immense heterogeneity found within tumors classified as glioblastoma (**Figs. 3.2** and **3.3**).

Recently, and importantly, Verhaak and colleagues[3] described a classification of high-grade gliomas into 4 distinct types according to genetic and molecular features based on genomic abnormalities found in The Cancer Genome Atlas Network. The investigators used the factor analysis method to integrate data from glioblastoma and normal brain samples on 3 different gene expression platforms. Consensus clustering and further validation ultimately yielded 4 subtypes that were named from their signature gene expression: proneural, neural, classic, and mesenchymal.

[a] Department of Neurosurgery, Hospital of the University of Pennsylvania, Silverstein 3, 3400 Spruce Street, Philadelphia, PA 19104, USA; [b] Department of Neurosurgery, The Emory Clinic, Building B, 2nd Floor, 1365 Clifton Road, North East, Suite 2200, Atlanta, GA 30322, USA
* Corresponding author.
E-mail address: Steven.Brem@uphs.upenn.edu

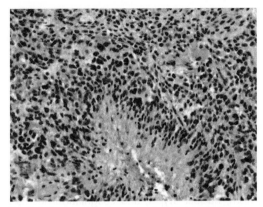

Fig. 3.1 Standard and prototypical histopathologic hematoxylin and eosin stain of glioblastoma. Clearly seen are necrotic foci (*pink*) surrounded by a pseudopalisading necrosis. H&E stain. (*Courtesy of* KGH, GNU free documentation license. Available at: https://commons.wikimedia.org/wiki/File:Glioblastoma_(1).jpg. Accessed April 28, 2016.)

The classic subtype consisted of chromosome 7 amplifications paired with chromosome 10 loss 100% of the time. In addition, high-level epidermal growth factor receptor (*EGFR*) amplification was found in 97% of the classic subtype, and infrequently in others. There was also a lack of *TP53* mutations despite *TP53* being a frequently mutated gene in glioblastoma. In the mesenchymal subtype, there were focal hemizygous deletions at region 17q11.2, which contained the gene *NF1*, and there were frequent comutations of *NF1* and *PTEN*

that intersected the AKT (protein kinase B) pathway. The proneural subtype was defined mostly by alterations of *PDGFRA* and *IDH1*, and most *TP53* mutations were found in the proneural subtype. The neural subtype had expression of several different neuronal markers that were ontologically consistent with genes involved in axonal and synaptic transmission as well as neuronal projection (**Fig. 3.4**).

After classification of subtypes was completed, the effect of level of treatment intensity was evaluated for each of the subtypes. Aggressive treatments reduced mortality in the classic, mesenchymal, and neural subtypes (trend toward, but not statistically significant), but not the proneural subtype (**Table 3.1**).

Primary and Secondary Glioblastoma

It has been recognized since the 1940s that 2 distinct clinical histories exist for glioblastoma. In the first, there is a rapidly progressive onset of disease without a preexisting low-grade tumor, occurring most frequently with older patients. In the second, there is the transformation of an existing low-grade tumor to glioblastoma in a younger patient and a comparable clinical course.[4] These two pathways have been evaluated and characterized by their molecular genetics and are referred to respectively as primary and secondary glioblastoma.

The ability to differentiate between these 2 different types of glioblastoma progression is

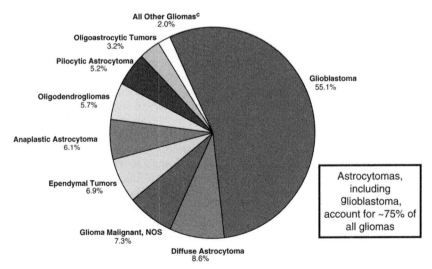

Fig. 3.2 Distribution of primary brain and central nervous system gliomas by histology subtypes (N = 97,910), Central Brain Tumor Registry of the United States Statistical Report: National Program of Cancer Registries and Surveillance, Epidemiology, and End Results, 2008 to 2012. [a] Percentages may not add up to 100% because of rounding. [b] International Classification of Diseases for Oncology, Third Edition, codes = 9380 to 9384, 9391 to 9460. [c] Includes histologies from unique astrocytoma variants, other neuroepithelial tumors, and neuronal and mixed neuronal-glial tumors. NOS, not otherwise specified.

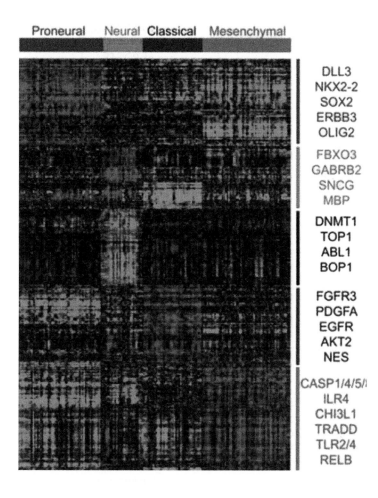

Proneural Neural **Classical** Mesenchymal

DLL3
NKX2-2
SOX2
ERBB3
OLIG2

FBXO3
GABRB2
SNCG
MBP

DNMT1
TOP1
ABL1
BOP1

FGFR3
PDGFA
EGFR
AKT2
NES

CASP1/4/5/
ILR4
CHI3L1
TRADD
TLR2/4
RELB

Fig. 3.3 Clustering gene expression subtypes based on 173 samples from The Cancer Genome Atlas. (*From* Verhaak RG, Hoadley KA, Purdom E, et al. Integrated genomic analysis identifies clinically relevant subtypes of glioblastoma characterized by abnormalities in PDGFRA, IDH1, EGFR, and NF1. Cancer Cell 2010;17:101; with permission.)

based on significant genetic and epidemiologic evidence. First and foremost, only approximately 5% of all cases of glioblastoma are thought to be manifestations of secondary glioblastoma,[5] an observation based on several population-based studies, including a landmark study by Ohgaki and colleagues[5] that examined 715 glioblastomas in Zürich, Switzerland, between 1980 and 1994. The study also examined age differences between diagnostic groups and found that the mean age of primary glioblastoma was 62 years, compared with a much younger 45 years for patients with secondary glioblastoma.

The molecular and genetic pathways to both primary and secondary glioblastoma also provide the opportunity to discuss the wayward progression of an astrocyte or precursor cell to a high-grade glioma (**Fig. 3.5**).

TP53 and MDM2
TP53 is a gene found on chromosome 17 that codes for a 53-kDa protein involved in various aspects of the cell cycle, including cell death, response of cells to DNA damage, differentiation,

and vascular phenomena. It is generally thought that *TP53* mutations are found more frequently in secondary glioblastoma because they are often the first detectable genetic alteration in up to two-thirds of low-grade astrocytomas, although they may occur in up to 30% of primary glioblastomas as well given the variety of functions enacted by *TP53* in the cell cycle.[5] After DNA damage, p53 is activated and induces a variety of genes, including p21, which is a cycle-independent kinase inhibitor. After induction of *p21*, *MDM2* (mouse double minute 2 homolog, an E3 ubiquitin-protein ligase whose key target is the p53 tumor suppressor) becomes involved in an autoregulatory feedback loop. *MDM2* is able to repress p53 by binding to and blocking the N-terminal transactivation domain of p53. *MDM2* binds to both the mutant and wild-type *TP53* proteins, inhibiting transcription of activation of wild-type *TP53*. As a component of this feedback loop, transcription of the MDM2 gene is induced by the wild-type *TP53*. As a result, the normal feedback loop, which would regulate the activity of the *TP53* protein and expression of *MDM2*, is

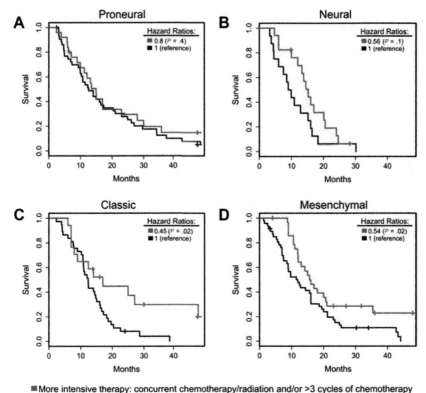

Fig. 3.4 Survival by treatment and tumor subtype. (*From* Verhaak RG, Hoadley KA, Purdom E, et al. Integrated genomic analysis identifies clinically relevant subtypes of glioblastoma characterized by abnormalities in PDGFRA, IDH1, EGFR, and NF1. Cancer Cell 2010;17:106; with permission.)

disrupted. Also involved in this loop is the role of a *p14* gene product, which binds to *MDM2* and inhibits *MDM2*-mediated *TP53* silencing and degradation.[6] As a result, loss of normal *TP53* function could follow altered expression from *TP53* itself, *MDM2*, or *p14* (**Fig. 3.6**).

Loss of Heterozygosity on Chromosome 10 and PTEN

The genetic concept of loss of heterozygosity (LOH) is a large-scale chromosomal event that ends in the loss of an entire gene and surrounding chromosome region. This event is relevant in many oncologic processes because it typically indicates the absence of a functional tumor suppressor gene. Although 1 chromosome of the original chromosome pair still remains, the remaining copy of the tumor suppression gene is left vulnerable to something as seemingly Lilliputian as an inactivation by a point mutation.[7]

LOH of chromosome 10, region q, is considered by many experts to be the most frequent genetic aberration in primary and secondary glioblastomas.[5,8] In the case of primary glioblastoma (and less frequently secondary glioblastoma) the

encoded region of 10q23-24 corresponds with the *PTEN* gene (phosphatase and tensin homolog, involved in regulating enzymatic activity, which further regulates cell proliferation and death and an upstream regulator of *PI3K*). Astrocytic cells with PTEN deficiencies in mouse models are susceptible to neoplastic transformation or malignant progression.[9] In addition, LOH at 10 P is present mostly in primary glioblastomas with common complete loss of chromosome 10.[10]

EGFR and PDGFRA

The EGFR is a transmembrane glycoprotein activated by a specific family of extracellular protein ligands. *EGFR* amplification and overexpression occur in approximately 40% of primary glioblastomas but very rarely in secondary glioblastomas. It also seems that EGFR amplification has a significant age correlation, with amplification typically detected in patients more than 35 years of age.[5] Overall it seems that 57% of samples from patients with glioblastoma contain *EGFR* mutations of some variety, although that includes mutation, splicing, or rearrangement of the gene.[11] It is postulated that activation of *EGFR* occurs through

TABLE 3.1
Glioblastoma molecular subclassifications

Classification	Characteristics
Classic	Chromosome 7 amplification Chromosome 10 loss EGFR amplifications Lack of TP53, NF1, PGFRA, or IDH1 mutations Expression of NES, Notch and Sonic hedgehog signaling pathways
Mesenchymal	NF1 deletions/mutations PTEN mutation Expression of mesenchymal markers (CHI3L1, MET) Genes of tumor necrosis factor family and NF-kB pathways
Proneural	PDGFRA alterations IDH1 mutations TP53 mutations Expression of development genes (PDGFRA, NKX2-2, OLIG2, SOX, DCX, DLL3, ASCL1, TCF4) Developmental disturbances
Neural	Overexpression of neuronal markers (NEFL, GABRA1, SYT1, SLC12A5) Neuron projection and axon and synaptic transmission disturbances

Abbreviation: NF-kB, nuclear factor kappa B.

receptor tyrosine kinase–mediated interactions at the cell surface or between mutated *EGFR* and the wild-type receptor.[12]

The most common mutation in the EGFR gene is the variant (v) III, which consists of a truncation of the extracellular domain from exons 2 to 7, and is thought to be constitutively activated in glioblastoma.[13] It is thought that constitutive activation of the vIII variant results in a more invasive glioblastoma phenotype. Note that although up to 60% of primary glioblastomas contain the EGFR variant III, there are several other mutations, deletions, and insertions that provide substantial heterogeneity to the concept of EGFR aberration. The roles of EGFR as a therapeutic target and prognostic biomarker are discussed in other chapters of this book.

Similarly to *EGFR*, *PDGFR* (platelet-derived growth factor receptor) encodes a tyrosine kinase cell surface receptor, and its most common

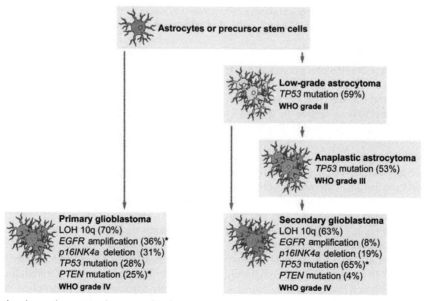

Fig. 3.5 Molecular and genetic alterations leading to primary and secondary glioblastoma. * Genetic alterations that significantly differ in frequency between primary and secondary glioblastoma. (*From* Ohgaki H, Kleihues P. Genetic pathways to primary and secondary glioblastoma. Am J Pathol 2007;170:1449; with permission.)

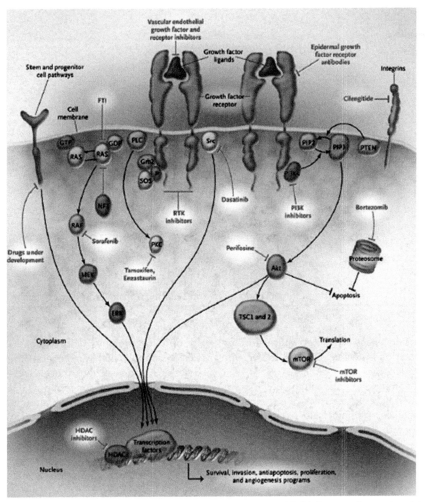

Fig. 3.6 Major signaling pathways in glioblastoma. (*From* Wen PY, Kesari S. Malignant gliomas in adults. N Engl J Med 2008;359:497. Copyright © 2008 Massachusetts Medical Society. Reprinted with permission from Massachusetts Medical Society.)

isoform is *PDGFRA* (*PDGFR* alpha polypeptide). It can be mutated in up to approximately one-third of glioblastomas and has been found to be both amplified and constitutively active in 23% and 40% of glioblastomas, respectively[14] (**Fig. 3.7**).

Isocitrate Dehydrogenase
Isocitrate dehydrogenase (IDH) is an enzyme that is best known from its role in the Krebs cycle, catalyzing the oxidative decarboxylation of isocitrate, resulting in alpha-ketoglutarate and carbon dioxide. The isoforms *IDH1* and *IDH2* encode a cytosolic and a mitochondrial protein, respectively. It is most commonly found in secondary glioblastoma, with an incidence of approximately 60% to 80%, and is much less commonly found in primary glioblastoma (on the order of 5% or less).[15] It is postulated that, given the ubiquitous nature of IDH1 and IDH2 mutation, alteration of

DNA methylation patterns and ultimately gene transcriptions in several downstream targets, including hypoxia monitoring and histone demethylation, form the basis of an early driving mutation of glioblastoma.[16,17]

It has been shown in several studies that IDH1/IDH2 mutations have prognostic significance.[18,19] In a study evaluating survival after administration of temozolomide in patients with secondary glioblastoma, IDH mutation was present in 73.4% of patients and was associated with prolonged progression-free survival and a higher rate of objective response to temozolomide.[19] In a recent study of 207 patients who underwent resection for glioblastoma, IDH1 status was independently associated with complete resection of enhancing disease (93% among IDH1 mutants vs 67% among wild type). So important is the IDH status in terms of the natural history of

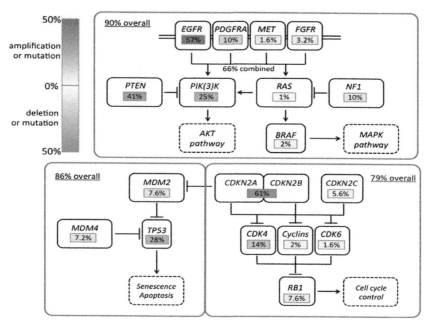

Fig. 3.7 Glioblastoma signaling pathways. (*From* Brennan CW, Verhaak RG, McKenna A, et al. The somatic genomic landscape of glioblastoma. Cell 2013;155(2):470; with permission.)

glioblastoma that the 2016 classification of CNS tumors by the World Health Organization defines glioblastomas that are IDH-mutant positive and those that are IDH-wildtype as two distinct entitites.[20]

MGMT Promoter Methylation

The most well-studied and clinically relevant promoter hypermethylation in glioblastoma is that of the promoter of MGMT, which encodes for 06-methylguanine DNA methyltransferase.[21,22] It is found in approximately 40% of patients with primary glioblastoma, and corresponds with the silencing of the MGMT gene. The role of MGMT is that of enzymatic DNA repair. The benefit of prolonged progression-free survival and overall survival in patients with the MGMT promoter methylation is probably explained by the ability of MGMT to restore guanine from 06-methylguanine. For example, temozolomide alkylates DNA at the N7 or O6 position of guanine, subsequently disrupting replication of DNA and initiating cell death.

Multiple randomized trials have supported the association of MGMT promoter hypermethylation and favorable response to temozolomide.[23–26] In 2005, the relationship between MGMT silencing and survival of patients enrolled in a randomized trial was evaluated by methylation-specific polymerase chain reaction analysis. MGMT promoter methylation was found in 45% of the 206 cases analyzed and was an independent favorable prognostic factor regardless of treatment. In patients with a methylated MGMT promoter, a significant survival benefit was conferred when they were treated with temozolomide and radiotherapy compared with patients who underwent radiotherapy alone (21.7 months vs 15.3 months). When methylation of the MGMT promoter did not occur there no statistically significant difference in survival between treatment groups. In a subgroup analysis of a randomized trial published by the European Organization for Research and Treatment of Cancer and the National Cancer Institute of Canada, MGMT promoter methylation status was again found to be a reliable predictor of positive outcome, not only in survival but in performance status and evaluation by the Mini Mental Status Examination, and the investigators recommended mandatory MGMT screening in all patients who were to undergo treatment by an alkylating chemotherapeutic (**Table 3.2**).

The Glioma Stem Cell Hypothesis

The scientific conceptualization of cancer stem cells is based on the ability of stem cells to differentiate and self-renew, possessing the same characteristics as normal stem cells but also being able to initiate a tumor mass consisting of a more heterogenous population of cells.[27,28] The cancer stem cells have been found in a variety of different solid and blood cancers, and are thought to be involved in tumorigenesis through differentiation

TABLE 3.2
Representative targeted therapies

Target	Drug	Current Trials in Glioblastoma
RTK Pathway		
EGFR	Afatinib (BIBW2992)	NCT00977431, NCT00727506
	Dacomitinib (PF-00299804)	NCT01520870, NCT01112527
	Erlotinib (OSI-744)	NCT00301418
	Gefitinib	—
	Lapatinib	NCT01591577
FGFR	BGJ398	NCT01975701
mTOR	CC214-1	—
	CC214-2	—
PDGFR	Dasatinib	NCT00892177, NCT00423735, NCT00869401
	Imatinib	—
PI3K	Buparlisib (BKM120)	NCT01934361, NCT01870726
	PX866	NCT01259869
	XL147 (SAR245408)	NCT01240460
PI3K/mTOR	PF-05212384 (PKI-587)	—
	XL765 (SAR245409)	NCT01240460
PI3/VEGF	Carboxyamidotriazole orotate	NCT01107522
VEGF	Aflibercept	—
	Cabozantinib	—
VEGF2	CT322	—
	XL184	—
VEGF/EGFR	AEE788	—
	Vandetanib (ZD6474)	NCT00821080, NCT00441142, NCT00995007
VEGF/PDGFR	Axitinib	NCT01562197, NCT01508117
	Cediranib	—
	Dovitinib (TK1258)	NCT01753715, NCT01972750
	Nintedanib (BIBF1120)	NCT01666600
	Sorafenib	NCT01817751, NCT01434602
	Sunitinib	—
P53 Pathway		
P53/MDM2	ISA27	—
	SM13	—
Cell Cycle Regulators		
Wee1	MK-1775	NCT01849146
Other		
IDH	AG-221	NCT02273739

Abbreviations: EGFR, epidermal growth factor receptor; FGFR, fibroblast growth factor receptor; MDM, murine double minute; mTOR, mammalian target of rapamycin; PDGFR, platelet-derived growth factor receptor; PI3K, phosphoinositide-3-kinase; RTK, receptor tyrosine kinase; VEGF, vascular endothelial growth factor.

and self-renewal. The cells seem to exist in both undifferentiated and differentiated states, and represent a subpopulation originating as neural stem cells transforming into glioma stem cells and driving gliomagenesis. Neural stem cells, transforming into glioma stem cells, and the putative precursors to glioma stem cells, are commonly found in the dentate gyrus of the

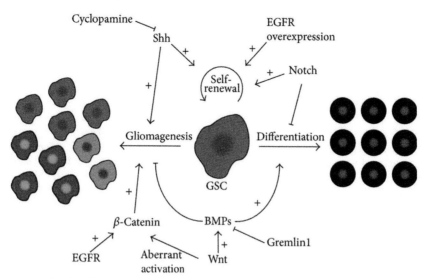

Fig. 3.8 Factors involved in glioma stem cell renewal. BMP, bone morphogenic protein; GSC, glioma stem cell. (*From* Liebelt BD, Shingu T, Zhou X, et al. Glioma stem cells: signaling, microenvironment, and therapy. Stem Cells Int 2016;2016:7849890.)

hippocampus, the subcortical white matter, and the subventricular zone.

The formation of neurospheres seems to be a critical step in the associated functions of glioma stem cells.[29] The isolation of glioma stem cells by the culturing of neurospheres is difficult, but extensive study into the traits and characteristic of neurospheres isolated from samples from patients with glioblastoma has helped to elucidate cellular and genetic pathways that provide clues to the driving forces behind transformation from neural stem cells to glioma stem cells. Yuan and colleagues[29] were able to identify self-renewing cells isolated from glioblastoma that generated daughter cells of different phenotypes from a single mother cell, and were subsequently able to differentiate into phenotypically diverse populations of cells similar to those found in the initial glioblastoma sample.

Implicated signaling pathways involved in glioma stem cell pathogenesis are often linked to normal neural development, and include bone morphogenic protein, nuclear factor kappa B, Wnt/beta catenin, Notch, Shh, and epidermal growth factor.[27] Vascular factors also seem to be heavily involved in glioma stem cell behavior. Medium from glioma stem cell cultures has been found to have levels of vascular endothelial growth factor 10 to 20 times higher than non-glioma stem cells[30] (Fig. 3.8).

The concept of a subpopulation of self-renewing cells with the capability to differentiate into glioblastoma is linked to the concept of glioma stem cells playing a key role in resistance to chemotherapy and radiation in the treatment of glioblastoma. Glioma stem cells are able to bypass changes induced by chemotherapy and radiation in several ways: modifications the cell cycle regulation, reduced drug accumulation within cells, DNA repair and processing, and continued renewal of a progenitor cell population. Importantly, some glioma cells seem to perpetually self-renew at a slow rate, making them less sensitive to the effects of chemoradiation intended to disrupt the cell cycle.[31] Among these elusive behaviors is a seemingly increased rate of *MGMT* expression in glioma stem cells compared with differentiated glioblastoma cells, resulting in enhanced DNA repair mechanisms and making the cells more adept at repairing base pair abnormalities, which include the temozolomide-induced 06-methylguanine aberration.[32] Glioma stem cells also seem to limit chemotherapeutic bioavailability via overexpression of ATP-binding cassette transporter channels and curate the cell cycle and base excision repair mechanisms exceptionally well. These factors work together to ensure glioma stem cell survival in the midst of chemotherapy and radiation.

SUMMARY

This chapter describes in broad terms the major elements of glioblastoma pathogenesis. Other chapters specifically describe the mechanisms of small molecule inhibitors, targets for therapeutics and their molecular basis, immune evasion, and mechanisms of angiogenesis and proliferation.

The landscape of molecular and genetic profiling of glioblastoma is continuously expanding, and, as these phenomena are increasingly well described, therapeutic targets with biological underpinnings may more accurately be tailored to care and treatment in the clinical realm.

REFERENCES

1. Louis DN, Ohgaki H, Wiestler OD, et al. The 2007 WHO classification of tumours of the central nervous system. Acta Neuropathol 2007;114:97–109.
2. Frosch M, Douglas A, Girolami U. The central nervous system. 8th edition. Philadelphia: Saunders/Elsevier; 2010.
3. Verhaak RG, Hoadley KA, Purdom E, et al. Integrated genomic analysis identifies clinically relevant subtypes of glioblastoma characterized by abnormalities in PDGFRA, IDH1, EGFR, and NF1. Cancer Cell 2010;17:98–110.
4. Ohgaki H, Kleihues P. Genetic pathways to primary and secondary glioblastoma. Am J Pathol 2007;170:1445–53.
5. Ohgaki H, Dessen P, Jourde B, et al. Genetic pathways to glioblastoma: a population-based study. Cancer Res 2004;64:6892–9.
6. Nakamura M, Watanabe T, Klangby U, et al. p14ARF deletion and methylation in genetic pathways to glioblastomas. Brain Pathol 2001;11:159–68.
7. Rasheed BK, McLendon RE, Friedman HS, et al. Chromosome 10 deletion mapping in human gliomas: a common deletion region in 10q25. Oncogene 1995;10:2243–6.
8. McNamara MG, Sahebjam S, Mason WP. Emerging biomarkers in glioblastoma. Cancers (Basel) 2013;5:1103–19.
9. Fraser MM, Zhu X, Kwon CH, et al. Pten loss causes hypertrophy and increased proliferation of astrocytes in vivo. Cancer Res 2004;64:7773–9.
10. Fujisawa H, Reis RM, Nakamura M, et al. Loss of heterozygosity on chromosome 10 is more extensive in primary (de novo) than in secondary glioblastomas. Lab Invest 2000;80:65–72.
11. Brennan CW, Verhaak RG, McKenna A, et al. The somatic genomic landscape of glioblastoma. Cell 2013;155:462–77.
12. Thorne AH, Zanca C, Furnari F. Epidermal growth factor receptor targeting and challenges in glioblastoma. Neuro Oncol 2016;18:914–8.
13. Humphrey PA, Wong AJ, Vogelstein B, et al. Amplification and expression of the epidermal growth factor receptor gene in human glioma xenografts. Cancer Res 1988;48:2231–8.
14. Ozawa T, Brennan CW, Wang L, et al. PDGFRA gene rearrangements are frequent genetic events in PDGFRA-amplified glioblastomas. Genes Dev 2010;24:2205–18.
15. Parsons DW, Jones S, Zhang X, et al. An integrated genomic analysis of human glioblastoma multiforme. Science 2008;321:1807–12.
16. Noushmehr H, Weisenberger DJ, Diefes K, et al. Identification of a CpG island methylator phenotype that defines a distinct subgroup of glioma. Cancer Cell 2010;17:510–22.
17. Koh J, Cho H, Kim H, et al. IDH2 mutation in gliomas including novel mutation. Neuropathology 2015;35:236–44.
18. Beiko J, Suki D, Hess KR, et al. IDH1 mutant malignant astrocytomas are more amenable to surgical resection and have a survival benefit associated with maximal surgical resection. Neuro Oncol 2014;16:81–91.
19. SongTao Q, Lei Y, Si G, et al. IDH mutations predict longer survival and response to temozolomide in secondary glioblastoma. Cancer Sci 2012;103:269–73.
20. Louis DN, Perry A, Reifenberger G, et al. The 2016 World Health Organization classification of tumors of the central nervous system: a summary. Acta Neuropathol 2016;131:803–20.
21. Aldape K, Zadeh G, Mansouri S, et al. Glioblastoma: pathology, molecular mechanisms and markers. Acta Neuropathol 2015;129:829–48.
22. Camara-Quintana JQ, Nitta RT, Li G. Pathology: commonly monitored glioblastoma markers: EFGR, EGFRvIII, PTEN, and MGMT. Neurosurg Clin N Am 2012;23:237–46, viii.
23. Hegi ME, Diserens AC, Gorlia T, et al. MGMT gene silencing and benefit from temozolomide in glioblastoma. N Engl J Med 2005;352:997–1003.
24. Wick W, Hartmann C, Engel C, et al. NOA-04 randomized phase III trial of sequential radiochemotherapy of anaplastic glioma with procarbazine, lomustine, and vincristine or temozolomide. J Clin Oncol 2009;27:5874–80.
25. Wick W, Platten M, Meisner C, et al. Temozolomide chemotherapy alone versus radiotherapy alone for malignant astrocytoma in the elderly: the NOA-08 randomised, phase 3 trial. Lancet Oncol 2012;13:707–15.
26. Gorlia T, van den Bent MJ, Hegi ME, et al. Nomograms for predicting survival of patients with newly diagnosed glioblastoma: prognostic factor analysis of EORTC and NCIC trial 26981-22981/CE.3. Lancet Oncol 2008;9:29–38.
27. Liebelt BD, Shingu T, Zhou X, et al. Glioma stem cells: signaling, microenvironment, and therapy. Stem Cells Int 2016;2016:7849890.
28. Lathia JD, Mack SC, Mulkearns-Hubert EE, et al. Cancer stem cells in glioblastoma. Genes Dev 2015;29:1203–17.

29. Yuan X, Curtin J, Xiong Y, et al. Isolation of cancer stem cells from adult glioblastoma multiforme. Oncogene 2004;23:9392–400.

30. Bao S, Wu Q, Sathornsumetee S, et al. Stem cell-like glioma cells promote tumor angiogenesis through vascular endothelial growth factor. Cancer Res 2006;66:7843–8.

31. Auffinger B, Spencer D, Pytel P, et al. The role of glioma stem cells in chemotherapy resistance and glioblastoma multiforme recurrence. Expert Rev Neurother 2015;15:741–52.

32. Liu G, Yuan X, Zeng Z, et al. Analysis of gene expression and chemoresistance of CD133+ cancer stem cells in glioblastoma. Mol Cancer 2006;5:67.

CHAPTER 4

Translating Molecular Biomarkers of Gliomas to Clinical Practice

Cheddhi J. Thomas, MD[a,1,2], Jean-Pierre Gagner, MD, PhD[b,1], Rabaa Baitalmal, MBBS[b,c], David Zagzag, MD, PhD[a,b,d,e,*]

Glioma classification and grading have traditionally been based on the histomorphology of the tumors. Recent advances have identified new molecular markers with diagnostic, prognostic, and/or predictive (ie, therapeutic) significance (**Box 4.1, Table 4.1**). Since the publication of the World Health Organization (WHO) guidelines in 2007, there has been a rapid expansion of molecular data on central nervous system (CNS) tumors that has improved clinicians' diagnostic, prognostic, and therapeutic abilities. Although most of this information has not yet been translated into tangible clinical advances, many changes have been implemented in the revised WHO guidelines for the classification of tumors of the CNS (2016) for gliomas.[1] This chapter reviews recently identified genetic markers that have had a significant impact on the molecular classification of gliomas. Many have been shown to be essential in better diagnosing CNS tumors, reliably determining the prognosis, and allowing better clinical management. Based on the revised WHO classification, each tumor type is discussed separately, accompanied by the relevant molecular profiles.

ADULT DIFFUSE GLIOMAS

Adult diffuse gliomas are infiltrating glial neoplasms that include astrocytomas and oligodendrogliomas. In the 2007 edition of the *WHO Classification of Tumours of the Central Nervous System*, these entities were diagnosed and classified as grade II (diffuse) or grade III (anaplastic) based on histologic features.[2] In cases in which a morphologic distinction between these two entities was not clear, a diagnosis of oligoastrocytoma was appropriate. Following major advances in our understanding of molecular gliomagenesis, the revised *WHO Classification of Tumours of the Central Nervous System* (2016) has refined the diagnostic criteria for astrocytomas and oligodendrogliomas by incorporating clinically relevant molecular information about the mutation status of isocitrate dehydrogenase 1/2 (*IDH1/2*), and alpha thalassemia/mental retardation syndrome X-linked (*ATRX*) genes and codeletion of chromosome arms 1p and 19q. After an initial *IDH* mutation, oligodendrogliomas are thought to develop via subsequent telomerase reverse transcriptase (*TERT*) promoter mutations and codeletion of 1p/19q, whereas *IDH*-mutant astrocytomas develop with subsequent alterations of TP53 and/or ATRX.[3] The diagnosis of oligoastrocytoma is now strongly discouraged (**Fig. 4.1**).

Point mutations in cytosolic IDH1 and mitochondrial IDH2 most commonly by substitution of arginine to histidine (R132H) or to lysine

Conflict of Interest: The authors declare no commercial or financial conflicts of interest.

[a] Division of Neuropathology, Department of Pathology, NYU Langone Medical Center, 550 First Avenue, New York, NY 10016, USA; [b] Microvascular and Molecular Neuro-Oncology Laboratory, Department of Pathology, NYU Langone Medical Center, 550 First Avenue, New York, NY 10016, USA; [c] Department of Pathology, Faculty of Medicine, King Abdulaziz University, Abdullah Sulayman Street, Jeddah 21589, Saudi Arabia; [d] Department of Neurosurgery, NYU Langone Medical Center, 550 First Avenue, New York, NY 10016, USA; [e] NYU Langone Laura and Isaac Perlmutter Cancer Center, 160 E. 34th Street, New York, NY 10016, USA

[1]Contributed equally to this chapter.

[2]Current address: Anatomic Pathology and Neuropathology, Incyte Diagnostics, 13103 East Mansfield Avenue, Spokane Valley, WA 99216, USA.

* Corresponding author. Department of Pathology, NYU Langone Medical Center, 550 First Avenue, New York, NY 10016.

E-mail address: david.zagzag@nyumc.org

but is limited because the specimens must contain at least 50% neoplastic cells to ensure reliability. Another method, pyrosequencing, has a higher sensitivity than Sanger sequencing because it can detect as little as 10% mutant alleles. Moreover, clinical efforts have been undertaken to determine whether IDH mutations can be detected indirectly, and magnetic resonance spectroscopy has been proposed as a reliable technique to achieve this goal by detecting the levels of 2-HG.[9–12]

Diffuse Astrocytomas

Diffuse astrocytomas are now defined based on their IDH status as (1) diffuse astrocytoma, *IDH* mutant (most common); (2) diffuse astrocytoma, *IDH* wild-type or (3) diffuse astrocytoma, not otherwise specified (NOS; given when *IDH* testing is unavailable or inconclusive). A characteristic feature of *IDH*-mutated astrocytomas is the presence of a mutation in *ATRX* and frequent mutation of *TP53*[3] (see **Fig. 4.1**; **Fig. 4.2**).

ATRX is a nuclear chromatin remodeling protein that is encoded by the *ATRX* gene on chromosome Xq21.1. Loss-of-function mutations in *ATRX* are associated with alterations in replication and activation of the alternative lengthening of telomeres (ALT) pathway.[13] In diffuse gliomas, *ATRX* mutation is a useful marker for astrocytic differentiation, and is frequently seen in combination with mutations of *IDH* and *TP53*. In contrast, *IDH*-mutant, 1p/19q codeleted oligodendrogliomas only rarely harbor concurrent mutations in *ATRX* to the point that they are considered to be mutually exclusive.[14] For these reasons, IHC or sequencing for ATRX has a role both in confirming a diagnosis of astrocytoma and in ruling out a diagnosis of oligodendroglioma (**Fig. 4.2C, D**). IHC is sensitive and able to detect 82% to 89% of mutants that are detectable by sequencing.[14] Importantly, although they often exist in tandem, the presence of an *ATRX* mutation does not confirm the presence of a concurrent *IDH* mutation.[13] The prognostic implications of *ATRX* mutation are limited, and are mostly related to increased accuracy in the diagnosis of diffuse gliomas as astrocytic versus oligodendroglial. In non–1p/19q-codeleted gliomas, *ATRX* mutation has been associated with better treatment outcomes.[14]

(R172K), respectively, alter their catalytic activity such that they produce high levels of the oncometabolite 2-hydroxyglutarate (2-HG), instead of α-ketoglutarate.[4] The presence of 2-HG results in disruption of tet methylcytosine dioxygenase 2 (TET2) activity, leading to aberrant histone regulation and development of the glioma–CpG island methylator phenotype (G-CIMP).[5]

G-CIMP is an epigenetic molecular profile that was noted and named after the observation of a subset of gliomas within The Cancer Genome Atlas (TCGA) database that showed concerted hypermethylation at a large number of loci.[6] In general, CIMP gliomas are lower-grade, often *IDH*-mutated, tumors. Mutation of *IDH* is the molecular basis for the G-CIMP phenotype.[7] Overall, *IDH*-mutant, G-CIMP high infiltrating gliomas are associated with a favorable prognosis compared with *IDH* wild-type tumors. IDH status is an even stronger predictor of patient outcome than histologic grade in infiltrating gliomas.[8]

IDH mutations can be detected by immunohistochemical analysis of formalin-fixed, paraffin-embedded (FFPE) tissue using the IDH1 R132H mutant-specific antibody (**Fig. 4.2A, B**). Direct Sanger sequencing, although requiring more tissue specimens, has the advantage over immunohistochemistry (IHC) of not only detecting IDH1 R132H but also detecting other noncanonical IDH mutations. This technique is highly sensitive,

Oligodendrogliomas

Changes to the diagnostic criteria of oligodendroglioma and anaplastic oligodendroglioma

TABLE 4.1
Overview of common chromosomal, genetic, epigenetic and phenotypic alterations in gliomas and their use as biomarkers

Gene/Phenotype[a]	Gene Family/Alternative Name	Chromosomal Location	Driver Gene[b]	Typical Mutation[c]	Copy Number Alteration	Translocation Partner	Detection Method	Adult Glioma Tumor Type	Pediatric Glioma Tumor Type	Biomarker Clinical Utility	References
Chromosomal											
—	—	1p/19q	—	—	Codeletion	—	FISH, LOH, MLPA, 450K-MA	OD, AOD	—	Diag, Prog, Pred (chemo + radiotherapy)	96,104
CIC	Transcription repressor	19q13.2	TSG	R215Q/W	Del	—	IHC (loss of staining), others	OD, AOD	—	Diag, Prog	23,105
FUBP1	DNA-binding protein	1p31.1	TSG	Many	Del	—	IHC (loss of staining), others	OD, AOD	—	Diag, Prog	23,105
—	—	7 or 7q	—	—	Single copy gain	—	FISH, others	DA, AA, GBM	—	—	84
—	—	10 or 10q	—	—	Single copy loss	—	FISH, others	GBM	—	—	84
Genetic											
ACVR1	RSTK	2q23-q24	TSG	Few	—	—	qRT-PCR, Seq	—	Midline HGG, DIPG	—	80
BRAF	RAF kinase	7q34	ONC	V600E	—	—	MS-IHC, qRT-PCR, Seq	PXA, EGBM	PA, PXA, cortical HGG	Diag	67,89
BRAF	—	—	—	—	Amp	KIAA1549, others	FISH, others; qRT-PCR, Seq	PA	PA, PMA	Diag	67,81

(continued on next page)

TABLE 4.1
(continued)

Gene/Phenotype[a]	Gene Family/Alternative Name	Chromosomal Location	Driver Gene[b]	Typical Mutation[c]	Copy Number Alteration	Translocation Partner	Detection Method	Adult Glioma Tumor Type	Pediatric Glioma Tumor Type	Biomarker Clinical Utility	References
CDKN2A	Kinase inhibitor/p14, p16	9p21	TSG	—	Del	—	FISH, MLPA, 450K-MA	OD, AOD, DA, AA, GBM	PXA	—	37,39
CDKN2B	Kinase inhibitor	9p21	—	—	Del	—	FISH, MLPA, 450K-MA	OD, AOD, DA, AA, GBM	PXA	—	39
EGFR	RTK	7p12	ONC	—	Amp	SEPT14	FISH, others; qRT-PCR, Seq	Classic GBM	Cortical HGG	Diag	40,41
EGFR	—	—	—	EGFRvIII, A289D/T/V	—	—	MS-IHC, qRT-PCR, Seq	Classic GBM	—	Diag	26,39
FGFR1	RTK/CD331	8p11.23-p11.22	—	K656E	—	TACC1	qRT-PCR, Seq; FISH, others	—	PA, midline HGG/DIPG	—	68,81
FGFR3	RTK/CD333	4p16.3	ONC	—	—	TACC3	FISH, qRT-PCR, Seq	GBM	—	—	82,83
IDH1	Dehydrogenase	2q34	ONC	R132H, others	—	—	MS-IHC, qRT-PCR, Seq	OD, AOD, DA, AA, GBM	Cortical HGG	Diag, Prog	26,104
IDH2	Dehydrogenase	15q26.1	ONC	R172K, others	—	—	qRT-PCR, Seq	OD, AOD, DA, AA, GBM	—	Diag, Prog	4,104
MDM2	Ubiquitin protein ligase	12q13-q14	ONC	Few	Amp	—	FISH, MLPA, 450K-MA	GBM	—	—	39
MDM4	p53 regulator	1q32	ONC	Few	Amp	—	FISH, MLPA, 450K-MA	GBM	—	—	39
MET	RTK	7q31	ONC	—	Amp	—	FISH, MLPA, 450K-MA	GBM	—	—	39,46
MYC	Transcription factor	8q24	ONC	—	Amp	—	FISH, MLPA, 450K-MA	Astrocytoma, GBM	—	—	57
NF1	RAS negative regulator	17q11.2	TSG	Many	Del	—	qRT-PCR, Seq; FISH, others	Mesenchymal GBM	PA, midline HGG	—	26

Gene	Function	Location	Class	Mutation	CNV	Other	Method	Subtype	Tumor type	Clinical	Ref
NOTCH1	receptor	9q34.3	TSG	F357del	Amp	—	qRT-PCR, Seq; FISH, others	OD	—	—	60
NTRK2	RTK	9q22.1	—	—	Amp	QKI	FISH, others; qRT-PCR, Seq	—	PA, non-brain-stem HGG	—	68,71
PDGFRA	RTK/CD140a	4q12	ONC	Many	Amp	KDR	qRT-PCR, Seq; FISH, others	Proneural GBM	Midline HGG, DIPG	Prog	26,42
PIK3CA	PI3 kinase	3q26.3	ONC	H1047L/R/Y	Amp	—	qRT-PCR, Seq; FISH, others	OD, AOD, GBM	Midline HGG, DIPG	—	39,53
PIK3R1	Regulatory subunit of PI3 kinase	5q13.1	TSG	G376R	Del	—	qRT-PCR, Seq; FISH, others	OD, AOD, GBM	Midline HGG, DIPG	—	39,53
PTEN	Phosphatase	10q23	TSG	R130[d]/Q	Del	—	qRT-PCR, Seq; FISH, others	Astrocytoma, classical GBM	—	Prog	30,39
PTPN11	Phosphatase	12q24.1	ONC	Many	—	—	qRT-PCR, Seq	—	PA	—	68
RB1	Ligand	13q14.2	TSG	R445[d], X445_splice	Del	—	qRT-PCR, Seq; FISH, others	Mesenchymal GBM	—	—	29,39
TERT	Telomerase	5p15.33	—	Promoter	—	—	qRT-PCR, Seq	OD, AOD, astrocytoma, GBM	—	Diag, Prog	25,104
TP53	Transcription factor	17p13.1	TSG	R273C/H/L, R248Q/W	—	—	(IHC), qRT-PCR, Seq	Astrocytoma, GBM	Midline/cortical HGG	—	30,39
Epigenetic											
ATRX	Chromatin remodeler	Xq21.1	TSG	F2113fs	—	—	IHC (loss of staining), others	DA, AA, GBM	Cortical HGG	Diag, Prog	8,105
DAXX	Chromatin remodeler	6p21.3	TSG	—	Amp	—	FISH, MLPA, 450K-MA	—	Cortical HGG	—	74

(continued on next page)

TABLE 4.1 (continued)

Gene/Phenotype[a]	Gene Family/ Alternative Name	Chromosomal Location	Driver Gene[b]	Typical Mutation[c]	Copy Number Alteration	Trans-location Partner	Detection Method	Adult Glioma Tumor Type	Pediatric Glioma Tumor Type	Biomarker Clinical Utility	References
HIST1H3B	Histone	6p22.2	ONC	H3.1 K27M	—	—	qRT-PCR, Seq		Midline HGG, DIPG	Diag, Prog	106,107
H3F3A	Histone	1q42.12	ONC	H3.3 K27M	—	—	MS-IHC, qRT-PCR, Seq	Midline HGG, DIPG	Midline HGG, DIPG	Diag, Prog	27,74
H3F3A	Histone	1q42.12	ONC	H3.3 G34R/V	—	—	MS-IHC, qRT-PCR, Seq	—	Cortical HGG	Diag, Prog	27,74
MGMT	DNA cysteine MT	10q26	—	Promoter methylation	—	—	MS-PCR, 450K-MA	GBM	—	Prog, Pred (temozolomide)	62,95
SETD2	Histone lysine MT	3p21.31	TSG	Many	Del	—	qRT-PCR, Seq; FISH, others	—	Cortical HGG	—	79
TET2	Demethylase	4q24	TSG	Few	—	—	qRT-PCR, Seq	GBM	—	—	5
Phenotypic											
2-HG	2-hydroxyglutarate	—	—	—	—	—	MRS, mass spectrometry	OD, AOD, DA, AA, GBM	—	—	9,99
G-CIMP	Glioma-CpG island methylator phenotype	—	—	—	—	—	450K-MA	OD, AOD, DA, AA, GBM	—	—	26

Abbreviations: AA, anaplastic astrocytoma; AOD, anaplastic oligodendroglioma; CD, cluster of differentiation; DA, diffuse astrocytoma; Diag, diagnostic biomarker; DIPG, diffuse intrinsic pontine glioma; EGBM, epithelioid glioblastoma; EGFR, epidermal growth factor receptor; EGFRvIII, deleted exons 2 to 7 EGFR; FISH, fluorescence in situ hybridization; fs, frame shift; GBM, glioblastoma; HGG, high-grade (III–IV) glioma; IHC, immunohistochemistry; LGG, low-grade (I–II) glioma; LOH, loss of heterozygosity; MLPA, multiplex ligation-dependent probe amplification; MRS, magnetic resonance spectroscopy; MS-IHC, mutation-specific immunohistochemistry; MS-PCR, methylation-specific polymerase chain reaction; MT, methyltransferase; OD, oligodendroglioma; ONC, oncogene; PA, pilocytic astrocytoma; PMA, pilomyxoid astrocytoma; Pred, predictive biomarker; Prog, prognostic biomarker; PXA, pleomorphic xanthoastrocytoma; qRT-PCR, quantitative reverse transcriptase polymerase chain reaction; RSTK, receptor serine/threonine kinase; RTK, receptor tyrosine kinase; Seq, targeted nucleotide sequencing; TSG, tumor suppressor gene; 450K-MA, 450K CpG methylation array.

^a Gene symbols, gene families, and chromosomal locations according to the Human Genome Organisation Gene Nomenclature Committee (www.genenames.org) and Catalogue of Somatic Mutations in Cancer (cancer.sanger.ac.uk).

^a Gene genes that contain driver gene mutations as defined by Vogelstein and colleagues.[101]

^b Driver genes that contain driver gene mutations as defined by Vogelstein and colleagues.[101]

^c Gene mutations and copy number alterations based on the Merged Cohort of LGG and GBM (The Cancer Genome Atlas [TCGA], 2016) database (1102 samples) generated by TCGA Research Network (http://www.cbioportal.org/index.do). In addition, the translocation partners for BRAF,[67,81] EGFR,[40] FGFR1,[82] NTRK2,[71] and PDGFRA[42] are listed.

^d Change to a termination codon (nonsense mutation).

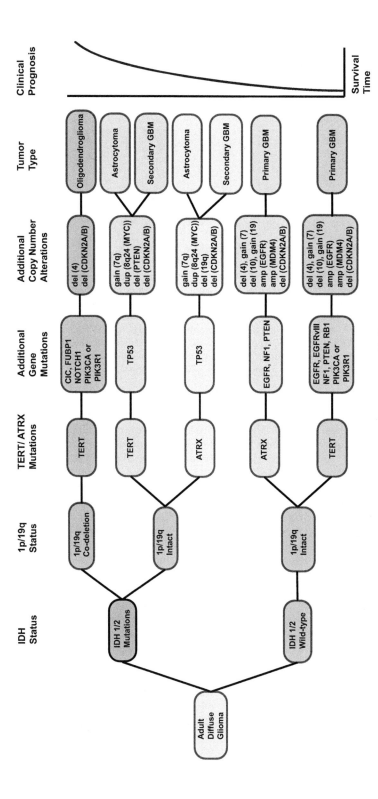

Fig. 4.1 Molecular classification model of adult diffuse gliomas based on the combined findings[102,103] of characteristic genomic alterations in astrocytic and oligodendroglial tumors.[3,24,104,105] The analysis of common mutations in *IDH1/2*, *ATRX* and the *TERT* promoter and codeletion of 1p/19q allows the classification of these tumors into 5 molecular subgroups that define the biological and clinical behavior of gliomas more accurately than the classification based solely on the histopathologic tumor types. Additional gene mutations and copy number alterations are associated with these subgroups.

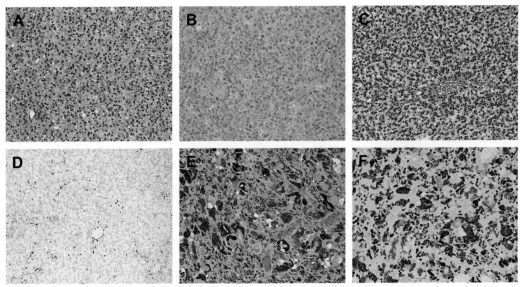

Fig. 4.2 Immunohistochemical assessment of IDH1, ATRX, and TP53 expression in gliomas. (A, B) Oligodendro-glioma, *IDH1* mutated, *ATRX* preserved (WHO grade II). Tumor cells show diffuse cytoplasmic immunoreactivity to IDH R132H. (C, D) Anaplastic astrocytoma, *ATRX* mutated, *IDH1* mutated, 1p/19q intact (WHO grade III). The nuclear expression of ATRX is not detected in tumor cells, but is retained in endothelial cells. A biphenotypic pattern of microgemistocytes and small round cells with scanty cytoplasm is seen on hematoxylin and eosin (H&E) staining. (E, F) Giant cell glioblastoma, *TP53* mutated, *IDH1* mutated (WHO grade IV). Tumor cells show strong, diffuse immu-noreactivity to TP53. Note the presence of bizarre-looking giant cells, including some multinucleated cells, and vascular proliferation on H&E staining (original magnification ×20 for all panels).

include the requirement of both an *IDH* mutation and a 1p/19q codeletion (see **Fig. 4.1**). There are 4 distinct types of oligodendroglioma tu-mors: (1) *IDH* mutant and 1p/19q codeleted, (2) NOS, (3) anaplastic *IDH* mutant and 1p/19q codeleted, and (4) anaplastic NOS (when only classic histology is available). The diagnosis of oligodendroglioma NOS should only be given after further analysis excludes potential diagno-ses such as dysembryoplastic neuroepithelial tu-mor, clear cell ependymoma, neurocytoma, pilocytic astrocytoma, and several other tumor types that are histologically similar to oligodendroglioma.

Loss of 1p/19q has more than just a diagnostic significance. It has been associated with a favorable prognosis and an increased sensitivity to chemotherapy.[15] Moreover, 1p/19q-codeleted anaplastic oligodendroglio-mas that show polysomy for chromosomes 1p and 19q have intermediate survival between 1p/19q-retained tumors and 1p/19q-codeleted oligodendrogliomas in a euploid background.[16,17] Codeletion of 1p/19q can be detected by fluorescence in situ hybridiza-tion (FISH), loss of heterozygosity (LOH) capil-lary gel electrophoresis, or as a change in copy number in the 450K CpG methylation

array (450K-MA) results[18,19] (**Figs. 4.3** and **4.4A**). However, only FISH allows the enumera-tion of absolute numbers of chromosomes and determination of ploidy status.

Several other recurrent molecular alterations can be found in oligodendrogliomas. *CIC* (Capi-cua transcriptional repressor), a gene that resides in chromosome 19q, plays a pivotal role in regu-lating RAS (rat sarcoma oncogene)/MAPK (mitogen-activated protein kinase) signaling.[20] Somatic mutations in *CIC* are present in as many as 69% of oligodendrogliomas.[21,22] *FUBP1* (far-upstream element binding protein) is a gene located on chromosome 1p. It has been suggested that inactivating somatic mutations in this gene (along with *CIC*) are also associated with the development of oligodendroglioma. Tumors with such alterations seem to cluster with 1p/19q-codeleted oligodendrogliomas.[23] Recent work has identified that TERT is overexpressed in oligodendrogliomas[24,25] (see **Fig. 4.1**). Oligodendrogliomas are therefore now recognized to contain at least 4 different recurrent molecular genetic correlates: *IDH* mutation, 1p/19q loss, *CIC* mutation, and *TERT* promoter mutation. Mutations in the *NOTCH1* gene (discussed later) were also observed in 31% of oligodendrogliomas.[3]

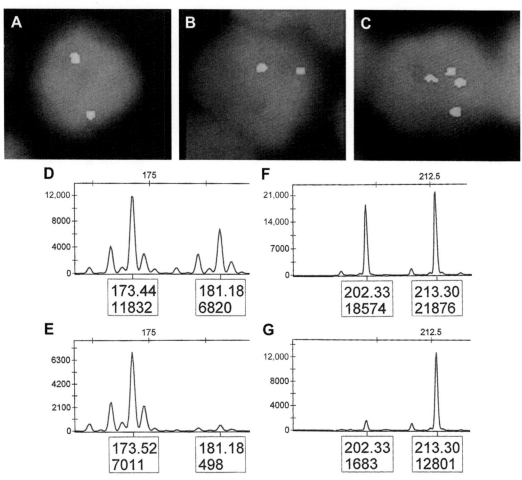

Fig. 4.3 FISH and LOH analyses of loss of chromosome arms 1p/19q in oligodendrogliomas. (*A–C*) FISH using probes for 1p or 19q (*red signal*) and control probes for 1q or 19p (*green*) with 4′,6-diamidino-2-phenylindole (DAPI) nuclear counterstain (*blue*) shows maintenance of 1p with 2 red and 2 green signals (*A*) and classic absolute loss of 1 copy of 1p, whereas 2 1q signals remain intact (*B*). In anaplastic oligodendroglioma, concurrent polysomy indicated by multiple 1q signals with ≈50% deletion of 1p/19q (*C*) is a marker of early recurrence.[16] Similar results were obtained for chromosome 19 (not shown). (*D–G*) Alternatively, LOH can be evaluated by comparing normal (blood) (*D, F*) and tumor DNA samples (*E, G*) for the presence of allelic loss of 1p and/or 19q using fluorescence-labeled polymorphic chromosomal markers for 1p (7 loci) (*D, E*) and 19q (4 loci) (*F, G*) followed by capillary gel electrophoresis. The blood sample shows 2 alleles for each heterozygous marker, but the decrease in peak height (bottom numbers in the boxes below the electropherograms) of 1 of the 2 alleles indicates that the tumor has undergone LOH for both 1p and 19q.

ADULT GLIOBLASTOMAS

Glioblastomas are high-grade, infiltrative astrocytomas with atypical nuclei, mitotic activity, extensive vascular proliferation, and/or necrosis. According to the revised WHO classification of CNS tumors, glioblastomas can be molecularly classified as *IDH* wild-type, *IDH*-mutant glioblastomas or NOS (see **Fig. 4.1**). Histologic IDH wild-type variants include giant cell (**Fig. 4.2E, F**), gliosarcoma, and the newly described epithelioid glioblastoma.[1] About 90% of glioblastomas (usually primary) present as *IDH* wild-type; glioblastomas are found to be *IDH* mutated in about 10% of cases, and these are most often secondary

glioblastomas that have progressed from lower-grade *IDH*-mutant gliomas.

Recent efforts to molecularly subclassify glioblastomas based on genetic and epigenetic expression profiling have consistently identified the classical, mesenchymal and proneural subtypes characterized by epidermal growth factor receptor (*EGFR*) amplification, neurofibromin 1 (*NF1*) loss, and platelet-derived growth factor receptor A (*PDGFRA*) amplification, respectively.[26] Notably, the proneural subtype was also associated with *IDH1/2* mutations, G-CIMP phenotype as well as *TP53* mutations. Additional mutations in histone H3F3A-K27 and H3F3A-G34 have defined

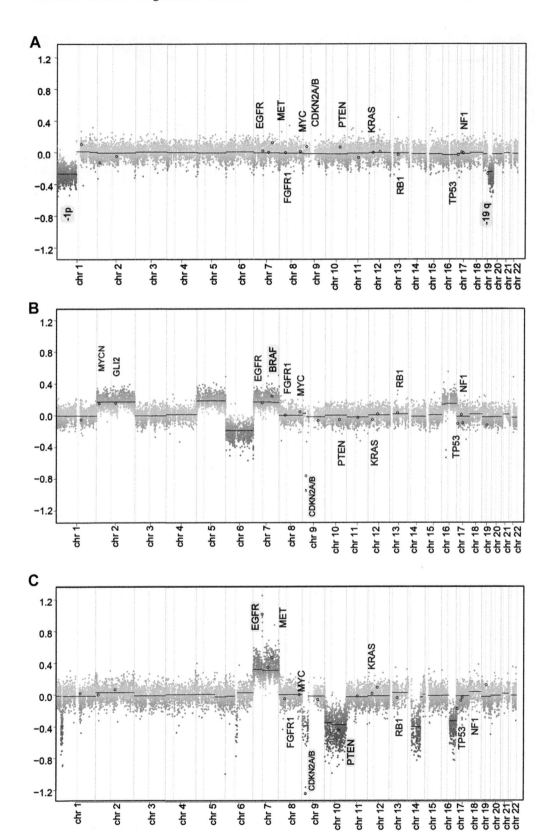

epigenetic subgroups of glioblastoma in young adult (and pediatric) patients, which are addressed later.[27]

IDH-mutated glioblastomas typically arise in younger patients following secondary transformation of a lower-grade astrocytoma. As such, the molecular features in IDH-mutant glioblastomas are often similar to those seen in IDH-mutant diffuse or anaplastic astrocytomas. IDH-mutant glioblastomas often harbor concurrent ATRX and TP53 mutations. Despite their high-grade histology, IDH-mutant glioblastomas show clinical behavior similar to that seen in lower-grade IDH-mutant astrocytomas. In contrast, IDH wild-type glioblastomas most commonly present as de novo tumors arising in patients older than 55 years. These tumors not only show vast histomorphologic heterogeneity but also harbor a wide variety of genetic alterations[28] (see **Fig. 4.1**; **Fig. 4.4C**). Data from TCGA show frequent alterations in 3 core signaling pathways: the CDK4/6-p16^{INK4a}-RB1-E2F, p14^{ARF}-MDM2-MDM4-p53, and RTK-RAS-PI3K pathways. These pathways and their common associated alterations are discussed below.

The CDK4/6-p16^{INK4a}-RB1-E2F Pathway

The CDK4/6-p16^{INK4a}-RB1-E2F pathway controls the expression of genes involved in the progression from the G1 to the S phase of the cell cycle. Cyclin-dependent kinase (CDK) 4/6 catalyzes the phosphorylation of the retinoblastoma (RB1) protein, which releases E2F transcription factor allowing downstream signaling. CDK4/6 activity is suppressed by the INK4 family of proteins; for example, p16^{INK4a}, which is encoded by the cyclin-dependent kinase inhibitor 2A (CDKN2A) gene.[29] CDKN2A also encodes p14^{ARF}, another tumor suppressor protein that stabilizes p53. As a result, inactivation of the CDKN2A locus can lead to dysregulation of both RB and p53 pathways.[30]

Data from the TCGA 2013 glioblastoma report showed that 79% of glioblastomas had 1 or more alterations affecting the RB pathway, with the most common being CDKN2A deletion in 76% of glioblastomas followed by amplification of CDK4/6 and RB1 mutation or deletion in 16% and 8% of cases, respectively[31] (see

Fig. 4.4C). In adults, deletion of CDKN2A is often seen in primary or recurrent glioblastomas.[32] Dysregulation of the RB signaling pathway has been found in 65% of anaplastic oligodendrogliomas. Simultaneous dysregulation of the RB1 and the TP53 pathways occurs in 45% of anaplastic oligodendrogliomas; whereas it is almost absent in WHO grade II oligodendrogliomas.[32,33] In low-grade diffuse gliomas, alterations of the RB pathway are more frequent (26%) in tumors lacking common genetic alterations of IDH1/2, TP53, and 1p/19q than in tumors that carry these common genetic alterations (11%).[34] Consistent with these results, a recent TCGA report showed that aberrations in the RB pathway are among the most common acquired copy number variations in histologically low-grade gliomas with IDH wild type: CDKN2A focal deletions in 63% of tumors (**Fig. 4.4B, C**), RB1 focal deletions in 25% of tumors, and CDK4 amplifications in 38% of tumors. Remarkably, similar frequencies of alterations among these loci were found in glioblastomas with IDH wild-type but not in other subtypes of low-grade gliomas. For example, the frequency of the homozygous deletions of CDKN2A/B (45%) in IDH wild-type low-grade gliomas is similar to (55%) in IDH wild-type glioblastomas.[3]

Alterations in any of the genes coding for components of the RB1 pathway have been associated with shorter survival in patients with glioblastoma,[35] anaplastic astrocytoma,[36] and low-grade diffuse gliomas.[34]

Deletions of CDKN2A can be reliably detected via FISH, polymerase chain reaction (PCR), or comparative genomic hybridization (CGH). Alternatively, loss of p16 expression by IHC can be used as a screening tool for detecting deletions.[37] Nonetheless, the diagnostic and prognostic utility of CDKN2A is limited. Preclinical studies have shown that RB1-deficient tumors are resistant to CDK4/6 inhibition. Therefore, testing for RB1 deficiency or loss of function may be useful in predicting therapeutic efficacy to CDK4/6 inhibitors. In addition, immunohistochemical detection of RB1 loss has been shown to reliably predict homozygous deletion.[29]

Fig. 4.4 Genomic copy number alterations in gliomas determined by methylation array. In addition to genome-wide DNA methylation patterns, the copy number dosages of investigated markers along chromosomes 1 to 22 are determined. Copy numbers greater than average are indicated in green, and copy numbers less than average in red. Typical copy number profiles of (A) oligodendroglioma with 1p/19q codeletion, (B) pleomorphic xanthoastrocytoma with deletion of CDKN2A/B on chromosome arm 9p21, and (C) glioblastoma with gain of chromosome 7 (EGFR), and loss of chromosome 9 (CDKN2A/B) and 10 (PTEN) are shown.

The p14^ARF-MDM2-MDM4-p53 Pathway

The protein p53 encoded by the gene *TP53* on chromosome 17p13.1 has essential roles in tumor suppression. In response to diverse stress signals such as DNA damage, p53 induces DNA repair, cell cycle arrest, and cell apoptosis. Most glioblastomas (86%) have dysregulation of the p53 pathway due to either mutation or deletion of *TP53* (28%), amplification of *MDM2/4* (15%; murine double minute 2 and 4, negative regulators of p53) and/or deletion or mutation of *CDKN2A* (58%; expresses p14^ARF, a negative regulator of MDM2/4).[31] Alterations of TP53 are mutually exclusive with MDM2/4 changes and are more common in secondary (68%) than in primary glioblastomas (28%). Loss of p14^ARF does not show predilection for a particular glioblastoma subtype.[38,39]

Despite many studies, the prognostic significance of p53 pathway mutation in glioblastomas remains unclear, probably because of the extensive diversity of mutations. Indeed, *p53* mutations are often found in *IDH*-mutant gliomas, which generally are associated with improved survival. In contrast, primary glioblastomas, which generally carry a worse prognosis, also frequently harbor mutations in *p53*.

The RTK-RAS-PI3K Pathway

A variety of cell surface tyrosine kinase receptors (RTKs) such as EGFR and PDGFRA have been found to be overexpressed in high-grade gliomas (90% have at least 1 phosphatidylinositol 3-kinase (PI3K) pathway alteration)[28] and show distinct alterations in the classic and proneural subtypes of glioblastoma, respectively.[26] The *EGFR* gene, located on chromosome 7p12, encodes an RTK that promotes cell proliferation through its effects on the MAPK and PI3K pathways. Approximately 50% of primary glioblastomas show EGFR overexpression because of amplification of the *EGFR* gene, which is essentially mutually exclusive with 1p/19q codeletion and *IDH* gene mutations. *EGFR* gene rearrangements, most commonly involving the EGFRvIII variant with an in-frame deletion of exons 2 to 7, result in constitutive activation of the mitogenic signaling pathways. In addition, recurrent translocations fuse portions of EGFR to several partners, EGFR-SEPT14 (septin 14) being the most common functional gene fusion.[40] These *EGFR* alterations strongly suggest the diagnosis of glioblastoma, specifically in older patients. However, there is insufficient evidence that either *EGFR* amplification or EGFRvIII mutation has prognostic value in patients with glioblastoma.[41] The *PDGFRA* gene, located on chromosome 4q12, encodes an RTK similar to

EGFR that is also involved in glioblastoma proliferation. *PDGFRA* is mutated in up to 30% of glioblastomas. Several rearrangements have been identified. The PDGFRAdelta[8,9] isoform (with a deletion of exons 8 and 9) is common and results in constitutive activation. Gene fusion between kinase insert domain receptor (*KDR*) and the *PDGFRA* gene shows constitutively increased tyrosine kinase activity.[42] *PDGFRA* amplification also occurs and shows a significant reduction in the median survival only in the *IDH1* mutation subgroup.[43] Despite the importance of PDGFR in glioblastoma proliferation, no definitive prognostic significance has been seen in clinical studies.

MET is a hypoxia-induced proto-oncogene and the RTK for hepatocyte growth factor.[44] Genomic amplification of *MET* is common in glioblastomas,[26] and single cell–level genomic studies showed that a small fraction of glioblastoma cells contain focal amplification of c-MET.[45] Several cellular processes, including cell proliferation, survival, and migration, in gliomas are regulated by MET.[44] MET overexpression has been associated with poor prognosis and enhanced tumor invasiveness in patients with glioblastoma.[46]

Phosphatase and tensin homolog (*PTEN*), a tumor suppressor gene residing on chromosome 10q23, encodes a protein that acts as a negative regulator of the PI3K/AKT/mammalian target of rapamycin (mTOR) signaling pathway.[32] Alterations of *PTEN* by deletions or mutations are common in adult primary glioblastoma,[31] but rare in pediatric malignant gliomas.[47] LOH of chromosome 10 is the most frequent chromosomal alteration in primary glioblastomas (up to 80%), with the *PTEN* locus deletion being among the most commonly deleted regions on this chromosome.[48] Loss of PTEN expression by IHC does not independently confer a worse prognosis in newly diagnosed glioblastoma cases treated with temozolomide (TMZ).[49] In contrast, LOH of chromosome 10 is predictive of shorter survival.[48] In a phase II clinical trial, intact PTEN by IHC correlated with O6-methylguanine-DNA methyltransferase (*MGMT*) promoter methylation and carried a survival advantage in newly diagnosed patients with glioblastoma treated with tyrosine kinase inhibitor (TKI) and TMZ combined with radiation therapy.[50] FISH can easily identify cytogenetic aberrations in *PTEN*, including both homozygous and hemizygous deletions, as well as entire loss of chromosome 10. Alternatively, PCR-based methods can be used. Assessment of PTEN loss by IHC is still unreliable.[32]

Phosphatidylinositol-4,5-bisphosphate 3-kinase represents a family of proteins with a wide variety of roles, including cell growth, survival, and differentiation. This PI3K family is subdivided into several classes of proteins. Class I proteins, such as PIK3CA and PIK3R1, have distinct catalytic and regulatory functions, respectively, as part of the PI3K/AKT/mTOR pathway. This signaling cascade is activated by RTKs such as EGFR and is inhibited by PTEN. Several members of this pathway, including RTK, PI3K, AKT, and mTOR, present prime targets for pharmacologic inhibition.[51] In glioblastomas, activation of the PI3K/AKT/mTOR pathway is associated with resistance to TMZ chemotherapy.[52] Activation of this pathway has been associated with a significantly decreased overall survival in patients with glioblastoma.[53]

Other Mutations in Glioblastomas

MYC (ie, c-MYC) and MYCN (neuroblastoma derived homolog of MYC) are members of the myelocytomatosis oncogene homolog (MYC) family of transcription factors, which play pivotal roles in metabolism, protein synthesis, proliferation, DNA repair, and apoptosis.[54] Several studies report amplification or overexpression of members of the MYC family in gliomas.[4] TCGA data showed enrichment of *MYCN* focal amplifications along with *ATRX* mutations in the G-CIMP-high glioblastoma subtype.[31] In glioblastoma with primitive neuronal component, *MYCN* and *MYC* amplifications were identified by FISH in 43% of cases and were restricted to the primitive neuronal component.[55] MYC is the most frequently amplified locus in *IDH*-mutant gliomas during malignant progression (22% of cases). Furthermore, using integrated genomic analysis approach, alterations in the MYC signaling pathway components FBXW7 (F-box and WD repeat domain containing 7), and MAX (MYC associated factor X) were found in 56% of *IDH*-mutant gliomas and were each independently associated with glioma progression.[56] The role of MYC as a prognostic marker remains to be established. However, it has been suggested that high levels of MYC expression detected by IHC correlate with prolonged overall survival in patients with glioblastoma.[57] The significance of MYC as a predictive marker is controversial. For example, recent preclinical studies showed that higher levels of MYC expression promote resistance to TMZ.[58] In contrast, a previous study showed that MYC is essential for inducing apoptosis in response to TMZ treatment independent of MGMT expression.[59]

The *NOTCH1* gene, located on chromosome 9q, encodes a transmembrane receptor that plays a pivotal role in cell proliferation, differentiation, and apoptosis. NOTCH1 mutations result in inactivation of Notch protein function and have been noted most often in lower-grade gliomas with an *IDH* mutation and 1p/19q codeletion.[3] Novel mutations in the Notch pathway genes (NOTCH1, NOTCH2, NOTCH4, NOTCH2NL), including recurrent NOTCH1 A465T mutation, have been noted in anaplastic astrocytoma.[60] The significance of NOTCH1 mutations as a biomarker is under investigation.

O6-Methylguanine-DNA Methyltransferase

MGMT is a DNA methyltransferase enzyme that has demonstrated valuable predictive significance in patients with glioblastoma who are being considered for treatment using TMZ. TMZ is a chemotherapeutic alkylating agent that is frequently used in the treatment of glioblastoma. Its mechanism of action involves methylation of the O6 position of guanine, which leads to DNA mismatch and double-strand breaks, resulting in the death of affected cells. When the MGMT enzyme is active, it prevents this cascade by removing the methyl group from the O6 guanine. MGMT promoter methylation results in decreased enzymatic activity of MGMT, leading to decreased DNA mismatch repair and an increased sensitivity to TMZ.[61,62] However, even in the absence of TMZ treatment, MGMT suggests a longer progression-free survival.[63] Methylation of the *MGMT* promoter is common in adult glioblastomas (~40%) and is frequently seen in *IDH*-mutant/CIMP-high gliomas. In contrast, *MGMT* promoter methylation is rarely seen in pediatric tumors. Some studies have shown that *MGMT* promoter methylation is associated with increased overall survival in pediatric glioblastomas and even better response to TMZ, but other studies have contradicted this finding.[64] Note that the interaction between *MGMT* promoter methylation status and TMZ is complex and can be affected by other factors. For instance, mutations and/or altered expression in mismatch repair (MMR) proteins (MSH2, MSH6, MLH1, PMS2) have been suggested as alternate mechanisms of resistance to TMZ.[65] In addition, different modalities of MGMT testing, including IHC, PCR techniques, and pyrosequencing, have yielded varying levels of correlation with clinical outcome.

ADULT AND PEDIATRIC WELL-CIRCUMSCRIBED ASTROCYTOMAS

The pilocytic astrocytoma (PA) and the pleomorphic xanthoastrocytoma (PXA) (see **Fig. 4.4**B) are generally well demarcated and occur almost exclusively in a younger population[66] (**Fig. 4.5**). Closely resembling PXA is the epithelioid glioblastoma, which also tends to occur in young patients. All of these tumors commonly harbor alterations of B-Raf proto-oncogene (BRAF). BRAF is a member of the Raf family of serine/threonine protein kinases that is encoded by the *BRAF* gene on chromosome 7q34. This receptor exerts its effect through activation of the MAPK (RAS-RAF-MEK-ERK) and the PI3K (PI3K-AKT-mTOR) signaling pathways and is involved in many cellular processes, including cell proliferation and differentiation. Somatic mutations in the *BRAF* gene have been implicated in the pathogenesis of several cancers, notably melanoma, and more recently glioma. *BRAF* is mutated in 3% of glioma cases, specifically in most low-grade pediatric gliomas and many adult gliomas. Two alterations in *BRAF* are most commonly observed in these patients. First, the BRAF V600E point mutation (**Fig. 4.6A, B**), which results in a substitution of a valine (V) to a glutamic acid (E), occurs within the ATP-binding site of the kinase domain and allows downstream constitutive activation of MEK and ERK even without RAS activation. This mutation is found in PAs, PXAs

and in epithelioid glioblastomas.[67] Second, the KIAA1549:BRAF truncated fusion gene has a partial copy of *BRAF* with the activation domain but with loss of an inhibitory domain, and is under the regulatory control of *KIAA1549*[68] (see **Fig. 4.5**). This mutation is commonly seen in PAs. Except for the presence of BRAF V600E in a high proportion of epithelioid glioblastomas in adults, the clinical utility of both BRAF V600E and KIAA1549:BRAF alterations as diagnostic and/or prognostic biomarkers has not yet been clearly defined.[68] The BRAF V600E mutation is a potential target for the new BRAF inhibitors, dabrafenib (Tafinlar) and vemurafenib (Zelboraf).[69] However, with regard to the KIAA1549:BRAF fusion, it is predicted that this mutant protein will be stimulated by BRAF inhibitors and that downstream MEK1/MEK2 inhibitors (eg, trametinib [Mekinist]), may be more appropriate agents for therapeutic intervention.

PAs have also been shown to harbor recurrent gain-of-function mutations in and overexpression of protein tyrosine phosphatase nonreceptor type 11 (*PTPN11*) gene (see **Fig. 4.5**), the protein product of which regulates the RAS/ERK/MAPK signaling pathway.[66,68] Additionally, 2 novel

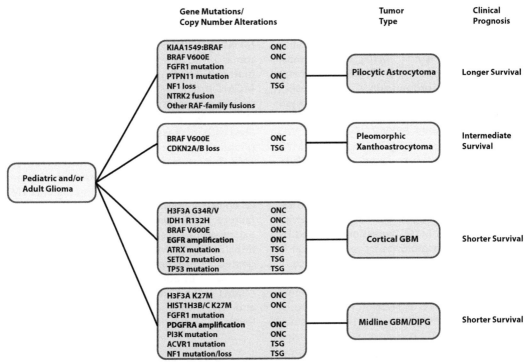

Fig. 4.5 Molecular classification model of pediatric and adult gliomas based on the combined findings of characteristic genomic alterations in these tumors.[106,107] The analysis of *KIAA1549:BRAF* fusion gene; BRAF V600E mutation; and mutations in histones H3.1 K27M, H3.3 K27M, H3.3 G34R/V, or *ATRX*, among others, is beginning to allow the classification of pediatric gliomas into molecular subgroups, with the pediatric high-grade gliomas showing neuroanatomical preferences.

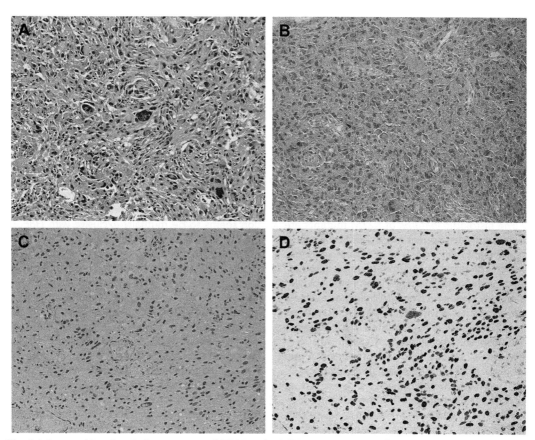

Fig. 4.6 Immunohistochemical assessment of BRAF and H3K27M expression in gliomas. (*A, B*) Pleomorphic xanthoastrocytoma, BRAF V600E mutated (WHO grade II). Tumor cells show cytoplasmic granular expression of BRAF V600E. Pleomorphic mononucleated or multinucleated cells with frequent nuclear inclusions are seen on H&E staining. (*C, D*) Glioblastoma, H3K27M mutated, *IDH1* wild type (WHO grade IV). Tumor cells show strong, positive nuclear staining for H3K27M. Both H3.1 K27M and H3.3 K27M antigens are recognized by the antibody (original magnification ×20 for all panels).

neurotrophic receptor tyrosine kinase 2 (*NTRK2*) gene fusions QKI:NTRK2 and NACC2:NTRK2 have been identified in PAs.[68] *NTRK* genes, including NTRK2, encodes the family of tropomyosin-receptor kinase (Trk) receptors, which together with their ligands, neurotrophins, play pivotal roles both in neural development and tumorigenesis.[70] Other fusions involving *NTRK* genes have also been reported in several glioma tumors, including pediatric HGGs.[70,71]

PEDIATRIC GLIOBLASTOMAS

Alterations of the H3.3-ATRX-DAXX (death domain–associated protein) chromatin remodeling pathway have recently been implicated in up to 44% of pediatric gliomas. H3.1 and H3.3 are both variants of histone subunit H3 and are key modulators of gene replication and transcription. H3.1, a replication-dependent histone, is encoded by the genes *HIST1H3B* and *HIST1H3C*

(among others), which are found on chromosome 6p22.2. H3.3 is a replication-independent histone encoded by 2 genes: *H3F3A* (1q42.12) and *H3F3B* (17q25.1). DAXX, a protein involved in chromatin remodeling, forms a heterodimer with ATRX (DAXX-ATRX), which recruits histone H3.3.[72] Mutations in this pathway are associated with altered lengthening of telomeres and changes in gene expression.[73] Mutations in the H3.3-ATRX-DAXX pathway are often associated with *TP53* mutations as well.[74]

The modulatory functions of histone subunits H3.1 and H3.3 rely on posttranslational trimethylation of a specific lysine residue (K27). In either subunit, missense mutations resulting in replacement of this residue by methionine (K27M) can cause a reduction in H3K27me3 leading to altered gene repression and tumorigenesis.[13] In general, *H3K27M* mutant tumors occur exclusively in midline locations, especially within the pons and thalamus but also within the spine,

3. The Cancer Genome Atlas Research Network. Comprehensive, integrative genomic analysis of diffuse lower-grade gliomas. N Engl J Med 2015; 372(26):2481–98.

4. Waitkus MS, Diplas BH, Yan H. Isocitrate dehydrogenase mutations in gliomas. Neuro Oncol 2016; 18(1):16–26.

5. Ito S, D'Alessio AC, Taranova OV, et al. Role of Tet proteins in 5mC to 5hmC conversion, ES-cell self-renewal and inner cell mass specification. Nature 2010;466(7310):1129–33.

6. Wang J, Su HK, Zhao HF, et al. Progress in the application of molecular biomarkers in gliomas. Biochem Biophys Res Commun 2015;465(1):1–4.

7. Duncan CG, Barwick BG, Jin G, et al. A heterozygous IDH1 R132H/WT mutation induces genome-wide alterations in DNA methylation. Genome Res 2012; 22(12):2339–55.

8. Wiestler B, Capper D, Holland-Letz T, et al. ATRX loss refines the classification of anaplastic gliomas and identifies a subgroup of IDH mutant astrocytic tumors with better prognosis. Acta Neuropathol 2013;126(3):443–51.

9. Dang L, White DW, Gross S, et al. Cancer-associated IDH1 mutations produce 2-hydroxyglutarate. Nature 2009;462(7274):739–44.

10. Hartmann C, Hentschel B, Tatagiba M, et al. Molecular markers in low-grade gliomas: predictive or prognostic? Clin Cancer Res 2011;17(13): 4588–99.

11. Juratli TA, Kirsch M, Robel K, et al. IDH mutations as an early and consistent marker in low-grade astrocytomas WHO grade II and their consecutive secondary high-grade gliomas. J Neurooncol 2012;108(3):403–10.

12. Sonoda Y, Kumabe T, Nakamura T, et al. Analysis of IDH1 and IDH2 mutations in Japanese glioma patients. Cancer Sci 2009;100(10):1996–8.

13. Tanboon J, Williams EA, Louis DN. The diagnostic use of immunohistochemical surrogates for signature molecular genetic alterations in gliomas. J Neuropathol Exp Neurol 2015;75(1):4–18.

14. Brandner S, von Deimling A. Diagnostic, prognostic and predictive relevance of molecular markers in gliomas. Neuropathol Appl Neurobiol 2015;41(6):694–720.

15. Wesseling P, van den Bent M, Perry A. Oligodendroglioma: pathology, molecular mechanisms and markers. Acta Neuropathol 2015;129(6): 809–27.

16. Snuderl M, Eichler AF, Ligon KL, et al. Polysomy for chromosomes 1 and 19 predicts earlier recurrence in anaplastic oligodendrogliomas with concurrent 1p/19q loss. Clin Cancer Res 2009;15(20): 6430–7.

17. Wiens AL, Cheng L, Bertsch EC, et al. Polysomy of chromosomes 1 and/or 19 is common and associated with less favorable clinical outcome in oligodendrogliomas: fluorescent in situ hybridization analysis of 84 consecutive cases. J Neuropathol Exp Neurol 2012;71(7):618–24.

18. Jansen M, Yip S, Louis DN. Molecular pathology in adult gliomas: diagnostic, prognostic, and predictive markers. Lancet Neurol 2010;9(7): 717–26.

19. Yip S, Butterfield YS, Morozova O, et al. Concurrent CIC mutations, IDH mutations, and 1p/19q loss distinguish oligodendrogliomas from other cancers. J Pathol 2012;226(1):7–16.

20. Tseng AS, Tapon N, Kanda H, et al. Capicua regulates cell proliferation downstream of the receptor tyrosine kinase/ras signaling pathway. Curr Biol 2007;17(8):728–33.

21. Bettegowda C, Agrawal N, Jiao Y, et al. Mutations in CIC and FUBP1 contribute to human oligodendroglioma. Science 2011;333(6048):1453–5.

22. Gravendeel LA, Kloosterhof NK, Bralten LB, et al. Segregation of non-p.R132H mutations in IDH1 in distinct molecular subtypes of glioma. Hum Mutat 2010;31(3):E1186–99.

23. Sahm F, Koelsche C, Meyer J, et al. CIC and FUBP1 mutations in oligodendrogliomas, oligoastrocytomas and astrocytomas. Acta Neuropathol 2012; 123(6):853–60.

24. Killela PJ, Reitman ZJ, Jiao Y, et al. TERT promoter mutations occur frequently in gliomas and a subset of tumors derived from cells with low rates of self-renewal. Proc Natl Acad Sci U S A 2013; 110(15):6021–6.

25. Arita H, Narita Y, Fukushima S, et al. Upregulating mutations in the TERT promoter commonly occur in adult malignant gliomas and are strongly associated with total 1p19q loss. Acta Neuropathol 2013;126(2):267–76.

26. Verhaak RG, Hoadley KA, Purdom E, et al. Integrated genomic analysis identifies clinically relevant subtypes of glioblastoma characterized by abnormalities in PDGFRA, IDH1, EGFR, and NF1. Cancer Cell 2010;17(1):98–110.

27. Sturm D, Witt H, Hovestadt V, et al. Hotspot mutations in H3F3A and IDH1 define distinct epigenetic and biological subgroups of glioblastoma. Cancer Cell 2012;22(4):425–37.

28. Aldape K, Zadeh G, Mansouri S, et al. Glioblastoma: pathology, molecular mechanisms and markers. Acta Neuropathol 2015;129(6): 829–48.

29. Goldhoff P, Clarke J, Smirnov I, et al. Clinical stratification of glioblastoma based on alterations in retinoblastoma tumor suppressor protein (RB1) and association with the proneural subtype. J Neuropathol Exp Neurol 2012;71(1):83–9.

30. Chow LM, Endersby R, Zhu X, et al. Cooperativity within and among Pten, p53, and Rb pathways

induces high-grade astrocytoma in adult brain. Cancer Cell 2011;19(3):305–16.

31. Brennan CW, Verhaak RG, McKenna A, et al. The somatic genomic landscape of glioblastoma. Cell 2013;155(2):462–77.

32. Pekmezci M, Perry A. Practical molecular pathologic diagnosis of infiltrating gliomas. Surg Pathol Clin 2015;8(1):49–61.

33. Watanabe T, Nakamura M, Yonekawa Y, et al. Promoter hypermethylation and homozygous deletion of the p14ARF and p16INK4a genes in oligodendrogliomas. Acta Neuropathol. 2001;101(3): 185–9.

34. Kim YH, Lachuer J, Mittelbronn M, et al. Alterations in the RB1 pathway in low-grade diffuse gliomas lacking common genetic alterations. Brain Pathol 2011;21(6):645–51.

35. Backlund LM, Nilsson BR, Goike HM, et al. Short postoperative survival for glioblastoma patients with a dysfunctional Rb1 pathway in combination with no wild-type PTEN. Clin Cancer Res 2003; 9(11):4151–8.

36. Backlund LM, Nilsson BR, Liu L, et al. Mutations in Rb1 pathway-related genes are associated with poor prognosis in anaplastic astrocytomas. Br J Cancer 2005;93(1):124–30.

37. Purkait S, Jha P, Sharma MC, et al. CDKN2A deletion in pediatric versus adult glioblastomas and predictive value of p16 immunohistochemistry. Neuropathology 2013;33(4):405–12.

38. Ohgaki H, Kleihues P. Genetic profile of astrocytic and oligodendroglial gliomas. Brain Tumor Pathol 2011;28(3):177–83.

39. The Cancer Genome Atlas Research Network. Comprehensive genomic characterization defines human glioblastoma genes and core pathways. Nature 2008;455(7216):1061–8.

40. Frattini V, Trifonov V, Chan JM, et al. The integrated landscape of driver genomic alterations in glioblastoma. Nat Genet 2013;45(10):1141–9.

41. Chen JR, Xu HZ, Yao Y, et al. Prognostic value of epidermal growth factor receptor amplification and EGFRvIII in glioblastoma: meta-analysis. Acta Neurol Scand 2015;132(5):310–22.

42. Ozawa T, Brennan CW, Wang L, et al. PDGFRA gene rearrangements are frequent genetic events in PDGFRA-amplified glioblastomas. Genes Dev 2010;24(19):2205–18.

43. Phillips JJ, Aranda D, Ellison DW, et al. PDGFRA amplification is common in pediatric and adult high-grade astrocytomas and identifies a poor prognostic group in IDH1 mutant glioblastomas. Brain Pathol 2013;23(5):565–73.

44. Trusolino L, Bertotti A, Comoglio PM. MET signalling: principles and functions in development, organ regeneration and cancer. Nat Rev Mol Cell Biol 2010;11(12):834–48.

45. Snuderl M, Fazlollahi L, Le LP, et al. Mosaic amplification of multiple receptor tyrosine kinase genes in glioblastoma. Cancer Cell 2011;20(6):810–7.

46. Kong DS, Song SY, Kim DH, et al. Prognostic significance of c-Met expression in glioblastomas. Cancer 2009;115(1):140–8.

47. Pollack IF, Hamilton RL, James CD, et al. Rarity of PTEN deletions and EGFR amplification in malignant gliomas of childhood: results from the Children's Cancer Group 945 cohort. J Neurosurg 2006;105(Suppl 5):418–24.

48. Ohgaki H. Genetic pathways to glioblastomas. Neuropathology 2005;25(1):1–7.

49. Carico C, Nuno M, Mukherjee D, et al. Loss of PTEN is not associated with poor survival in newly diagnosed glioblastoma patients of the temozolomide era. PLoS One 2012;7(3): e33684.

50. Prados MD, Chang SM, Butowski N, et al. Phase II study of erlotinib plus temozolomide during and after radiation therapy in patients with newly diagnosed glioblastoma multiforme or gliosarcoma. J Clin Oncol 2009;27(4):579–84.

51. Li X, Wu C, Chen N, et al. PI3K/Akt/mTOR signaling pathway and targeted therapy for glioblastoma. Oncotarget 2016;7(22):33440–50.

52. Stupp R, Mason WP, van den Bent MJ, et al. Radiotherapy plus concomitant and adjuvant temozolomide for glioblastoma. N Engl J Med 2005;352(10): 987–96.

53. Chakravarti A, Zhai G, Suzuki Y, et al. The prognostic significance of phosphatidylinositol 3-kinase pathway activation in human gliomas. J Clin Oncol 2004;22(10):1926–33.

54. Swartling FJ. Myc proteins in brain tumor development and maintenance. Ups J Med Sci 2012; 117(2):122–31.

55. Perry A, Miller CR, Gujrati M, et al. Malignant gliomas with primitive neuroectodermal tumorlike components: a clinicopathologic and genetic study of 53 cases. Brain Pathol 2009;19(1):81–90.

56. Bai H, Harmanci AS, Erson-Omay EZ, et al. Integrated genomic characterization of IDH1-mutant glioma malignant progression. Nat Genet 2016; 48(1):59–66.

57. Cenci T, Martini M, Montano N, et al. Prognostic relevance of c-Myc and BMI1 expression in patients with glioblastoma. Am J Clin Pathol 2012; 138(3):390–6.

58. Luo H, Chen Z, Wang S, et al. c-Myc-miR-29c-REV3L signalling pathway drives the acquisition of temozolomide resistance in glioblastoma. Brain 2015;138(Pt 12):3654–72.

59. De Salvo M, Maresca G, D'Agnano I, et al. Temozolomide induced c-Myc-mediated apoptosis via Akt signalling in MGMT expressing glioblastoma cells. Int J Radiat Biol 2011;87(5):518–33.

60. Killela PJ, Pirozzi CJ, Reitman ZJ, et al. The genetic landscape of anaplastic astrocytoma. Oncotarget 2014;5(6):1452–7.

61. Hegi ME, Diserens AC, Gorlia T, et al. MGMT gene silencing and benefit from temozolomide in glioblastoma. N Engl J Med 2005;352(10): 997–1003.

62. Chen C, Wang F, Cheng Y, et al. Predictive value of MGMT promoter methylation status in Asian and Caucasian patients with malignant gliomas: a meta-analysis. Int J Clin Exp Med 2015;8(4): 6553–62.

63. Wick W, Hartmann C, Engel C, et al. NOA-04 randomized phase III trial of sequential radiochemotherapy of anaplastic glioma with procarbazine, lomustine, and vincristine or temozolomide. J Clin Oncol 2009;27(35):5874–80.

64. Rizzo D, Ruggiero A, Martini M, et al. Molecular biology in pediatric high-grade glioma: impact on prognosis and treatment. Biomed Res Int 2015;2015:215135.

65. Parker NR, Khong P, Parkinson JF, et al. Molecular heterogeneity in glioblastoma: potential clinical implications. Front Oncol 2015;5:55.

66. Collins VP, Jones DT, Giannini C. Pilocytic astrocytoma: pathology, molecular mechanisms and markers. Acta Neuropathol 2015;129(6): 775–88.

67. Penman CL, Faulkner C, Lowis SP, et al. Current understanding of BRAF alterations in diagnosis, prognosis, and therapeutic targeting in pediatric low-grade gliomas. Front Oncol 2015;5:54.

68. Jones DT, Hutter B, Jager N, et al. Recurrent somatic alterations of FGFR1 and NTRK2 in pilocytic astrocytoma. Nat Genet 2013;45(8):927–32.

69. Robinson GW, Orr BA, Gajjar A. Complete clinical regression of a BRAF V600E-mutant pediatric glioblastoma multiforme after BRAF inhibitor therapy. BMC Cancer 2014;14:258.

70. Amatu A, Sartore-Bianchi A, Siena S. NTRK gene fusions as novel targets of cancer therapy across multiple tumour types. ESMO Open 2016;1(2):e000023.

71. Wu G, Diaz AK, Paugh BS, et al. The genomic landscape of diffuse intrinsic pontine glioma and pediatric non-brainstem high-grade glioma. Nat Genet 2014;46(5):444–50.

72. Appin CL, Brat DJ. Biomarker-driven diagnosis of diffuse gliomas. Mol Aspects Med 2015;45:87–96.

73. Gielen GH, Gessi M, Buttarelli FR, et al. Genetic analysis of diffuse high-grade astrocytomas in infancy defines a novel molecular entity. Brain Pathol 2015;25(4):409–17.

74. Schwartzentruber J, Korshunov A, Liu XY, et al. Driver mutations in histone H3.3 and chromatin remodelling genes in paediatric glioblastoma. Nature 2012;482(7384):226–31.

75. Solomon DA, Wood MD, Tihan T, et al. Diffuse midline gliomas with histone H3-K27M mutation: a series of 47 cases assessing the spectrum of morphologic variation and associated genetic alterations. Brain Pathol 2015. http://dx.doi.org/10.1111/bpa.12336.

76. Zhang RQ, Shi Z, Chen H, et al. Biomarker-based prognostic stratification of young adult glioblastoma. Oncotarget 2016;7(4):5030–41.

77. Hochart A, Escande F, Rocourt N, et al. Long survival in a child with a mutated K27M-H3.3 pilocytic astrocytoma. Ann Clin Transl Neurol 2015;2(4): 439–43.

78. Bjerke L, Mackay A, Nandhabalan M, et al. Histone H3.3. mutations drive pediatric glioblastoma through upregulation of MYCN. Cancer Discov 2013;3(5):512–9.

79. Fontebasso AM, Schwartzentruber J, Khuong-Quang DA, et al. Mutations in SETD2 and genes affecting histone H3K36 methylation target hemispheric high-grade gliomas. Acta Neuropathol 2013;125(5):659–69.

80. Buczkowicz P, Hoeman C, Rakopoulos P, et al. Genomic analysis of diffuse intrinsic pontine gliomas identifies three molecular subgroups and recurrent activating ACVR1 mutations. Nat Genet 2014;46(5):451–6.

81. Becker AP, Scapulatempo-Neto C, Carloni AC, et al. KIAA1549: BRAF gene fusion and FGFR1 hotspot mutations are prognostic factors in pilocytic astrocytomas. J Neuropathol Exp Neurol 2015; 74(7):743–54.

82. Singh D, Chan JM, Zoppoli P, et al. Transforming fusions of FGFR and TACC genes in human glioblastoma. Science 2012;337(6099):1231–5.

83. Di Stefano AL, Fucci A, Frattini V, et al. Detection, characterization, and inhibition of FGFR-TACC fusions in IDH wild-type glioma. Clin Cancer Res 2015;21(14):3307–17.

84. Masui K, Mischel PS, Reifenberger G. Molecular classification of gliomas. Handb Clin Neurol 2016;134:97–120.

85. Chi AS, Batchelor TT, Kwak EL, et al. Rapid radiographic and clinical improvement after treatment of a MET-amplified recurrent glioblastoma with a mesenchymal-epithelial transition inhibitor. J Clin Oncol 2012;30(3): e30–33.

86. Nikiforova MN, Hamilton RL. Molecular diagnostics of gliomas. Arch Pathol Lab Med 2011;135(5): 558–68.

87. Kato Y. Specific monoclonal antibodies against IDH1/2 mutations as diagnostic tools for gliomas. Brain Tumor Pathol 2015;32(1):3–11.

88. Maire CL, Ligon KL. Molecular pathologic diagnosis of epidermal growth factor receptor. Neuro Oncol 2014;16(Suppl 8):viii1–6.

89. Ritterhouse LL, Barletta JA. BRAF V600E mutation-specific antibody: a review. Semin Diagn Pathol 2015;32(5):400–8.

90. Bechet D, Gielen GG, Korshunov A, et al. Specific detection of methionine 27 mutation in histone 3 variants (H3K27M) in fixed tissue from high-grade astrocytomas. Acta Neuropathol 2014; 128(5):733–41.

91. Ikemura M, Shibahara J, Mukasa A, et al. Utility of ATRX immunohistochemistry in diagnosis of adult diffuse gliomas. Histopathology 2016;69(2):260–7.

92. Takami H, Yoshida A, Fukushima S, et al. Revisiting TP53 mutations and immunohistochemistry—a comparative study in 157 diffuse gliomas. Brain Pathol 2015;25(3):256–65.

93. van den Bent MJ, Gao Y, Kerkhof M, et al. Changes in the EGFR amplification and EGFRvIII expression between paired primary and recurrent glioblastomas. Neuro Oncol 2015;17(7):935–41.

94. Wick W, Weller M, van den Bent M, et al. MGMT testing—the challenges for biomarker-based glioma treatment. Nat Rev Neurol 2014;10(7): 372–85.

95. Bady P, Sciuscio D, Diserens AC, et al. MGMT methylation analysis of glioblastoma on the Infinium methylation BeadChip identifies two distinct CpG regions associated with gene silencing and outcome, yielding a prediction model for comparisons across datasets, tumor grades, and CIMP-status. Acta Neuropathol 2012;124(4): 547–60.

96. Franco-Hernandez C, Martinez-Glez V, de Campos JM, et al. Allelic status of 1p and 19q in oligodendrogliomas and glioblastomas: multiplex ligation-dependent probe amplification versus loss of heterozygosity. Cancer Genet Cytogenet 2009;190(2):93–6.

97. Sahm F, Schrimpf D, Jones DT, et al. Next-generation sequencing in routine brain tumor diagnostics enables an integrated diagnosis and identifies actionable targets. Acta Neuropathol 2015;131(6): 903–10.

98. Nikiforova MN, Wald AI, Melan MA, et al. Targeted next-generation sequencing panel (GlioSeq) provides comprehensive genetic profiling of central nervous system tumors. Neuro Oncol 2016;18(3): 379–87.

99. Emir UE, Larkin SJ, de Pennington N, et al. Noninvasive quantification of 2-hydroxyglutarate in human gliomas with IDH1 and IDH2 mutations. Cancer Res 2016;76(1):43–9.

100. Biomarkers Definitions Working Group. Biomarkers and surrogate endpoints: preferred definitions and conceptual framework. Clin Pharmacol Ther 2001; 69(3):89–95.

101. Vogelstein B, Papadopoulos N, Velculescu VE, et al. Cancer genome landscapes. Science 2013; 339(6127):1546–58.

102. Ellison DW. Multiple molecular data sets and the classification of adult diffuse gliomas. N Engl J Med 2015;372(26):2555–7.

103. Foote MB, Papadopoulos N, Diaz LA Jr. Genetic classification of gliomas: refining histopathology. Cancer Cell 2015;28(1):9–11.

104. Eckel-Passow JE, Lachance DH, Molinaro AM, et al. Glioma groups based on 1p/19q, IDH, and TERT promoter mutations in tumors. N Engl J Med 2015;372(26):2499–508.

105. Jiao Y, Killela PJ, Reitman ZJ, et al. Frequent ATRX, CIC, FUBP1 and IDH1 mutations refine the classification of malignant gliomas. Oncotarget 2012;3(7): 709–22.

106. Fontebasso AM, Gayden T, Nikbakht H, et al. Epigenetic dysregulation: a novel pathway of oncogenesis in pediatric brain tumors. Acta Neuropathol 2014;128(5):615–27.

107. Jones C, Baker SJ. Unique genetic and epigenetic mechanisms driving paediatric diffuse high-grade glioma. Nat Rev Cancer 2014;14(10):651–61.

ACKNOWLEDGMENTS

The authors are grateful to their NYU Langone Medical Center colleagues Matija Snuderl, MD, for contributing illustrated cases of cytogenetics analysis and methylation array; Cyrus Hedvat, MD, PhD, for providing an illustrated case of loss of heterozygosity analysis; and Elad Mashiach for assisting with the preparation of images and diagrams, and the editing of the chapter.

CHAPTER 5

Multimodality Targeting of Glioma Cells

Zhenqiang He, MD[a,b], Richard Alan Mitteer Jr, MS[a], Yonggao Mou, MD[b],
Yi Fan, MD, PhD[a,c,*]

Glioma is the most common malignant primary tumor in the central nervous system, accounting for about 80% of total malignant brain tumors.[1,2] The World Health Organization (WHO) classification divides glioma into 4 grades according to the degree of malignancy: anaplastic astrocytoma (WHO grade III) and well-differentiated astrocytoma (WHO grade I/II) have various median survivals from 2 to 7 years[2,3]; glioblastoma (GBM; WHO grade IV), which constitutes 54.9% of all gliomas, is the most serious and malignant form of glioma, with a median overall survival of 12 to 15 months.[4,5]

Despite the aggressive standard-of-care treatment, which includes surgical resection, fractionated radiation, and temozolomide-based chemotherapy, the relapse of high-grade glioma is essentially universal, and the 5-year survival rate of patients with GBM is less than 10%.[6–9] Multiple mechanisms contribute to treatment inefficacy: complete surgical removal is nearly impossible because of its location and infiltrative nature; the use of fractionated radiation is restricted because of the potential damage to normal brain tissue; the blood-brain barrier (BBB) blocks most chemotherapy drugs; and glioma cells develop primary and acquired resistance to chemotherapy. Therefore, the development of new therapies is urgently needed.

Angiogenesis, the formation of new blood vessels, plays a critical role in the growth and spread of cancer. Antiangiogenic therapy that primarily targets vascular endothelial growth factor (VEGF) has been an efficient therapeutic strategy in treating non–small cell lung, colorectal, renal, and ovarian cancers.[10] Glioma is among the most vascularized tumors in humans. Recent studies show that bevacizumab, a monoclonal antibody against VEGF, increased progression-free survival (PFS) but not overall survival (OS) in newly diagnosed GBM,[11–13] which may indicate some initial therapeutic efficacy that did not translate to long-term outcomes. In contrast, targeted molecular therapy has recently achieved remarkable success in various cancer types, including non–small cell lung cancer, breast cancer, and leukemia.[14,15] Recent advances in identifying oncogenic signal pathways and deciphering metabolic, genomic, and epigenetic regulation in glioma cells have provided deep insights into the molecular pathogenesis of the malignancy, and more importantly, have shed light on the development of new targeted therapies in patients with glioma. This chapter discusses the potential targets of glioma therapy and their clinical efficacy, the potential therapeutic barriers, and the new direction and promise, with a focus on antiangiogenic and targeted molecular therapies.

ANTIANGIOGENIC THERAPY

Therapeutic Targets and Treatment Efficacy

Angiogenesis proceeds by endothelial cell (EC) sprouting and outgrowth from existing vessels.[16,17] This process is subjected to spatiotemporal regulation: triggered by binding of angiogenic factors to their receptors and executed by sequent activation of downstream signal pathways. These signaling events eventually induce Rho GTPase–mediated and phosphatidylinositol 3-kinase (PI3K)–mediated

[a] Department of Radiation Oncology, University of Pennsylvania Perelman School of Medicine, 3400 Civic Center Boulevard, Philadelphia, PA 19104, USA; [b] Department of Neurosurgery, Sun Yat-sen University Cancer Center, State Key Laboratory of Oncology in South China, Collaborative Innovation Center for Cancer Medicine, 651 Dong-Feng East Road, Guangzhou 510000, China; [c] Department of Neurosurgery, University of Pennsylvania Perelman School of Medicine, 3400 Civic Center Boulevard, Philadelphia, PA 19104, USA
* Corresponding author. Department of Radiation Oncology, University of Pennsylvania Perelman School of Medicine, 3400 Civic Center Boulevard, SCTR 8-132, Philadelphia, PA 19104.
E-mail address: fanyi@uphs.upenn.edu

cell migration and invasion, and lead to genetic and metabolic reprogramming to promote cell growth and proliferation.[17,18] These ligands, receptors, kinases, and transcriptional factors in the regulatory network can serve as potential targets for antiangiogenic therapy (**Fig. 5.1**).

Angiogenic factors

The most widely preferred approach for antiangiogenesis currently is the blockade of the pathways of angiogenic factors, including VEGF, basic fibroblast growth factor (bFGF), platelet-derived growth factor (PDGF), hepatocyte growth factor/scatter factor (HGF/SF), and angiopoietins.[19,20] Several of these factors are described here.

Vascular endothelial growth factor. VEGF and its receptor VEGFR2 have served as the primary therapeutic targets for antiangiogenic therapy in last 3 decades.[21–24] Bevacizumab, the most widely used humanized VEGF antibody, has been approved for treating metastatic colorectal carcinoma, non–small cell lung cancer, metastatic renal cell carcinoma, breast cancer (in the European Union [EU]), ovarian cancer (in the EU), and recurrent GBM.[25] Ranibizumab is another neutralizing antibody against VEGF, with a similar binding affinity. Bevacizumab, used as monotherapy or in combination with chemotherapy, slightly improved PFS but not OS in most clinical trials including patients with GBM.[23,26] Ziv-aflibercept is a recombinant fusion protein consisting of VEGF-binding portions from the extracellular domains of VEGF1/2, therefore binding to circulating VEGF like a trap.

Ziv-aflibercept has approximately 100-fold higher affinity than either bevacizumab or ranibizumab, showing markedly more potent blockade of VEGFR-1 or VEGFR-2 activation.[20,27] Clinical trials showed that Ziv-aflibercept plus FOLFIRI (folinic acid, fluorouracil and irinotecan) improved PFS and OS in metastatic colorectal carcinoma with a median OS of 13.5 months, compared with a median OS of 12.06 months with FOLFIRI alone.[28,29] The efficacy of Ziv-aflibercept needs further evaluation in patients with glioma.

Basic fibroblast growth factor. bFGF/fibroblast growth factor receptor (FGFR) induces angiogenesis by promoting extracellular matrix degradation, altering intercellular adhesion, enhancing cell motility, and stimulating cell growth in ECs.[30] Pazopanib is a second-generation tyrosine kinase inhibitor that targets FGFR, VEGFR, platelet-derived growth factor receptor (PDGFR), and c-Kit. Pazopanib has been approved by the US Food and Drug Administration (FDA) for treating soft tissue sarcoma. Pazopanib did not prolong PFS but showed in situ biological activities indicated by radiographic responses in a phase II trial for patients with recurrent GBM.[31] The combination of pazopanib and lapatinib (epidermal growth factor receptor [EGFR] inhibitor) was evaluated in a phase I/II trial, but was terminated early because of the poor 6-month PFS rate.[32] Other clinical trials are ongoing to evaluate the combination of pazopanib with temozolomide in newly diagnosed GBM (NCT02331498) and the combination of pazopanib with topotecan in recurrent GBM (NCT01931098).

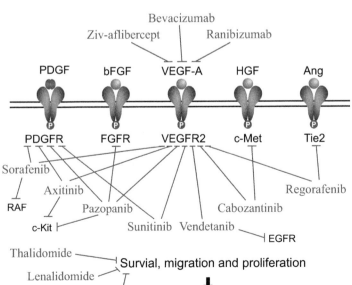

Fig. 5.1 Antiangiogenic therapeutic targets and agents. VEGF and its receptor VEGFR2 have served as the primary targets for antiangiogenic therapy. Shown are currently used agents and therapeutic targets for antiangiogenesis in clinics. Ang, Angiopoietins; bFGF, basic fibroblast growth factor; EGFR, epidermal growth factor receptor; FGFR, fibroblast growth factor receptor; HGF, hepatocyte growth factor; PDGF, platelet-derived growth factor; RAF, rapidly activated fibrosarcoma.

Platelet-derived growth factor. Aberrant activation of PDGF/PDGFR signaling is one of the hallmarks of glioma biology. Overexpression of PDGF/PDGFR has been found in glioma cells and surrounding ECs; coexpression of ligand receptor in these cells allows both autocrine and paracrine forms of activation, resulting in vessel formation and glioma cell migration, survival, and invasion.[33] Both sorafenib and sunitinib are multitargeted angiogenesis inhibitors that target PDGFR, VEGFR, mast/stem cell growth factor (c-Kit) and FMS-like tyrosine kinase 3 (FLT-3). They have been approved for the treatment of multiple cancer types, including renal cell carcinoma, hepatocellular carcinoma, pancreatic neuroendocrine tumor, and gastrointestinal stromal tumors. A phase II trial of sunitinib alone in recurrent anaplastic astrocytoma and recurrent GBM failed to show significant antitumor activity; no partial responses (PRs) or complete responses (CRs) were observed in the cohort.[34] A phase I trial of the combination of sorafenib with temozolomide and radiation therapy showed that sorafenib was well tolerated.[35] Combination of sorafenib and temsirolimus (mammalian target of rapamycin [mTOR] inhibitor) showed poor efficacy with a 6-month PFS rate of 0%.[36] Further clinical trials of different combinations of sorafenib with other agents are now under study (NCT01434602, NCT01817751).

Hepatocyte growth factor. HGF is often highly expressed in GBM, which may lead to increased glioma cell invasion.[37] HGF/c-Met also stimulates EC proliferation and migration and induces angiogenesis.[38–40] Cabozantinib is an orally bioavailable inhibitor that targets HGF, c-Met, rearranged during transfection (RET), and VEGFR2. Cabozantinib has been approved for treating medullary thyroid cancer. A phase I trial of cabozantinib with temozolomide and radiotherapy in newly diagnosed patients with GBM showed that cabozantinib was well tolerated at a dose of 40 mg daily. Several phase II trials of cabozantinib in patients with malignant gliomas were completed (NCT01068782, NCT00704288), but the results have not been published yet.

Angiopoietins. Angiopoietins and their receptor Tie2 are important for angiogenesis induction.[41,42] Regorafenib is an oral multikinase inhibitor that targets several protein kinases, including those involved in the regulation of tumor angiogenesis (VEGFR, Tie2, PDGFR, and FGFR) and oncogenesis (c-Kit, RET, rapidly activated fibrosarcoma 1 (RAF1), BRAF, and BRAF^{V600E}).[43] Regorafenib has been approved for treating metastatic colorectal cancer and gastrointestinal stromal tumor. Large randomized clinical trials revealed that regorafenib provides a significantly improved PFS in metastatic gastrointestinal stromal tumors.[44,45] Although the antitumor efficacy of regorafenib in malignant glioma cells was shown in a preclinical study,[43] the clinical effects of regorafenib have not been validated in patients with glioma.

Antivascular agents

Thalidomide and its derivatives, lenalidomide and pomalidomide, are synthetic derivatives of glutamic acid with multiple properties, including immunomodulatory, antiinflammatory, and antiangiogenesis effects.[46,47] These agents can inhibit EC proliferation, block biological functions induced by proangiogenic factors such as VEGF and bFGF, and induce antitumor activity.[47–49] They have been approved for treating multiple myeloma. Clinical trials revealed that thalidomide had a limited efficacy in patients with recurrent or newly diagnosed GBM.[50,51] Combinations of thalidomide with irinotecan or carmustine or conventional therapy have also failed to achieve sufficient efficacy in several phase II trials.[52–54] Furthermore, phase I trials showed that lenalidomide was tolerable in both pediatric and adult patients with glioma.[55–57] A phase II trial is ongoing to evaluate the antitumor effects of lenalidomide in patients with glioma (NCT01553149). Pomalidomide shows effective anticancer activities in hematologic malignancies such as multiple myeloma and acute myeloid leukemia, but the efficacy of pomalidomide in malignant glioma has not been fully investigated. A phase I trial of pomalidomide in recurrent gliomas is ongoing (NCT02415153). The antiangiogenic effects of these agents in gliomas needs further evaluation in clinical trials.

Potential Therapeutic Barriers

Antiangiogenic therapy, albeit initially groundbreaking, has encountered difficulties and failures in most malignant cancers. Current angiogenic therapies that mainly target VEGF pathways fail to produce a permanent response in most patients, usually showing a transient response initially with impressive radiographic responses followed by tumor regrowth and disease progression.[58,59] Moreover, certain patients show no response after the antiangiogenic treatment in multiple cancer types, including GBM,[58,60] suggesting both primary (intrinsic) and acquired (treatment-induced) mechanisms existing for the treatment resistance.

Primary resistance

Angiogenic pathway redundancy. There is a plethora of proangiogenic factors expressed in solid tumors inducing persistent, simultaneous activation of multiple RTK-mediated signal pathways. This abundance may explain why current therapies that target VEGF or several other angiogenic factors, such as PDGF and bFGF, individually have limited efficacy. This limited efficacy may be overcome by a combination of multiple angiogenic inhibitors. Molecular diagnosis that examines the activation panel of signal pathways specific to vascular ECs of tumor biopsy samples may further ensure the success of the combined therapies in individual patients.

Microenvironment-dependent protection. It has become increasingly recognized that the stromal cells including circulation-derived progenitor cells and myeloid cells in the tumor microenvironment contribute to the treatment resistance in ECs.[61–64] CD11b[+]Gr1[+] myeloid cells that express proangiogenic factors and other cytokines can infiltrate the tumor, which is critical for the anti-VEGF resistance in ECs. Studies show that targeting these cells by either antibody-based deletion or PI3K inhibition significantly reverses the treatment resistance in immunocompetent preclinical models of RT2 primitive neuroectodermal tumor and other murine cancers.[62,65] Recent studies showed that macrophages are a critical determinant for glioma progression.[66,67] These results suggest that targeting tumor-associated macrophage may serve as a promising strategy to sensitize antiangiogenic treatment in glioma.

Vascular transformation. Our recent work reveals that GBM-associated ECs undergo mesenchymal transformation to acquire fibroblast phenotypes, including enhanced cell migration and proliferation, leading to aberrant angiogenesis.[68] This new concept is different from the previously proposed endothelial-mesenchymal transition in a breast cancer model: instead of EC generation of tumor-associated fibroblasts de novo,[69] transformed ECs still retain vascular functions, including vessel formation and absorption of acylated low-density lipoprotein (acLDL). More importantly, transformation-induced downregulation of VEGFR2, and possibly its downstream signaling, renders the EC resistant to anti-VEGF treatment. Therefore, this newly identified mechanism may provide an explanation for primary resistance to anti-VEGF therapy and serve as an alternative target for antiangiogenic therapy in gliomas.

Acquired resistance
Compensatory activation of angiogenic pathways. Among other cancer types, GBM relapse after antiangiogenic therapy with the VEGFR

inhibitor cediranib was associated with the reactivation of tumor angiogenesis, suggesting the tumor development of resistance mechanisms to evade the VEGF/VEGFR2 blockade. Compensatory upregulation of the other angiogenic factor pathways may contribute to this resistance, as indicated by increased bFGF/FGFR system in experimental tumor models and in patients with cancer.[70,71] Therefore, an efficient antiangiogenic therapy may require the temporally precise targeting of multiple angiogenic pathways.

Pericyte-mediated vessel protection. Pericytes play a critical role in supporting EC function under physiologic conditions and inducing vascular abnormalities in cancer settings.[72–75] Previous studies show that VEGF inhibition reduces vascularity and selectively eliminates the ECs that have no pericyte coverage,[76,77] suggesting a protective role for pericytes. A further study reveals that tumor-associated pericytes secrete angiogenic factors, including VEGF, to support EC survival after antiangiogenic treatment.[78] As such, targeting pericytes seems to enhance the efficacy of antiangiogenic therapy in a mouse model of pancreatic islet cancer,[76] which needs to be clinically evaluated in patients with glioma.

Hypoxia-induced treatment resistance. Theoretically, antiangiogenic therapy designed to destroy the tumor vasculature can induce vascular shutdown, leading to hypoxia caused by lack of sufficient oxygen. Hypoxia stimulates tumor progression through a hypoxia-inducible factor (HIF) 1α/2α–dependent mechanism, by which HIFs transcribe multiple growth factors to enhance angiogenesis and tumor cell survival as well as metabolic enzymes to allow tumor cells to adapt to the poorly oxygenated environment.[79–81] Furthermore, hypoxia promotes the stemness of cancer stem cells, which is critical for their self-renewal and survival, and contributes to cancer recurrence and tumor resistance to cytotoxicity treatment.[82,83] In addition, HIF-1α is also activated in GBM-associated ECs,[84] likely contributing to the acquired resistance in tumor ECs to antiangiogenic therapy. Thus, combination with HIF-targeted therapy may offer new opportunities for overcoming the resistance of ECs to antiangiogenic therapy and tumor cells to chemotherapy. However, the concept of antiangiogenesis-induced tumor hypoxia is still controversial. In contrast, antiangiogenesis therapy targeting VEGF and VEGFR2 alleviates hypoxia, because of its vessel normalization effects.[23,85] Clinical data in patients with glioma show that anti-VEGF treatment induces transiently enhanced tumor blood perfusion and oxygenation.[60] Note that patients with recurrent and newly diagnosed GBM who show increased tumor oxygenation response to anti-VEGF therapy survive 6 to 9 months longer than those showing no responses,[86,87] suggesting that vessel normalization may induce survival benefits. This could be, at least partially, explained by the role of VEGF in vascular abnormalities. Further examination of the vessel normalization function of antiangiogenesis by using thalidomide, or its derivatives, and the inhibitors targeting other angiogenic factors in preclinical models and patients with cancer is needed.

New Direction and Promise
Endothelial metabolism
Emerging evidence indicates endothelial metabolism as a new and promising target for antiangiogenic therapy.[88,89] ECs are quiescent for years but sprout to generate new vasculature (ie, angiogenesis) after receiving angiogenic stimulation; a metabolic switch seems requisite for this angiogenic activation.[90] A recent study identified 6-phosphofructo-2-kinase/fructose-2,6-biphosphatase 3 (PFKFB3) as a major glycolytic enzyme in ECs, which regulates lamellipodia formation and cell migration, and is therefore critical for sprouting angiogenesis.[91] Consistently, PFKFB3 inhibition by 3-(3-pyridinyl)-1-(4-pyridinyl)-2-propen-1-one efficiently blocks inflammation-induced angiogenesis. Furthermore, peroxisome proliferator–activated receptor gamma coactivator-1 alpha (PGC-1α) inhibits notch activity in ECs, maintaining EC quiescence and inhibiting sprouting angiogenesis in diabetes.[92] A recent study revealed that carnitine palmitoyltransferase 1 (CPT1A), a rate-limiting enzyme of fatty acid oxidation, is required for EC proliferation and vascular sprouting.[93] These works have identified several promising metabolic targets, including PFKFB3, PGC-1α, and CPT1A, for the inhibition of sprouting angiogenesis, which may skew the vasculature toward a homeostatic, quiescent state. However, the roles of these metabolic targets in tumor angiogenesis remain largely unclear.

Vascular detransformation
Our recent work reveals endothelial-mesenchymal transformation as a driving force for vascular abnormalities and aberrant vascularization in gliomas.[68] As proof of principle, inhibition of the mesenchymal transformation by *Met* deletion in ECs reduces vascularity, normalizes vessels, and sensitizes tumors to temozolomide chemotherapy in a genetically engineered murine GBM model. These results suggest that vascular detransformation may serve as a new strategy for

antiangiogenesis and vessel normalization therapy. The authors expect that detransformation may not only structurally normalize tumor-associated vessels but may also recondition the abnormal tumor microenvironment, considering the increasingly recognized importance of ECs as a major source of growth factors and cytokines in the microenvironment. Therefore, vascular detransformation therapy may break the tumor resistance barrier and allow the reactivation of the host tumor immunity. Identification of the critical regulatory mechanisms is necessary for further evaluation of its therapeutic potential in preclinical models and patients with glioma.

TARGETED MOLECULAR THERAPY
Therapeutic Targets and Treatment Efficacy
Multiple pathways have served as potential therapeutic targets for treating glioma, including EGF, PDGF, and transforming growth factor-beta (TGF-β) pathways (**Fig. 5.2**) and developmental signal pathways (**Fig. 5.3**).

Receptor tyrosine kinases
Receptor tyrosine kinases (RTKs) control fundamental cellular events, including cell survival, proliferation, migration, metabolism, differentiation, and apoptosis.[94] RTKs are frequently mutated in gliomas, and the constitutively active mutations drive activation of oncogenic pathways leading to uncontrolled cell growth and tumorigenesis. Recent studies have revealed a critical role of RTKs, including EGFR, EGFR variant III (EGFR vIII), PDGFR, c-Met, and erythropoietin-producing human hepatocellular carcinoma (Eph) in glioma cell proliferation and invasion.[95] Among these RTKs, EGFR, EGFR vIII, and platelet-derived growth factor receptor (PDGFR)-A are frequently activated in patients with glioma: EGFR gene amplification occurs in about 40% of patients with GBM and the EGFR vIII mutant is found in approximately 30% to 50% of these EGFR-amplified gliomas[96]; PDGFRA gene amplification is observed in about 16% patients with GBM.[97] These mutation-mediated activations of RTKs induce the recruitment of PI3K and rat sarcoma (RAS) to the cell membrane, triggering downstream pro-oncogenic signal transduction cascades, eventually leading to cell malignancy.[98] The Cancer Genome Atlas (TCGA) data reveal that up to 88% of patients with GBM harbor genetic mutations of the RTK/RAS/PI3K pathway.[94] These RTKs therefore represent promising targets for antineoplastic treatment in glioma (see **Fig. 5.2**).

Epidermal growth factor receptor. Extensive studies have shown that activated EGFR and

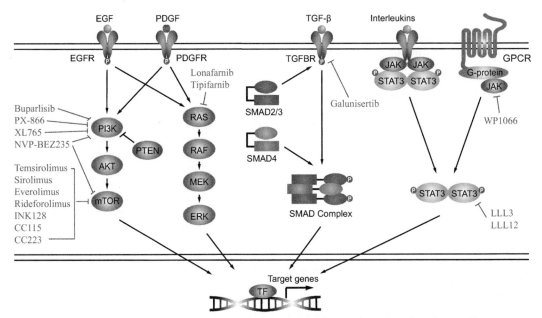

Fig. 5.2 Molecular targets in glioma. Multiple signal pathways are aberrantly activated in gliomas. Shown are potential targets and agents for targeted molecular therapies. EGFR inhibitors: gefitinib, erlotinib, lapatinib, cetuximab, and nimotuzumab. PDGFR inhibitors: imatinib, dasatinib (ABL, c-Kit, and PDGFR), sunitinib, sorafenib (VEGFR and PDGFR). Akt, Protein kinase B/Akt kinase; GPCR, G protein-coupled receptor; PTEN, phosphatase and tensin homolog; SMAD, small body size/mothers against decapentaplegic homology; TF, transcription factor.

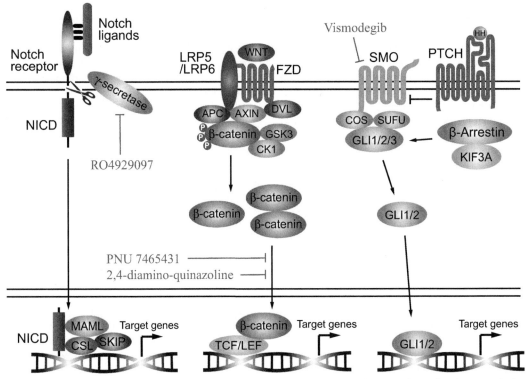

Fig. 5.3 Developmental pathways and their therapeutic targets in glioma. Developmental signal pathways including Wnt, Notch, and Hedgehog serve as therapeutic targets for gliomas. Potential therapeutic targets and agents for targeted molecular therapies are shown. APC, adenomatous polyposis coli; CK1, casein kinase 1; COS, Costal; CSL, CBF1-Su(H)-LAG1; DVL, dishevelled; FZD, frizzled; GSK3, glycogen synthase kinase 3; LEF, lymphoid enhancer-binding factor; LRP, LDL receptor related protein; MAML, mastermind-like; NICD, Notch intracellular domain; PTCH, Patched transmembrane receptor; SKIP, ski-interacting protein; SMO, smoothened; SUFU, suppressor of fused; TCF, T-cell-specific transcription factor.

mutant EGFR vIII promote pro-oncogenic signal transduction and induce tumor progression.[99] EGFR-targeted therapies have proved effective in other cancers, including lung cancer.[14] The effectiveness of the anti-EGFR agents has recently been evaluated in gliomas, both preclinically and clinically.[96,100] (1) Gefitinib is the first EGFR inhibitor that was tested in recurrent GBM. In a phase II trial, 55 patients with GBM were recruited for treatment with gefitinib. The results show a median PFS of only 8.1 weeks and a median OS of 39 weeks.[101] There was no significant improvement in the clinical outcomes compared with the historical control data. (2) Erlotinib is another orally available EGFR inhibitor that shows good permeability across the BBB. In several phase II trials, patients with recurrent GBM received erlotinib treatment. These patients had a PFS of 6 months (3%–20%) and an OS of 6 to 8.6 months.[102,103] No significant survival benefits were observed. Although the clinical efficacy of these EGFR inhibitors was limited, other pharmacologic inhibitors, including lapatinib, are under evaluation in patients with GBM in ongoing clinical trials (NCT00727506; NCT00977431). (3) Cetuximab is a chimeric monoclonal antibody against EGFR. An open-label phase II trial showed that, in 55 patients with recurrent GBM treated with cetuximab, those patients with EGFR gene amplification tended to have a longer OS, but the difference was insignificant.[104] (4) Nimotuzumab is an irreversible EGFR antibody. A randomized controlled study revealed that patients with malignant glioma who received nimotuzumab in addition to radiation and chemotherapy had a significantly longer OS of 16.5 months compared with 10.5 months in the control group.[105] These data suggest for the possibility of antibody neutralization treatment of EGFR in gliomas.

Platelet-derived growth factor receptor. The amplified or mutated PDGFR induces activation of the PI3K/mTOR and RAS/MAPK pathways, therefore serving as an important therapeutic target in glioma.[97] Imatinib is a well-known small-molecule inhibitor of PDGFR, c-KIT, and breakpoint cluster region fused with Abl1 (BCR-ABL). Imatinib has been successfully used to treat various cell types, including chronic myeloid lymphoma.[15] However, the results of trials for GBM have not been promising. A multicenter, randomized, phase III clinical trial showed that combined treatment with imatinib and hydroxyurea in patients with recurrent GBM only achieved a limited 6-month PFS rate (5%) and median OS (5.3 months), and had no survival benefit compared with those treated with hydroxyurea

alone.[106] Another PDGFR-targeted agent named dasatinib, which also inhibits c-KIT, ABL, and Src family kinase, showed no significant effect in monotherapy or combined with lomustine.[107] The combinations of dasatinib with standard chemoradiotherapy or bevacizumab are being evaluated in ongoing clinical trials (NCT00869401 and NCT00892177).

Phosphatidylinositol 3-kinase/Akt/mammalian target of rapamycin pathway

The PI3K/Akt/mTOR signal pathway is critical for cell survival, growth, migration, and metabolism, which is aberrantly activated in most patients with GBM,[94] because of the activation of upstream RTKs and/or a loss-of-function mutation of phosphatase and tensin homolog (PTEN) and phosphatase. Activated PI3K pathway is associated with increased proliferation and survival in glioma cells.[98]

Phosphatidylinositol 3-kinase. Buparlisib is a pan-PI3K inhibitor. Monotherapy with buparlisib showed no significant benefit in a phase II clinical trial in patients with recurrent GBM.[108] However, the efficacy of the combinations of buparlisib with bevacizumab or carboplatin plus lomustine are currently under investigation in clinical trials (NCT01349660, NCT01934361). PX-866 is a semisynthetic derivative of wortmannin, which can irreversibly inhibit PI3K. In a phase II trial with PX-866, 33 patients with recurrent GBM showed that PX-866 was well tolerated, and the 6-month PFS rate is 17%. Although 28% of patients showed stable disease (SD), the outcome was modest.[109]

Mammalian target of rapamycin. mTOR is a major downstream target of the PI3K pathway.[110] Multiple mTOR inhibitors, including temsirolimus, sirolimus, everolimus, and ridaforolimus, have been investigated in several trials.[111–114] Although these agents were well tolerated by patients, monotherapies failed to show any clinical benefit in patients with malignant glioma. There are several novel inhibitors, including INK128, CC115, and CC223, that can inhibit both mammalian target of rapamycin complex 1 (mTORC1) and mTORC2, showing great potential in preclinical studies.[115–117] Clinical trials with these agents are currently in progress (NCT02133183, NCT01353625, and NCT01177397). Furthermore, recent studies indicated that novel inhibitors, including NVP-BEZ235 and XL765, which dually target PI3K and mTOR, displayed robust antitumor activities in glioma cells, glioma stem cells, and animal models,[118] but further clinical investigation is needed of their efficacy in patients with glioma.

Rat sarcoma/rapidly activated fibrosarcoma/mitogen-activated erk kinase/extracellular signal-regulated kinase pathway

Rat sarcoma (RAS) belongs to a class of small GTPases. RAS is usually activated by RTKs and/or by the inactivation of neurofibromatosis 1 (NF1), followed by the downstream signal transduction of rapidly activated fibrosarcoma (RAF), mitogen-activated erk kinase (MEK), and extracellular signal-regulated kinase (ERK).[119] Farnesyl transferase (FT) posttranslationally modifies RAS proteins to activate their downstream signal transduction, serving as an important therapeutic target. Tipifarnib is an FT inhibitor. In a phase II trial with 67 patients with recurrent GBM treated with tipifarnib, only 7% of patients had a radiographic response and the 6-month PFS was 9%.[120] Similar results were observed with another FT inhibitor, lonafarnib. A phase Ib trial with 34 patients with recurrent GBM treated with lonafarnib combined with temozolomide showed that the CR and PR rate was 24% and the 6-month PFS was 38%.[121]

Transforming growth factor-beta pathway

The TGF-β pathway is essential for glioma cell proliferation, invasion, differentiation, and survival.[122–124] Trabedersen (AP12009) is a synthetic antisense phosphorothioate oligodeoxynucleotide complementary to the messenger RNA of the human TGF-β2 gene. In a phase IIb trial, 145 patients with recurrent/refractory GBM or anaplastic glioma were treated with trabedersen or standard chemotherapy. Patients treated with 2.48mg/cycle trabedersen had significantly better 14-month survival rates compared with other groups.[125] Galunisertib (LY2157299) is a novel kinase inhibitor of TGF-β1.[126] A first-in-human dose study showed that galunisertib was well tolerated and no adverse cardiac events were observed. Seven of 56 patients with malignant glioma achieved CR or PR and 5 patients had stable disease (SD) greater than or equal to 6 cycles of treatment.[127] Further clinical trials with galunisertib are ongoing (NCT02304419, NCT02304419).

Janus kinase/signal transducer and activator of transcription pathway

The Janus kinase (JAK) signal transducer and activator of transcription (STAT) signal pathway play an important role in preventing apoptosis and promoting the proliferation and the invasion of tumor cells.[128,129] WP1066 is an orally bioavailable inhibitor of JAK2 with potential antineoplastic activity. A preclinical study revealed that systemic intraperitoneal administration of WP1066 inhibited the growth of subcutaneous malignant glioma xenografts in mice.[130] A clinical trial of WP1066 is ongoing (NCT01904123). LLL3 and LLL12 are STAT3 inhibitors that directly inhibit the phosphorylation of STAT3 and expression of downstream STAT3-target genes. Both agents inhibited growth of glioma cells and GBM xenografts,[131,132] which needs further clinical investigation for their efficacy in patients with glioma.

Notch pathway

Notch signaling is activated via transmembrane ligands and receptors such as Delta-like ligand 1 (DLL1), DLL3, and DLL4, followed by the release of the intracellular domains into the nucleus and transcription activation in a gamma-secretase–dependent manner. The Notch pathway is critical for maintenance of stemness properties in cancer stem cells and tumor angiogenesis.[133–135] RO4929097 is a gamma-secretase inhibitor. Preclinical data showed that RO4929097 had limited effects as a single agent, but enhanced efficacy was observed when combined with DNA-interfering agents in GBM xenografts.[136] Clinical trials designed to investigate the clinical efficacy of RO4929097 as monotherapy or combined therapy with chemoradiation in patients with glioma are underway (NCT01269411, NCT01122901, and NCT01119599).

Hedgehog pathway

The hedgehog (HH) ligands bind to the patched (PTCH) transmembrane receptors to release Smoothened (SMO), leading to the activation of transcriptional factors, including glioma-associated oncogene homologue (GLI) 1 and GLI2. Most of the target genes, such as GLI1, GLI2, and PTCH1, are essential for self-renewal and the survival of cancer stem cells.[137,138] Vismodegib is a Hedgehog inhibitor that blocks the activities of the Hedgehog-ligand cell surface receptors PTCH and/or SMO. Vismodegib was proved to be clinically effective in patients with Recurrent Sonic Hedgehog–subgroup medulloblastoma.[139] The clinical trial with vismodegib in treating patients with recurrent GBM is ongoing (NCT00980343).

WNT/beta-catenin pathway

WNT/beta-catenin is the canonical WNT pathway. Translocation of beta-catenin induces activation of beta-catenin–T cell–specific transcription factor (TCF)/lymphoid enhancer–binding factor (LEF) complex, which is vital for tumor development, progression, and invasion.[138,140] WNT/beta-catenin is important for stemness functions in glioma cancer stem cells. Several small-molecule inhibitors of this pathway, including PNU 7465431 and 2,4-diamino-quinazoline, have recently been identified by high-throughput screening,[140,141] but their antitumor activities in gliomas remain unclear.

Isocitrate dehydrogenase 1/2

Tumor sequencing studies have identified high frequencies of isocitrate dehydrogenase 1 (IDH1)/IDH2 mutation in most secondary GBMs and approximately 60% to 70% of grade II and grade III gliomas.[142] Wild-type (IDH mutant negative) promotes oncogenic activity. Mutated IDH1 (mIDH1) was identified in 46% of the patients and was significantly correlated to a good survival in both univariate (HR 0.24, 95% CI 0.11 - 0.53) and in multivariate analysis (HR 0.40, 95% CI 0.17 - 0.91).[143] AGI-5198 is a novel inhibitor of the IDH1 mutant, which selectively inhibits IDH-1 R132H and depletes 2-HG production. A recent study showed that AGI-5198 reduced glioma cell growth in vitro.[144] A similar effect on glioma cells was induced by AG 120, another IDH inhibitor.[145] The clinical trial with AG 120 in IDH1-mutated multiple solid tumors, including glioma, is ongoing (NCT02073994).

Proteasome

The ubiquitin proteasome system is an essential metabolic constituent that controls intracellular protein concentrations and tightly regulates multiple cellular functions, including cell growth, survival, and metabolism and the cell cycle.[146] Proteasome inhibition has proved effective in myeloma.[147] Bortezomib is a proteasome inhibitor that has been evaluated in malignant gliomas. A phase I trial of bortezomib showed limited benefit in survival time (6 months median OS) in patients with recurrent high-grade gliomas.[148] Another phase I trial of bortezomib combined with temozolomide and radiotherapy showed that patients with newly diagnosed GBM treated with bortezomib had a median OS of 16.9 months, slightly longer than the historical control (14.4 months).[149] More phase II studies are needed to evaluate the therapeutic effect of proteasome inhibitors.

Histone deacetylase

Aberrant epigenetic function leads to altered gene expression and malignant cellular transformation, contributing to cancer development and progression. Central to epigenetic regulation is the histone acetylation mainly controlled by histone deacetylases (HDACs) and acetyltransferases. Inhibition of HDAC seems to reduce cell division and promote cancer cell apoptosis.[150]

The FDA has approved 2 HDAC inhibitors, vorinostat and romidepsin, as anticancer agents. Phase I trials of vorinostat combined with temozolomide or chemoradiation showed that vorinostat was well tolerated.[151,152] A phase II trial evaluated the monotherapy of vorinostat in patients with recurrent GBM and showed modest activity with a median OS of 5.7 months.[153] A phase II trial of combined therapy in newly diagnosed GBM is ongoing (NCT00731731).

Potential Therapeutic Barriers

Despite recent breakthroughs in glioma biology, most of the current targeted molecular therapies for malignant gliomas show only poor to modest therapeutic effects in clinical trials. There are several therapeutic barriers that limit their clinical efficacy.

Treatment-resistant glioma cancer stem cells

Cancer stem cells (CSCs), also known as tumor-initiating cells or tumor-propagating cells, are highly tumorigenic and able to differentiate asymmetrically to orchestrate a heterogeneous tumor mass. Importantly, CSCs are refractory to radiation and chemotherapy, and therefore contribute significantly to therapy resistance and tumor relapse.[154–156] Recent studies have identified a prominent population of CSCs in brain tumors, including GBM, which are pluripotent and radioresistant and have the ability to repopulate tumors.[157,158] Radiation induces robust enrichment of the CD133+ CSC population in human GBM and mouse xenograft tumors.[158,159] Multiple mechanisms generally contribute to the treatment resistance in CSCs, including cell dormancy, increased drug efflux and detoxification, activation of antiapoptotic signal pathways, and enhanced activities for DNA repair.[160]

Intratumoral heterogeneity

Gliomas, including GBM, are well characterized by a high degree of intratumoral heterogeneity, which contributes to the tumor resistance to molecular targeted therapies. Malignant gliomas consist of cells with different phenotypes, genotypes, and epigenetic states.[161,162] According to the TCGA gene expression data, GBM has been classified into 4 molecular subtypes: proneural, neural, classic, and mesenchymal.[163] Although each subtype shows a different mutated gene expression pattern, single-cell RNA sequencing revealed that the established GBM subtype classifiers are variably expressed across individual cells within a single tumor. Coamplification of 3 RTKs (EGFR, MET, PDGFRA) was observed in different cells of 34 GBM samples (7.3% TCGA GBM).[164]

This may contribute significantly to the resistance to monotargeted therapy because other RTKs could compensate by maintaining the pathway activation when only 1 RTK is inhibited. The complex intratumoral heterogeneity may be the major reason for the failure of most targeted therapies in malignant gliomas.

Signaling pathway redundancy

Redundancy of multiple signaling pathways may be another possible explanation for the limited efficacy of the targeted agents. Major pathways identified by TCGA data, including RTK/RAS/PI3K, p53, and Rb, have complicated interplay networks.[94] Crosstalk and feedback loops were also found in the aforementioned pathways.[165–167] A single inhibitor may not be able to suppress the signal transduction of the pathway because of the interactive network.

Blood-brain barrier

The BBB is an anatomic and biochemical barrier that protects the brain from potentially harmful substances. The BBB ECs are characterized by the absence of fenestrations, more extensive tight junctions, and sparse pinocytic vesicular transport. EC tight junctions limit the paracellular flux of hydrophilic molecules across the BBB. Although disruption of the BBB can be found in most patients with GBM, there are still regions of the tumor with an intact BBB.[168] Most lipophilic small-molecule inhibitors are thought to be able to penetrate the BBB by passive diffusion, but tight junctions hold the ECs together on the BBB and limit the delivery of targeted agents into the tumor.[168,169]

New Direction and Promise
New molecular targets

Discovery of new therapeutic targets will be crucial for next-generation therapies in gliomas. For example, the FGFR-ATCC fusion gene, expressed in about 3% of GBM, promotes tumor progression.[170,171] An FGFR inhibitor significantly prolonged the survival of mice harboring intracranial GBM xenografts.[170] BGJ398, a pan FGFR inhibitor, is under evaluation in a phase II clinical trial for patients with FGFR-ATCC⁺ recurrent GBM (NCT01975701). Importantly, the development of new therapies that are effective at eradicating glioma CSCs is urgently needed. The combination of traditional cytotoxic chemotherapy and inhibition of the aforementioned developmental signal pathways (see **Fig. 5.3**) may offer opportunities to eliminate both CSCs and glioma cells. Recent studies have revealed several potential therapeutic targets for CSC-focused treatment, including

BMP/Gremlin1,[172,173] Ephrins,[174,175] iNOS,[176] iron transporter,[177] MELK,[178,179] TGF-β,[180–182] transcription factors Ascl1[183] and Myc,[184] and the epigenetic modifier MLL.[185] Therapeutic strategies that target these molecules have great promise to overcome CSC-mediated treatment resistance to radiation and chemotherapy and to prevent glioma relapse.

Combined targeted molecular therapies

The development of combination antiretroviral therapy (cART) to combat acquired immune deficiency syndrome (AIDS) has been one of the most impressive achievements in medical sciences.[186] The combination regimen of different inhibitors of nucleoside analogue reverse transcriptase successfully reduces human immunodeficiency virus infection to a manageable chronic disease.[186,187] As indicated by the cART in AIDS treatment, the combination of targeted molecular therapies with other novel therapeutic modalities may represent a promising way to significantly prolong the survival of patients with glioma and reduce gliomas to chronic diseases.

Single-agent treatment. There are several pharmacologic inhibitors that can target multiple kinases or signaling pathways. Vandetanib, the dual EGFR and VEGFR inhibitor, when combined with temozolomide, has been shown to shrink glioma xenografts.[188] However, the phase I trial showed a marginal effect of vandetanib in patients with recurrent GBM with a median OS of 6.3 months after vandetanib treatment.[189] Both sunitinib and sorafenib target VEGFR, PDGFR, c-KIT, and FLT-3. Sunitinib failed to show a significant outcome in a phase II clinical trial,[34] but a phase I trial of sorafenib in primary or recurrent high-grade gliomas showed a significant effect with a median OS of 18 months.[35] Further clinical evaluation of these agents with multiple targets is needed.

Multiple-agent treatment. Combinations of different targeted agents are expected to have synergistic effects. However, phase II clinical trials of 2 combinations, gefitinib plus everolimus and erlotinib plus sirolimus, had negligible efficacy in patients with recurrent GBM, with median OS of 5.8 months and 8.5 months, respectively.[113,190] Other combinations, including dasatinib plus erlotinib, vorinostat plus bortezomib, and pazopanib plus lapatinib, also showed limited clinical efficacy in different trials.[32,191,192] A new combination of perifosine (AKT inhibitor) and temsirolimus (mTOR inhibitor) is under investigation in a phase I/II clinical trial (NCT01051557). These results suggest that an appropriate combination may be crucial for a favorable outcome, which should be based on the genetic and epigenetic diagnosis of individual tumors.

Combination of multiple therapeutic modalities

Antiangiogenesis plus targeted molecular therapy. Antiangiogenesis therapy that targets VEGF/VEGFR can normalize tumor-associated blood vessels within a certain therapeutic window, which may promote vessel-based drug delivery to the tumor and therefore enhance the outcome of targeted molecular therapy.[85,193] Moreover, vessel normalization can reduce intratumoral hypoxia by temporally increasing perfusion, leading to less hypoxia-dependent treatment resistance to the targeted molecular therapy.[85,194] Considering the important role of tumor ECs as a niche for CSCs and glioma cells, antiangiogenic therapy may recondition the tumor microenvironment to make it less malignancy permissive for glioma cells, enhancing the efficacy of the targeted molecular therapy. Cumulatively, a significantly better clinical outcome is expected for combined antiangiogenesis plus targeted molecular therapy in patients with glioma.

Immunotherapy plus targeted molecular therapy. Recent studies have highlighted the potential of immunotherapy for glioma treatment.[195–197] Cancer immunotherapy includes passive immunotherapy such as administration of antibodies or activated immune cells, and active immunotherapy that attempts to stimulate the immune system by presenting antigens in a way that triggers an immune response; both show promising results for glioma therapy in preclinical models. Monoclonal antibodies against immune modulators such as ipilimumab (CTLA-4 inhibitor) and nivolumab (PD-1 inhibitor) are currently being evaluated in a phase II clinical trial for patients with recurrent GBM (NCT02017717). However, most immunotherapy targets specific antigens or certain subgroups of tumor cells. Combined targeted molecular therapy can work as a complementary treatment, when designed to kill additional off-target cells based on the molecular signature of the tumor.

Proton radiation plus targeted molecular therapy. Proton therapy is one of the newer radiation treatment modalities and, compared with conventional x-ray photon radiation, proton beams can be applied to small, precise areas with minimal lateral scattering in tissue, ensuring that little to no radiation is delivered to healthy tissue surrounding the tumor.[198] This property makes proton therapy an excellent option for treating gliomas in order to minimize neurocognitive deficits in normal brain tissue.[199–201] Clinical trials investigating the therapeutic effect of proton therapy in different grades of glioma are ongoing (NCT02671981 and NCT01358058). Note that recent studies by others and our group show that proton radiation causes significantly greater cytotoxic damage in the radiation-resistant, stem cell–like tumor cells in non–small cell lung cancer and GBM than conventional photon radiation.[202,203] Therefore, proton therapy may further enhance the efficacy of targeted molecular therapy by eliminating CSCs that are refractory to conventional targeted treatments, improving the survival of patients with glioma.

Improvement of drug delivery through the blood-brain barrier

Drug penetration of the BBB is a major challenge for targeted molecular therapy in gliomas. There are several potential strategies that help these agents penetrate the BBB. Focus ultrasonography can temporally open the tight conjunctions between ECs by transcranial delivery of low-frequency ultrasound waves, thereby enhancing delivery of therapeutic agents into the brain.[204–206] Certain compounds, such as histamine, leukotrienes, and bradykinin, can disrupt tight junctions in BBB ECs by transiently increasing cytosolic Ca^{2+} levels and inducing cytoskeleton reorganization. Furthermore, elacridar, a dual inhibitor of drug efflux transporters P-gp and ATP-binding cassette sub-family G member 2 (ABCG2), when combined with other potential targeted agents, may improve drug delivery through the BBB ECs.[168,207,208] Together, these BBB-targeting approaches in combination with targeted molecular therapy may improve drug delivery to tumors, leading to better clinical outcomes.

REFERENCES

1. de Robles P, Fiest KM, Frolkis AD, et al. The worldwide incidence and prevalence of primary brain tumors: a systematic review and meta-analysis. Neuro Oncol 2015;17:776–83.
2. Ostrom QT, Gittleman H, Fulop J, et al. CBTRUS statistical report: primary brain and central nervous system tumors diagnosed in the United States in 2008-2012. Neuro Oncol 2015;17(Suppl 4):iv1–62.
3. Shibahara I, Sonoda Y, Shoji T, et al. Malignant clinical features of anaplastic gliomas without IDH mutation. Neuro Oncol 2015;17:136–44.

4. Weller M, Wick W, Aldape K, et al. Glioma. Nat Rev Dis Primers 2015;1:15017.

5. Stupp R, Mason WP, van den Bent MJ, et al. Radiotherapy plus concomitant and adjuvant temozolomide for glioblastoma. N Engl J Med 2005;352:987–96.

6. Eyupoglu IY, Buchfelder M, Savaskan NE. Surgical resection of malignant gliomas-role in optimizing patient outcome. Nat Rev Neurol 2013;9:141–51.

7. Weller M, van den Bent M, Hopkins K, et al. FANO guideline for the diagnosis and treatment of anaplastic gliomas and glioblastoma. Lancet Oncol 2014;15:e395–403.

8. Wen PY, Kesari S. Malignant gliomas in adults. N Engl J Med 2008;359:492–507.

9. Cuddapah VA, Robel S, Watkins S, et al. A neurocentric perspective on glioma invasion. Nat Rev Neurosci 2014;15:455–65.

10. Kerbel RS. Tumor angiogenesis. N Engl J Med 2008;358:2039–49.

11. Chinot OL, Wick W, Mason W, et al. Bevacizumab plus radiotherapy-temozolomide for newly diagnosed glioblastoma. N Engl J Med 2014;370:709–22.

12. Friedman HS, Prados MD, Wen PY, et al. Bevacizumab alone and in combination with irinotecan in recurrent glioblastoma. J Clin Oncol 2009;27:4733–40.

13. Gilbert MR, Dignam JJ, Armstrong TS, et al. A randomized trial of bevacizumab for newly diagnosed glioblastoma. N Engl J Med 2014;370:699–708.

14. Jett JR, Carr LL. Targeted therapy for non-small cell lung cancer. Am J Respir Crit Care Med 2013;188:907–12.

15. O'Hare T, Zabriskie MS, Eiring AM, et al. Pushing the limits of targeted therapy in chronic myeloid leukaemia. Nat Rev Cancer 2012;12:513–26.

16. Folkman J. Angiogenesis: an organizing principle for drug discovery? Nat Rev Drug Discov 2007;6:273–86.

17. Weis SM, Cheresh DA. Tumor angiogenesis: molecular pathways and therapeutic targets. Nat Med 2011;17:1359–70.

18. Carmeliet P, Jain RK. Molecular mechanisms and clinical applications of angiogenesis. Nature 2011;473:298–307.

19. Ferrara N, Kerbel RS. Angiogenesis as a therapeutic target. Nature 2005;438:967–74.

20. Gacche RN, Meshram RJ. Angiogenic factors as potential drug target: efficacy and limitations of anti-angiogenic therapy. Biochim Biophys Acta 2014;1846:161–79.

21. Carmeliet P. VEGF as a key mediator of angiogenesis in cancer. Oncology 2005;69(Suppl 3):4–10.

22. Ferrara N, Gerber HP, LeCouter J. The biology of VEGF and its receptors. Nat Med 2003;9:669–76.

23. Jain RK. Antiangiogenesis strategies revisited: from starving tumors to alleviating hypoxia. Cancer Cell 2014;26:605–22.

24. Ellis LM, Hicklin DJ. VEGF-targeted therapy: mechanisms of anti-tumour activity. Nat Rev Cancer 2008;8:579–91.

25. Shih T, Lindley C. Bevacizumab: an angiogenesis inhibitor for the treatment of solid malignancies. Clin Ther 2006;28:1779–802.

26. Welti J, Loges S, Dimmeler S, et al. Recent molecular discoveries in angiogenesis and antiangiogenic therapies in cancer. J Clin Invest 2013;123:3190–200.

27. Papadopoulos N, Martin J, Ruan Q, et al. Binding and neutralization of vascular endothelial growth factor (VEGF) and related ligands by VEGF Trap, ranibizumab and bevacizumab. Angiogenesis 2012;15:171–85.

28. Van Cutsem E, Tabernero J, Lakomy R, et al. Addition of aflibercept to fluorouracil, leucovorin, and irinotecan improves survival in a phase III randomized trial in patients with metastatic colorectal cancer previously treated with an oxaliplatin-based regimen. J Clin Oncol 2012;30:3499–506.

29. Patel A, Sun W. Ziv-aflibercept in metastatic colorectal cancer. Biologics 2014;8:13–25.

30. Cross MJ, Claesson-Welsh L. FGF and VEGF function in angiogenesis: signalling pathways, biological responses and therapeutic inhibition. Trends Pharmacol Sci 2001;22:201–7.

31. Iwamoto FM, Lamborn KR, Robins HI, et al. Phase II trial of pazopanib (GW786034), an oral multitargeted angiogenesis inhibitor, for adults with recurrent glioblastoma (North American Brain Tumor Consortium study 06-02). Neuro Oncol 2010;12:855–61.

32. Reardon DA, Groves MD, Wen PY, et al. A phase I/II trial of pazopanib in combination with lapatinib in adult patients with relapsed malignant glioma. Clin Cancer Res 2013;19:900–8.

33. Hoelzinger DB, Demuth T, Berens ME. Autocrine factors that sustain glioma invasion and paracrine biology in the brain microenvironment. J Natl Cancer Inst 2007;99:1583–93.

34. Pan E, Yu D, Yue B, et al. A prospective phase II single-institution trial of sunitinib for recurrent malignant glioma. J Neurooncol 2012;110:111–8.

35. Den RB, Kamrava M, Sheng Z, et al. A phase I study of the combination of sorafenib with temozolomide and radiation therapy for the treatment of primary and recurrent high-grade gliomas. Int J Radiat Oncol Biol Phys 2013;85:321–8.

36. Lee EQ, Kuhn J, Lamborn KR, et al. Phase I/II study of sorafenib in combination with temsirolimus for recurrent glioblastoma or gliosarcoma: North American Brain Tumor Consortium study 05-02. Neuro Oncol 2012;14:1511–8.

37. Koochekpour S, Jeffers M, Rulong S, et al. Met and hepatocyte growth factor/scatter factor expression in human gliomas. Cancer Res 1997;57:5391–8.

38. Bussolino F, Di Renzo MF, Ziche M, et al. Hepatocyte growth factor is a potent angiogenic factor which stimulates endothelial cell motility and growth. J Cell Biol 1992;119:629–41.

39. Shojaei F, Lee JH, Simmons BH, et al. HGF/c-Met acts as an alternative angiogenic pathway in sunitinib-resistant tumors. Cancer Res 2010;70:10090–100.

40. Tomita N, Morishita R, Taniyama Y, et al. Angiogenic property of hepatocyte growth factor is dependent on upregulation of essential transcription factor for angiogenesis, ets-1. Circulation 2003;107:1411–7.

41. Felcht M, Luck R, Schering A, et al. Angiopoietin-2 differentially regulates angiogenesis through TIE2 and integrin signaling. J Clin Invest 2012;122:1991–2005.

42. Fagiani E, Christofori G. Angiopoietins in angiogenesis. Cancer Lett 2013;328:18–26.

43. Wilhelm SM, Dumas J, Adnane L, et al. Regorafenib (BAY 73-4506): a new oral multikinase inhibitor of angiogenic, stromal and oncogenic receptor tyrosine kinases with potent preclinical antitumor activity. Int J Cancer 2011;129:245–55.

44. Demetri GD, Reichardt P, Kang Y-K, et al. Efficacy and safety of regorafenib for advanced gastrointestinal stromal tumours after failure of imatinib and sunitinib (GRID): an international, multicentre, randomised, placebo-controlled, phase 3 trial. Lancet 2013;381:295–302.

45. Grothey A, Cutsem EV, Sobrero A, et al. Regorafenib monotherapy for previously treated metastatic colorectal cancer (CORRECT): an international, multicentre, randomised, placebo-controlled, phase 3 trial. Lancet 2013;381:303–12.

46. Zhu YX, Kortuem KM, Stewart AK. Molecular mechanism of action of immune-modulatory drugs thalidomide, lenalidomide and pomalidomide in multiple myeloma. Leuk Lymphoma 2013;54:683–7.

47. D'Amato RJ, Loughnan MS, Flynn E, et al. Thalidomide is an inhibitor of angiogenesis. Proc Natl Acad Sci U S A 1994;91:4082–5.

48. Pan B, Lentzsch S. The application and biology of immunomodulatory drugs (IMiDs) in cancer. Pharmacol Ther 2012;136:56–68.

49. Bartlett JB, Dredge K, Dalgleish AG. The evolution of thalidomide and its IMiD derivatives as anticancer agents. Nat Rev Cancer 2004;4:314–22.

50. Turner CD, Chi S, Marcus KJ, et al. Phase II study of thalidomide and radiation in children with newly diagnosed brain stem gliomas and glioblastoma multiforme. J Neurooncol 2007;82:95–101.

51. Fine HA, Figg WD, Jaeckle K, et al. Phase II trial of the antiangiogenic agent thalidomide in patients with recurrent high-grade gliomas. J Clin Oncol 2000;18:708.

52. Alexander BM, Wang M, Yung WK, et al. A phase II study of conventional radiation therapy and thalidomide for supratentorial, newly-diagnosed glioblastoma (RTOG 9806). J Neurooncol 2013;111:33–9.

53. Giglio P, Dhamne M, Hess KR, et al. Phase 2 trial of irinotecan and thalidomide in adults with recurrent anaplastic glioma. Cancer 2012;118:3599–606.

54. Fine HA, Wen PY, Maher EA, et al. Phase II trial of thalidomide and carmustine for patients with recurrent high-grade gliomas. J Clin Oncol 2003;21:2299–304.

55. Warren KE, Goldman S, Pollack IF, et al. Phase I trial of lenalidomide in pediatric patients with recurrent, refractory, or progressive primary CNS tumors: Pediatric Brain Tumor Consortium study PBTC-018. J Clin Oncol 2011;29:324–9.

56. Drappatz J, Wong ET, Schiff D, et al. A pilot safety study of lenalidomide and radiotherapy for patients with newly diagnosed glioblastoma multiforme. Int J Radiat Oncol Biol Phys 2009;73:222–7.

57. Fine HA, Kim L, Albert PS, et al. A phase I trial of lenalidomide in patients with recurrent primary central nervous system tumors. Clin Cancer Res 2007;13:7101–6.

58. Bergers G, Hanahan D. Modes of resistance to anti-angiogenic therapy. Nat Rev Cancer 2008;8:592–603.

59. Jain RK. Antiangiogenic therapy for cancer: current and emerging concepts. Oncology (Williston Park) 2005;19:7–16.

60. Batchelor TT, Sorensen AG, di Tomaso E, et al. AZD2171, a pan-VEGF receptor tyrosine kinase inhibitor, normalizes tumor vasculature and alleviates edema in glioblastoma patients. Cancer Cell 2007;11:83–95.

61. De Palma M, Venneri MA, Galli R, et al. Tie2 identifies a hematopoietic lineage of proangiogenic monocytes required for tumor vessel formation and a mesenchymal population of pericyte progenitors. Cancer Cell 2005;8:211–26.

62. Shojaei F, Wu X, Malik AK, et al. Tumor refractoriness to anti-VEGF treatment is mediated by CD11b+Gr1+ myeloid cells. Nat Biotechnol 2007;25:911–20.

63. Shojaei F, Ferrara N. Refractoriness to antivascular endothelial growth factor treatment: role of myeloid cells. Cancer Res 2008;68:5501–4.

64. Rivera LB, Bergers G. Intertwined regulation of angiogenesis and immunity by myeloid cells. Trends Immunol 2015;36:240–9.

65. Rivera LB, Meyronet D, Hervieu V, et al. Intratumoral myeloid cells regulate responsiveness and

resistance to antiangiogenic therapy. Cell Rep 2015;11:577–91.

66. Pyonteck SM, Akkari L, Schuhmacher AJ, et al. CSF-1R inhibition alters macrophage polarization and blocks glioma progression. Nat Med 2013; 19:1264–72.

67. Zhou W, Ke SQ, Huang Z, et al. Periostin secreted by glioblastoma stem cells recruits M2 tumour-associated macrophages and promotes malignant growth. Nat Cell Biol 2015;17:170–82.

68. Huang M, Liu T, Ma P, et al. c-Met-mediated endothelial plasticity drives aberrant vascularization and chemoresistance in glioblastoma. J Clin Invest 2016;126(5):1801–14.

69. Zeisberg EM, Potenta S, Xie L, et al. Discovery of endothelial to mesenchymal transition as a source for carcinoma-associated fibroblasts. Cancer Res 2007;67:10123–8.

70. Casanovas O, Hicklin DJ, Bergers G, et al. Drug resistance by evasion of antiangiogenic targeting of VEGF signaling in late-stage pancreatic islet tumors. Cancer Cell 2005;8:299–309.

71. Brower V. How well do angiogenesis inhibitors work? Biomarkers of response prove elusive. J Natl Cancer Inst 2009;101:846–7.

72. Allt G, Lawrenson JG. Pericytes: cell biology and pathology. Cells Tissues Organs 2001;169:1–11.

73. Armulik A, Abramsson A, Betsholtz C. Endothelial/pericyte interactions. Circ Res 2005;97:512–23.

74. Gerhardt H, Betsholtz C. Endothelial-pericyte interactions in angiogenesis. Cell Tissue Res 2003; 314:15–23.

75. Bergers G, Song S. The role of pericytes in blood-vessel formation and maintenance. Neuro Oncol 2005;7:452–64.

76. Bergers G, Song S, Meyer-Morse N, et al. Benefits of targeting both pericytes and endothelial cells in the tumor vasculature with kinase inhibitors. J Clin Invest 2003;111:1287–95.

77. Mancuso MR, Davis R, Norberg SM, et al. Rapid vascular regrowth in tumors after reversal of VEGF inhibition. J Clin Invest 2006;116:2610–21.

78. Song S, Ewald AJ, Stallcup W, et al. PDGFRbeta+ perivascular progenitor cells in tumours regulate pericyte differentiation and vascular survival. Nat Cell Biol 2005;7:870–9.

79. Semenza GL. Regulation of hypoxia-induced angiogenesis: a chaperone escorts VEGF to the dance. J Clin Invest 2001;108:39–40.

80. Keith B, Simon MC. Hypoxia-inducible factors, stem cells, and cancer. Cell 2007;129:465–72.

81. Semenza GL. Hypoxia-inducible factors in physiology and medicine. Cell 2012;148:399–408.

82. Semenza GL. Dynamic regulation of stem cell specification and maintenance by hypoxia-inducible factors. Mol Aspects Med 2016;47-48:15–23.

83. Heddleston JM, Li Z, Lathia JD, et al. Hypoxia inducible factors in cancer stem cells. Br J Cancer 2010;102:789–95.

84. Fan Y, Potdar AA, Gong Y, et al. Profilin-1 phosphorylation directs angiocrine expression and glioblastoma progression through HIF-1alpha accumulation. Nat Cell Biol 2014;16:445–56.

85. Carmeliet P, Jain RK. Principles and mechanisms of vessel normalization for cancer and other angiogenic diseases. Nat Rev Drug Discov 2011;10:417–27.

86. Emblem KE, Mouridsen K, Bjornerud A, et al. Vessel architectural imaging identifies cancer patient responders to anti-angiogenic therapy. Nat Med 2013;19:1178–83.

87. Sorensen AG, Emblem KE, Polaskova P, et al. Increased survival of glioblastoma patients who respond to antiangiogenic therapy with elevated blood perfusion. Cancer Res 2012;72:402–7.

88. Verdegem D, Moens S, Stapor P, et al. Endothelial cell metabolism: parallels and divergences with cancer cell metabolism. Cancer Metab 2014;2:19.

89. Rivera LB, Bergers G. Angiogenesis. Targeting vascular sprouts. Science 2014;344:1449–50.

90. Ghesquiere B, Wong BW, Kuchnio A, et al. Metabolism of stromal and immune cells in health and disease. Nature 2014;511:167–76.

91. De Bock K, Georgiadou M, Schoors S, et al. Role of PFKFB3-driven glycolysis in vessel sprouting. Cell 2013;154:651–63.

92. Sawada N, Jiang A, Takizawa F, et al. Endothelial PGC-1alpha mediates vascular dysfunction in diabetes. Cell Metab 2014;19:246–58.

93. Schoors S, Bruning U, Missiaen R, et al. Fatty acid carbon is essential for dNTP synthesis in endothelial cells. Nature 2015;520:192–7.

94. Cancer Genome Atlas Research Network. Comprehensive genomic characterization defines human glioblastoma genes and core pathways. Nature 2008;455:1061–8.

95. Nakada M, Nakada S, Demuth T, et al. Molecular targets of glioma invasion. Cell Mol Life Sci 2007; 64:458–78.

96. Hatanpaa KJ, Burma S, Zhao D, et al. Epidermal growth factor receptor in glioma: signal transduction, neuropathology, imaging, and radioresistance. Neoplasia 2010;12:675–84.

97. Nazarenko I, Hede SM, He X, et al. PDGF and PDGF receptors in glioma. Ups J Med Sci 2012; 117:99–112.

98. Engelman JA. Targeting PI3K signalling in cancer: opportunities, challenges and limitations. Nat Rev Cancer 2009;9:550–62.

99. Inda MM, Bonavia R, Mukasa A, et al. Tumor heterogeneity is an active process maintained by a mutant EGFR-induced cytokine circuit in glioblastoma. Genes Dev 2010;24:1731–45.

100. van den Bent MJ, Brandes AA, Rampling R, et al. Randomized phase II trial of erlotinib versus temozolomide or carmustine in recurrent glioblastoma: EORTC brain tumor group study 26034. J Clin Oncol 2009;27:1268–74.

101. Rich JN, Reardon DA, Peery T, et al. Phase II trial of gefitinib in recurrent glioblastoma. J Clin Oncol 2004;22:133–42.

102. Raizer JJ, Abrey LE, Lassman AB, et al, North American Brain Tumor Consortium. A phase II trial of erlotinib in patients with recurrent malignant gliomas and nonprogressive glioblastoma multiforme postradiation therapy. Neuro Oncol 2010; 12:95–103.

103. Yung WK, Vredenburgh JJ, Cloughesy TF, et al. Safety and efficacy of erlotinib in first-relapse glioblastoma: a phase II open-label study. Neuro Oncol 2010;12:1061–70.

104. Neyns B, Sadones J, Joosens E, et al. Stratified phase II trial of cetuximab in patients with recurrent high-grade glioma. Ann Oncol 2009;20(9):1596–603.

105. Hong J, Peng Y, Liao Y, et al. Nimotuzumab prolongs survival in patients with malignant gliomas: a phase I/II clinical study of concomitant radiochemotherapy with or without nimotuzumab. Exp Ther Med 2012;4:151–7.

106. Dresemann G, Weller M, Rosenthal MA, et al. Imatinib in combination with hydroxyurea versus hydroxyurea alone as oral therapy in patients with progressive pretreated glioblastoma resistant to standard dose temozolomide. J Neurooncol 2010;96:393–402.

107. Franceschi E, Stupp R, van den Bent MJ, et al. EORTC 26083 phase I/II trial of dasatinib in combination with CCNU in patients with recurrent glioblastoma. Neuro Oncol 2012;14:1503–10.

108. Wen, PY, Yung W, Mellinghoff IK, et al. Phase II trial of the phosphatidyinositol-3 kinase (PI3K) inhibitor buparlisib (BKM120) in recurrent glioblastoma. In: ASCO Annual Meeting Proceedings. Chicago (IL), May 30 - June 3, 2014.

109. Pitz MW, Eisenhauer EA, MacNeil MV, et al. Phase II study of PX-866 in recurrent glioblastoma. Neuro-oncology 2015;17:1270–4.

110. Pachow D, Wick W, Gutmann DH, et al. The mTOR signaling pathway as a treatment target for intracranial neoplasms. Neuro Oncol 2015;17:189–99.

111. Hainsworth JD, Shih KC, Shepard GC, et al. Phase II study of concurrent radiation therapy, temozolomide, and bevacizumab followed by bevacizumab/everolimus as first-line treatment for patients with glioblastoma. Clin Adv Hematol Oncol 2012;10:240–6.

112. Sarkaria JN, Galanis E, Wu W, et al. Combination of temsirolimus (CCI-779) with chemoradiation in newly diagnosed glioblastoma multiforme (GBM)(NCCTG trial N027D) is associated with increased infectious risks. Clin Cancer Res 2010; 16:5573–80.

113. Reardon DA, Desjardins A, Vredenburgh JJ, et al. Phase 2 trial of erlotinib plus sirolimus in adults with recurrent glioblastoma. J Neurooncol 2010; 96:219–30.

114. Reardon DA, Wen PY, Alfred Yung WK, et al. Ridaforolimus for patients with progressive or recurrent malignant glioma: a perisurgical, sequential, ascending-dose trial. Cancer Chemother Pharmacol 2011;69:849–60.

115. Janes MR, Vu C, Mallya S, et al. Efficacy of the investigational mTOR kinase inhibitor MLN0128/INK128 in models of B-cell acute lymphoblastic leukemia. Leukemia 2013;27:586–94.

116. Thijssen R, van Bochove G, Derks IA, et al. Combined inhibition of mTOR and DNA-PK blocks survival, adhesion, proliferation and chemoresistance in primary chronic lymphocytic leukemia (CLL) cells. Blood 2014;124:1981.

117. Mortensen DS, Fultz KE, Xu S, et al. CC-223, a potent and selective inhibitor of mTOR kinase: in vitro and in vivo characterization. Mol Cancer Ther 2015;14:1295–305.

118. Nawroth R, Stellwagen F, Schulz WA, et al. S6K1 and 4E-BP1 are independent regulated and control cellular growth in bladder cancer. PLoS One 2011;6:e27509.

119. Downward J. Targeting RAS signalling pathways in cancer therapy. Nat Rev Cancer 2003;3:11–22.

120. Cloughesy TF, Wen PY, Robins HI, et al. Phase II trial of tipifarnib in patients with recurrent malignant glioma either receiving or not receiving enzyme-inducing antiepileptic drugs: a North American Brain Tumor Consortium study. J Clin Oncol 2006;24:3651–6.

121. Yust-Katz S, Liu D, Yuan Y, et al. Phase 1/1b study of lonafarnib and temozolomide in patients with recurrent or temozolomide refractory glioblastoma. Cancer 2013;119:2747–53.

122. Pickup M, Novitskiy S, Moses HL. The roles of TGFbeta in the tumour microenvironment. Nat Rev Cancer 2013;13:788–99.

123. Wakefield LM, Hill CS. Beyond TGFbeta: roles of other TGFbeta superfamily members in cancer. Nat Rev Cancer 2013;13:328–41.

124. Sun J, Liu SZ, Lin Y, et al. TGF-beta promotes glioma cell growth via activating Nodal expression through Smad and ERK1/2 pathways. Biochem Biophys Res Commun 2014;443:1066–72.

125. Bogdahn U, Hau P, Stockhammer G, et al. Targeted therapy for high-grade glioma with the TGF-beta2 inhibitor trabedersen: results of a randomized and controlled phase IIb study. Neuro Oncol 2011;13:132–42.

126. Gueorguieva I, Cleverly AL, Stauber A, et al. Defining a therapeutic window for the novel

TGF-beta inhibitor LY2157299 monohydrate based on a pharmacokinetic/pharmacodynamic model. Br J Clin Pharmacol 2014;77:796–807.

127. Rodon J, Carducci MA, Sepulveda-Sánchez JM, et al. First-in-human dose study of the novel transforming growth factor-β receptor I kinase inhibitor LY2157299 monohydrate in patients with advanced cancer and glioma. Clin Cancer Res 2015;21(3):553–60.

128. Yu H, Lee H, Herrmann A, et al. Revisiting STAT3 signalling in cancer: new and unexpected biological functions. Nat Rev Cancer 2014;14: 736–46.

129. Zheng Q, Han L, Dong Y, et al. JAK2/STAT3 targeted therapy suppresses tumor invasion via disruption of the EGFRvIII/JAK2/STAT3 axis and associated focal adhesion in EGFRvIII-expressing glioblastoma. Neuro Oncol 2014;16:1229–43.

130. Iwamaru A, Szymanski S, Iwado E, et al. A novel inhibitor of the STAT3 pathway induces apoptosis in malignant glioma cells both in vitro and in vivo. Oncogene 2007;26:2435–44.

131. Fuh B, Sobo M, Cen L, et al. LLL-3 inhibits STAT3 activity, suppresses glioblastoma cell growth and prolongs survival in a mouse glioblastoma model. Br J Cancer 2009;100:106–12.

132. Lin L, Hutzen B, Li P-K, et al. A novel small molecule, LLL12, inhibits STAT3 phosphorylation and activities and exhibits potent growth-suppressive activity in human cancer cells. Neoplasia 2010;12: 39–50.

133. Ranganathan P, Weaver KL, Capobianco AJ. Notch signalling in solid tumours: a little bit of everything but not all the time. Nat Rev Cancer 2011;11:338–51.

134. Andersson ER, Lendahl U. Therapeutic modulation of Notch signalling–are we there yet? Nat Rev Drug Discov 2014;13:357–78.

135. Dell'albani P, Rodolico M, Pellitteri R, et al. Differential patterns of NOTCH1-4 receptor expression are markers of glioma cell differentiation. Neuro Oncol 2014;16:204–16.

136. Fan X, Khaki L, Zhu TS, et al. NOTCH pathway blockade depletes CD133-positive glioblastoma cells and inhibits growth of tumor neurospheres and xenografts. Stem Cells 2010;28:5–16.

137. Amakye D, Jagani Z, Dorsch M. Unraveling the therapeutic potential of the Hedgehog pathway in cancer. Nat Med 2013;19:1410–22.

138. Takebe N, Miele L, Harris PJ, et al. Targeting Notch, Hedgehog, and Wnt pathways in cancer stem cells: clinical update. Nature Reviews. Clin Oncol 2015;12:445–64.

139. Robinson GW, Orr BA, Wu G, et al. Vismodegib exerts targeted efficacy against recurrent sonic hedgehog-subgroup medulloblastoma: results from phase II Pediatric Brain Tumor Consortium studies PBTC-025B and PBTC-032. J Clin Oncol 2015;33:2646–54.

140. Anastas JN, Moon RT. WNT signalling pathways as therapeutic targets in cancer. Nat Rev Cancer 2013;13:11–26.

141. Takahashi-Yanaga F, Kahn M. Targeting Wnt signaling: can we safely eradicate cancer stem cells? Clin Cancer Res 2010;16:3153–62.

142. van den Bent MJ, Dubbink HJ, Marie Y, et al. IDH1 and IDH2 mutations are prognostic but not predictive for outcome in anaplastic oligodendroglial tumors: a report of the European Organization for Research and Treatment of Cancer Brain Tumor Group. Clin Cancer Res 2010;16:1597–604.

143. Dahlrot RH, Kristensen BW, Hjelmborg J, et al. A population-based study of low-grade gliomas and mutated isocitrate dehydrogenase 1 (IDH1). J Neurooncol 2013;114:309–17.

144. Rohle D, Popovici-Muller J, Palaskas N, et al. An inhibitor of mutant IDH1 delays growth and promotes differentiation of glioma cells. Science 2013;340:626–30.

145. Clark O, Yen K, Mellinghoff IK. Molecular pathways: isocitrate dehydrogenase mutations in cancer. Clin Cancer Res 2016;22(8):1837–42.

146. Vlachostergios PJ, Voutsadakis IA, Papandreou CN. The ubiquitin-proteasome system in glioma cell cycle control. Cell Division 2012;7:1.

147. Chauhan D, Hideshima T, Mitsiades C, et al. Proteasome inhibitor therapy in multiple myeloma. Mol Cancer Ther 2005;4:686–92.

148. Phuphanich S, Supko JG, Carson KA, et al. Phase 1 clinical trial of bortezomib in adults with recurrent malignant glioma. J Neurooncol 2010;100:95–103.

149. Kubicek GJ, Werner-Wasik M, Machtay M, et al. Phase I trial using proteasome inhibitor bortezomib and concurrent temozolomide and radiotherapy for central nervous system malignancies. Int J Radiat Oncol Biol Phys 2009;74:433–9.

150. Shabason JE, Tofilon PJ, Camphausen K. Grand rounds at the National Institutes of Health: HDAC inhibitors as radiation modifiers, from bench to clinic. J Cell Mol Med 2011;15:2735–44.

151. Lee EQ, Puduvalli VK, Reid JM, et al. Phase I study of vorinostat in combination with temozolomide in patients with high-grade gliomas: North American Brain Tumor Consortium study 04-03. Clin Cancer Res 2012;18:6032–9.

152. Iwamoto FM, Lamborn KR, Kuhn JG, et al. A phase I/II trial of the histone deacetylase inhibitor romidepsin for adults with recurrent malignant glioma: North American Brain Tumor Consortium study 03-03. Neuro Oncol 2011;13:509–16.

153. Galanis E, Jaeckle KA, Maurer MJ, et al. Phase II trial of vorinostat in recurrent glioblastoma multiforme: a north central cancer treatment group study. J Clin Oncol 2009;27:2052–8.

154. Reya T, Morrison SJ, Clarke MF, et al. Stem cells, cancer, and cancer stem cells. Nature 2001;414:105–11.

155. Beck B, Blanpain C. Unravelling cancer stem cell potential. Nat Rev Cancer 2013;13:727–38.

156. Nguyen LV, Vanner R, Dirks P, et al. Cancer stem cells: an evolving concept. Nat Rev Cancer 2012;12:133–43.

157. Singh SK, Hawkins C, Clarke ID, et al. Identification of human brain tumour initiating cells. Nature 2004;432:396–401.

158. Bao S, Wu Q, McLendon RE, et al. Glioma stem cells promote radioresistance by preferential activation of the DNA damage response. Nature 2006;444:756–60.

159. Tamura K, Aoyagi M, Wakimoto H, et al. Accumulation of CD133-positive glioma cells after high-dose irradiation by Gamma Knife surgery plus external beam radiation. J Neurosurg 2010;113:310–8.

160. Dean M, Fojo T, Bates S. Tumour stem cells and drug resistance. Nat Rev Cancer 2005;5:275–84.

161. Szerlip NJ, Pedraza A, Chakravarty D, et al. Intratumoral heterogeneity of receptor tyrosine kinases EGFR and PDGFRA amplification in glioblastoma defines subpopulations with distinct growth factor response. Proc Natl Acad Sci U S A 2012;109:3041–6.

162. Patel AP, Tirosh I, Trombetta JJ, et al. Single-cell RNA-seq highlights intratumoral heterogeneity in primary glioblastoma. Science 2014;344:1396–401.

163. Verhaak RG, Hoadley KA, Purdom E, et al. Integrated genomic analysis identifies clinically relevant subtypes of glioblastoma characterized by abnormalities in PDGFRA, IDH1, EGFR, and NF1. Cancer Cell 2010;17:98–110.

164. Snuderl M, Fazlollahi L, Le LP, et al. Mosaic amplification of multiple receptor tyrosine kinase genes in glioblastoma. Cancer Cell 2011;20:810–7.

165. Dotto GP. Crosstalk of Notch with p53 and p63 in cancer growth control. Nat Rev Cancer 2009;9:587–95.

166. Chen J, McKay RM, Parada LF. Malignant glioma: lessons from genomics, mouse models, and stem cells. Cell 2012;149:36–47.

167. Furnari FB, Cloughesy TF, Cavenee WK, et al. Heterogeneity of epidermal growth factor receptor signalling networks in glioblastoma. Nat Rev Cancer 2015;15:302–10.

168. Oberoi RK, Parrish KE, Sio TT, et al. Strategies to improve delivery of anticancer drugs across the blood-brain barrier to treat glioblastoma. Neuro Oncol 2016;18:27–36.

169. Nakada M, Kita D, Watanabe T, et al. The mechanism of chemoresistance against tyrosine kinase inhibitors in malignant glioma. Brain Tumor Pathol 2014;31(3):198–207.

170. Singh D, Chan JM, Zoppoli P, et al. Transforming fusions of FGFR and TACC genes in human glioblastoma. Science 2012;337:1231–5.

171. Di Stefano AL, Fucci A, Frattini V, et al. Detection, characterization, and inhibition of FGFR-TACC fusions in IDH wild-type glioma. Clin Cancer Res 2015;21:3307–17.

172. Yan K, Wu Q, Yan DH, et al. Glioma cancer stem cells secrete Gremlin1 to promote their maintenance within the tumor hierarchy. Genes Dev 2014;28:1085–100.

173. Piccirillo SG, Reynolds BA, Zanetti N, et al. Bone morphogenetic proteins inhibit the tumorigenic potential of human brain tumour-initiating cells. Nature 2006;444:761–5.

174. Binda E, Visioli A, Giani F, et al. The EphA2 receptor drives self-renewal and tumorigenicity in stem-like tumor-propagating cells from human glioblastomas. Cancer Cell 2012;22:765–80.

175. Day BW, Stringer BW, Al-Ejeh F, et al. EphA3 maintains tumorigenicity and is a therapeutic target in glioblastoma multiforme. Cancer Cell 2013;23:238–48.

176. Eyler CE, Wu Q, Yan K, et al. Glioma stem cell proliferation and tumor growth are promoted by nitric oxide synthase-2. Cell 2011;146:53–66.

177. Schonberg DL, Miller TE, Wu Q, et al. Preferential iron trafficking characterizes glioblastoma stem-like cells. Cancer Cell 2015;28:441–55.

178. Gu C, Banasavadi-Siddegowda YK, Joshi K, et al. Tumor-specific activation of the C-JUN/MELK pathway regulates glioma stem cell growth in a p53-dependent manner. Stem Cells 2013;31:870–81.

179. Joshi K, Banasavadi-Siddegowda Y, Mo X, et al. MELK-dependent FOXM1 phosphorylation is essential for proliferation of glioma stem cells. Stem Cells 2013;31:1051–63.

180. Ikushima H, Todo T, Ino Y, et al. Autocrine TGF-beta signaling maintains tumorigenicity of glioma-initiating cells through Sry-related HMG-box factors. Cell Stem Cell 2009;5:504–14.

181. Penuelas S, Anido J, Prieto-Sanchez RM, et al. TGF-beta increases glioma-initiating cell self-renewal through the induction of LIF in human glioblastoma. Cancer Cell 2009;15:315–27.

182. Anido J, Saez-Borderias A, Gonzalez-Junca A, et al. TGF-beta receptor inhibitors target the CD44(high)/Id1(high) glioma-initiating cell population in Human glioblastoma. Cancer Cell 2010;18:655–68.

183. Rheinbay E, Suva ML, Gillespie SM, et al. An aberrant transcription factor network essential for Wnt signaling and stem cell maintenance in glioblastoma. Cell Rep 2013;3:1567–79.

184. Zheng H, Ying H, Yan H, et al. p53 and Pten control neural and glioma stem/progenitor cell renewal and differentiation. Nature 2008;455:1129–33.

185. Gallo M, Ho J, Coutinho FJ, et al. A tumorigenic MLL-homeobox network in human glioblastoma stem cells. Cancer Res 2013;73:417–27.

186. Laskey SB, Siliciano RF. A mechanistic theory to explain the efficacy of antiretroviral therapy. Nature Reviews. Microbiology 2014;12:772–80.

187. McCutchan JA, Wu JW, Robertson K, et al. HIV suppression by HAART preserves cognitive function in advanced, immune-reconstituted AIDS patients. AIDS 2007;21:1109–17.

188. Jo M-Y, Kim YG, Kim Y, et al. Combined therapy of temozolomide and ZD6474 (vandetanib) effectively reduces glioblastoma tumor volume through anti-angiogenic and anti-proliferative mechanisms. Mol Med Rep 2012;6:88–92.

189. Kreisl TN, McNeill KA, Sul J, et al. A phase I/II trial of vandetanib for patients with recurrent malignant glioma. Neuro Oncol 2012;14:1519–26.

190. Kreisl TN, Lassman AB, Mischel PS, et al. A pilot study of everolimus and gefitinib in the treatment of recurrent glioblastoma (GBM). J Neurooncol 2009;92:99–105.

191. Reardon DA, Vredenburgh JJ, Desjardins A, et al. Phase 1 trial of dasatinib plus erlotinib in adults with recurrent malignant glioma. J Neurooncol 2012;108:499–506.

192. Friday BB, Anderson SK, Buckner J, et al. Phase II trial of vorinostat in combination with bortezomib in recurrent glioblastoma: a North Central Cancer Treatment Group study. Neuro Oncol 2011;14(2):215–21.

193. Jain RK. Normalizing tumor vasculature with anti-angiogenic therapy: a new paradigm for combination therapy. Nat Med 2001;7:987–9.

194. Jain RK. Normalization of tumor vasculature: an emerging concept in antiangiogenic therapy. Science 2005;307:58–62.

195. Bregy A, Wong TM, Shah AH, et al. Active immunotherapy using dendritic cells in the treatment of glioblastoma multiforme. Cancer Treat Rev 2013;39:891–907.

196. Reardon DA, Freeman G, Wu C, et al. Immunotherapy advances for glioblastoma. Neuro Oncol 2014;16:1441–58.

197. Schumacher T, Bunse L, Pusch S, et al. A vaccine targeting mutant IDH1 induces antitumour immunity. Nature 2014;512:324–7.

198. Durante M, Loeffler JS. Charged particles in radiation oncology. Nature Reviews. Clin Oncol 2010;7:37–43.

199. Lundkvist J, Ekman M, Ericsson SR, et al. Proton therapy of cancer: potential clinical advantages and cost-effectiveness. Acta Oncol 2005;44:850–61.

200. Allen AM, Pawlicki T, Dong L, et al. An evidence based review of proton beam therapy: the report of ASTRO's emerging technology committee. Radiother Oncol 2012;103:8–11.

201. Mendenhall NP, Malyapa RS, Su Z, et al. Proton therapy for head and neck cancer: rationale, potential indications, practical considerations, and current clinical evidence. Acta Oncol 2011;50:763–71.

202. Zhang X, Lin SH, Fang B, et al. Therapy-resistant cancer stem cells have differing sensitivity to photon versus proton beam radiation. J Thorac Oncol 2013;8:1484–91.

203. Alan Mitteer R, Wang Y, Shah J, et al. Proton beam radiation induces DNA damage and cell apoptosis in glioma stem cells through reactive oxygen species. Sci Rep 2015;5:13961.

204. Liu HL, Hua MY, Chen PY, et al. Blood-brain barrier disruption with focused ultrasound enhances delivery of chemotherapeutic drugs for glioblastoma treatment. Radiology 2010;255:415–25.

205. Hynynen K, McDannold N, Vykhodtseva N, et al. Noninvasive MR imaging-guided focal opening of the blood-brain barrier in rabbits. Radiology 2001;220:640–6.

206. Etame AB, Diaz RJ, Smith CA, et al. Focused ultrasound disruption of the blood-brain barrier: a new frontier for therapeutic delivery in molecular neurooncology. Neurosurg Focus 2012;32:E3.

207. Hendricks BK, Cohen-Gadol AA, Miller JC. Novel delivery methods bypassing the blood-brain and blood-tumor barriers. Neurosurg Focus 2015;38:E10.

208. Zhang F, Xu CL, Liu CM. Drug delivery strategies to enhance the permeability of the blood-brain barrier for treatment of glioma. Drug Des Devel Ther 2015;9:2089–100.

ACKNOWLEDGMENTS

This work was supported by National Institutes of Health grants R00HL103792 and R01NS094533, University of Pennsylvania Neuro-oncology Innovation Award, and McCabe Award (to Y. Fan).

CHAPTER 6

Current Standards of Care in Glioblastoma Therapy

Andreas F. Hottinger, MD, PhD[a],*, Kalil G. Abdullah, MD[b], Roger Stupp, MD[c]

INTRODUCTION

With an incidence of 3 to 5 per 100,000, glioblastoma fulfills the criteria of a rare cancer. Despite this, glioblastoma is the most common and most aggressive primary brain tumor and accounts for 12% to 15% of all intracranial neoplasms and 45% to 50% of all gliomas. Patients of any age may be affected, but it is most commonly observed in individuals over the age of 50 years.[1] The suspicion of the presence of a glioblastoma is typically raised if a patient presents with neurologic symptoms and an imaging study shows the presence of a suspect lesion. On computed tomography (CT), the lesion typically appears as a contrast-enhancing lesion with peritumoral edema. However, smaller lesions may be missed. MRI is significantly more sensitive than CT and represents the modality of choice. Glioblastoma appears as a heterogeneous enhancing lesion with or without necrotic core. The margins are usually diffuse as a reflection of the infiltrative nature of the lesion. There is typically prominent peritumoral edema.

At present, despite aggressive treatment, the prognosis of glioblastoma remains dismal, with overall an estimated median life expectancy of only 14-16 months following diagnosis.[2] Two-year and 5-year survival rates remain around 30% and 10% respectively.[3,4] With these outcomes, it is essential to tailor the treatments for each individual patient to offer the best possible outcome with the optimal quality of life.

The initiation of therapy for glioblastoma therefore depends on many factors. These factors include, but are not limited to, the patient's preoperative level of function, performance status, age, and the resources available to the patient and the treating physicians. This chapter describes the standard of care for newly diagnosed glioblastoma and provides a brief overview of the evidence that supports these treatment paradigms.

SURGICAL INTERVENTION

With radiographic and clinical findings suggestive of glioblastoma, referral to a neurosurgeon and specialized neuro-oncology team for evaluation is warranted. In those patients deemed capable of tolerating a neurosurgical intervention, safe maximal resection is typically preferred rather than biopsy. The decision to proceed with resection accomplishes several goals. The first is to provide an accurate initial diagnosis with a specific tumor grading, which functions as an important step in the initiation of a chemoradiation regimen. The analysis of molecular markers also provides essential molecular information about the tumor, which will assist with possible prognostic and treatment implications. Moreover, in the presence of significant neurologic deficits linked to an important mass that compresses surrounding tissue, a neurosurgical resection may also offer the possibility to improve the symptoms of the patient.

A biopsy should be performed in patients for whom an extensive resection cannot be performed safely. The main goal of the biopsy is to confirm the diagnosis of glioblastoma. The amount of tissue collected should also be sufficient to be able to perform some of the essential molecular marker analyses, especially the determination of the status of methylation of O6-methylguanine-methyl transferase (MGMT) gene promoter. This information is essential because these patients often present with poor performance status and treatment with temozolomide or radiation therapy alone might be

---

[a] Department of Clinical Neurosciences, Lausanne University Hospital, Rue du Bugnon 46, Lausanne 1011, Switzerland; [b] Department of Neurosurgery, Hospital of the University of Pennsylvania, Philadelphia, PA, USA; [c] Department of Oncology, Zurich University Hospital, Rämistrasse 100, Zurich CH 8091, Switzerland
* Corresponding author.
E-mail address: andreas.hottinger@gmail.com

important options to minimize further clinical deterioration (discussed later). However, note that the diagnosis established on biopsy might not represent the most aggressive part of the tumor: In 2001, Jackson and colleagues[5] examined a consecutive series of 81 patients with imaging findings suggestive of glioma who underwent stereotactic biopsy followed by resection, and found that diagnosis based on biopsy or resection in the same patient differed in 30% of the cases reviewed. Woodworth and colleagues[6] reviewed the histology of 21 stereotactic biopsies and found that although stereotactic biopsy samples correctly represented glioma in 91% of cases, 14% of cases were unable to be sufficiently graded for more definitive classification.

Surgical resection has been suggested to be an independent favorable prognostic factor for increases in Karnofsky Performance Scale (KPS), overall survival, and progression-free survival (PFS).[7]

Beyond simply the decision to undergo surgical resection as opposed to biopsy, Sanai and colleagues[8] showed that the extent of tumor resection and its correlation with survival could be estimated, based on retrospective data. They examined 500 consecutive newly diagnosed patients with supratentorial glioblastomas who underwent resection followed by chemoradiation. A significant survival advantage was imparted in those patients who had 78% extent of resection or greater (Fig. 6.1). The strongest evidence to suggest that the extent of resection can determine the outcome of patients stems from the work of Stummer and colleagues,[9] who evaluated the potential role of 5 aminolevulinic acid (5-ALA), an orally administered amino acid that allows neurosurgeons to visualize the tumor intraoperatively when illuminated with fluorescent blue light and to maximize surgical resection. This prospective randomized phase III trial included only patients for whom the neurosurgeon thought that a (near) complete resection could be achieved. Those with no residual tumor after the surgery showed a statistically significant improvement in overall survival compared with patients with poorer resections (Fig. 6.2).[9]

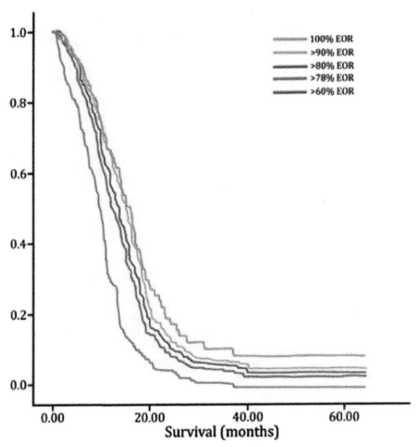

Fig. 6.1 Stepwise benefits in survival based on extent of resection (EOR). (*From* Sanai N, Polley MY, McDermott MW, et al. An extent of resection threshold for newly diagnosed glioblastomas. J Neurosurg 2011;115:3–8; with permission.)

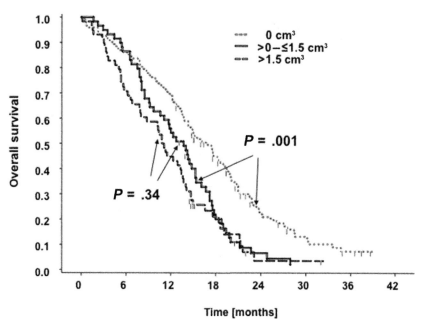

Fig. 6.2 Correlation between amount of residual tumor volume and median overall survival. (*From* Stummer W, Pichlmeier U, Meinel T, et al. Fluorescence-guided surgery with 5-aminolevulinic acid for resection of malignant glioma: a randomised controlled multicentre phase III trial. Lancet Oncol 2006;7:392–401; with permission.)

Carmustine wafers (Gliadel Wafer, Arbor Pharmaceuticals, LLC, Atlanta, GA) were first approved as adjunctive therapy by the US Food and Drug Administration (FDA) for recurrent glioblastoma in 1996, and then subsequently for de novo glioblastoma in 2003 based on trials conducted before the availability of temozolomide. Despite its approval by the FDA, carmustine wafers are not readily used as first-line treatment at many centers, partially because of cost and availability, but conflicting evidence from 2 recent meta-analyses has also questioned the modest survival benefit: both studies confirmed a statistically significant but modest survival advantage (16.2 months in the group in which carmustine wafers were added to adjuvant chemoradiotherapy vs 14 months in the standard treatment group) but also highlighted the complication profile (cited as high as 42.7%) for the use of carmustine wafers as routine treatment in de novo glioblastoma.[10,11] Moreover, because of the difficulty in interpretation of postoperative MRI in the presence of carmustine wafers, their use is a contraindication to inclusion in most clinical trials. Unfortunately, carmustine wafers were never formally tested and compared within or against temozolomide-containing regimens.

CHEMOTHERAPY AND RADIATION

Because glioblastomas are very infiltrative, neurosurgical resection cannot be considered as curative and additional treatments must be considered. These treatment decisions should ideally be defined by a multidisciplinary tumor board involving representatives from neurosurgery, radiation therapy, oncology, neuropathology, neuroradiology, and neurology. This approach should allow optimizing the management of every patient, based on the clinical situation, performance status, molecular markers, and other considerations. Management consists of a combination of radiation therapy to the site of tumor resection and residual tumor, usually with a safety margin of 2 cm, for a total of 58 to 60 Gy in fractions of 1.8 to 2.0 Gy.[12] During this course of radiation therapy, the oral alkylating agent temozolomide is given daily at a dosage of 75 mg/m^2/d to increase the radiosensitivity of the tumor.

After a break of 4 weeks, a new MRI is performed and temozolomide maintenance therapy is started for a maximum of 6 cycles (150 mg/m^2 on days 1–5 every 28 days in the first cycle, increased to 200 mg/m^2 in subsequent cycles in the absence of significant bone marrow and liver toxicity; **Fig. 6.3**).

Historically, the addition of temozolomide to a radiation regimen became standard of care in 2005 following a multicentric trial of 573 patients who were randomized to receiving either radiotherapy alone or radiotherapy with daily temozolomide followed by 6 cycles of adjuvant

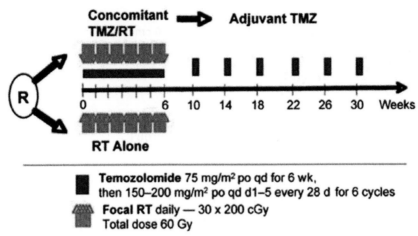

Fig. 6.3 Standard regimen of radiation and chemotherapy following surgical resection of glioblastoma. Trial design of EORTC 22981 study. R, randomization; RT, radiotherapy; TMZ, temozolomide. (*From* Hottinger AF, Stupp R, Homicsko K. Standards of care and novel approaches in the management of glioblastoma multiforme. Chin J Cancer 2014;33:32–9; with permission.)

temozolomide.[2] At a median follow-up of 20 months, the median overall survival was 14.6 months in the radiotherapy plus temozolomide group versus 12.1 months in the radiotherapy-alone group (hazard ratio [HR], 0.63; 95% confidence interval [CI], 0.52–0.75; P<.001) translating in a 2-year survival of 27% (**Fig. 6.4**).

27.2% in patients treated with radiotherapy and temozolomide versus 10.9% with radiotherapy alone were alive at 2 years. The respective 5-year survival rates were 10% and 2%.[4] As shown in a retrospective molecular analysis of a representative subgroup of patients of the trial, for which sufficient tissue was available, the benefit of temozolomide is mainly observed in patients

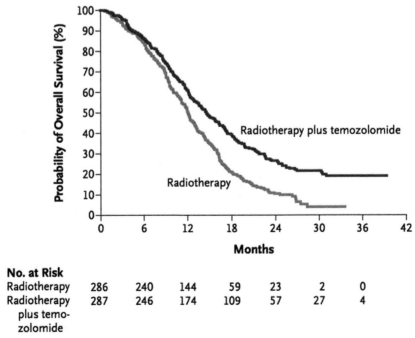

Fig. 6.4 Estimates of overall survival according to treatment group. (*From* Stupp R, Mason WP, van den Bent MJ, et al. Radiotherapy plus concomitant and adjuvant temozolomide for glioblastoma. N Engl J Med 2005;352:987–96; with permission.)

who have a methylated promoter of the gene *MGMT*. This enzyme is a ubiquitous DNA repair protein that can reverse the damages to the DNA induced by alkylating agents, including temozolomide. Methylation of the gene promoter silences the expression of the protein and thus renders the tumor more susceptible to alkylating agent therapy. This methylation of the promoter is observed in approximately 40% of all patients.

Considerations for Specific Patient Subgroups

Often the question remains open as to whether findings of a clinical trial can be extended to patients who would not have met the inclusion criteria of the trial; for instance, because they present a poorer performance status or are older and therefore also more likely to develop more frequent and severe side effects from the treatments. For glioblastoma, clinical trials have generally included patients between the ages of 18 and 70 years with an adequate performance status (Eastern Cooperative Oncology Group 0 and 1; KPS ≥70). In an effort to determine a standardized regimen for patients older than 70 years of age, 85 elderly patients with performance scores of greater than 70 with either anaplastic astrocytoma or glioblastoma, were randomly assigned to either supportive care alone or supportive care with radiotherapy (focal radiation in daily fractions of 1.8 Gy given 5 days per week, for a total dose of 50 Gy).[13] The median survival for the patients receiving radiotherapy in addition to supportive care was 29.1 weeks, versus 16.9 weeks for those who received supportive care alone. Quality of life and cognitive evaluations did not differ significantly between groups.

More recently, 2 trials compared the use of temozolomide and radiotherapy in elderly patients with glioblastoma. In a randomized study by Malmström and colleagues,[14] standard radiotherapy was associated with poor outcomes in a subset of patients older than 70 years (median survival, 5.2 months), and temozolomide (9 months) and hypofractionated radiotherapy (7 months) were superior. Similarly, Wick and colleagues[15] found that temozolomide alone was not inferior to radiotherapy alone in patients older than 65 years with a KPS greater than or equal to 60. In both studies, methylation of the MGMT promoter was identified as a significant prognostic factor for longer overall survival. A randomized trial investigating the possibility of combination therapy with radiotherapy and temozolomide is currently ongoing. Recent results from a randomized phase 3 trial, presented at ASCO 2016, show that elderly patients derive the same benefit from the combination of RT and TMZ than younger patients.[16] For these reasons, patients more than 65 or 70 years of age must be assessed even more carefully than younger patients to appraise their current performance score, goals of care and expectations, and evaluation of markers such as MGMT to establish the best treatment option, especially if they present with poor performance status.

NEWER TREATMENT STRATEGIES

The current standard regimen was determined in 2005 by Stupp and colleagues[2] and has remained valid despite numerous attempts to improve this approach, including targeted therapies, antiangiogenic agents, and vaccines. However, all these attempts have failed to show any improvement in overall survival when tested in phase III randomized trials.[17–19] The results obtained with the antiangiogenic agent bevacizumab exemplify the problems faced by neuro-oncologists and are detailed here as an example.

Bevacizumab is the most thoroughly evaluated of the antiangiogenic agents available for potential use in glioblastoma. At present, its use is not recommended as a standard component of treatment in newly diagnosed glioblastoma. Initial evaluations of bevacizumab took place in recurrent glioblastoma, for which several phase II trials, usually evaluating the combination of bevacizumab with a classic cytotoxic agent versus bevacizumab alone, typically showed similar or slightly improved PFS in the combination arm but no statistical difference when considering overall survival.[20,21] Two placebo-controlled phase III studies (RTOG 0825[3] and AVAglio[19] trials), produced similar results regarding the effectiveness of bevacizumab in de novo glioblastoma. In the RTOG 0825 study, 637 newly diagnosed patients were randomized to either standard TMZ/RT→TMZ and bevacizumab (10 mg/kg) every other week or the standard chemoradiation and placebo. Although PFS was longer in the bevacizumab group (10.7 months vs 7.3 months), there was no significant difference in overall survival between groups. In addition, there were increased rates of complications in the bevacizumab group along with decreased quality of life and neurocognitive function. The very similarly designed AVAglio study (in AvaGlio bevacizumab/placebo was initiated on day one of radiation, while in RTOG0825 bevacizumab/placebo was to begin only in the fourth week of irradiation) also found PFS benefit (10.6 months with bevacizumab and 6.2 months without) but a similar overall survival of 2 years in the

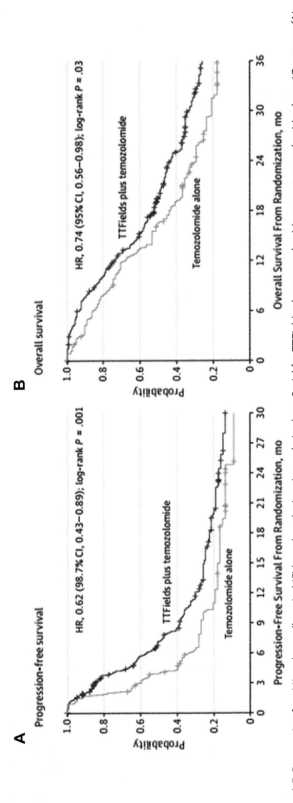

Fig. 6.5 Progression-free (A) and overall survival (B) based on the interim analysis phase 3 trial for TTFields plus temozolomide versus temozolomide alone. (Courtesy of Novocure, Portsmouth, NH, with permission; and *From* Stupp R, Taillibert S, Kanner AA, et al. Maintenance therapy with tumor-treating fields plus temozolomide versus temozolomide alone for glioblastoma: A Randomized Clinical Trial. JAMA 2015;314:2535–43, with permission.)

treatment and control groups (33.9% vs 30.1%). In both trials steroid requirement was decreased in bevacizumab-treated patients, while some adverse events were increased in frequency and severity.

Some promising approaches are starting to be integrated into the standard management of patients with glioblastoma. Tumor-treating fields (TTFields) consist of alternating low-intensity electrical fields applied via transducing arrays placed directly on the patient's shaved scalp. The physical forces exerted by the induced dipole will disrupt the tubulins and spindle apparatus, thus targeting replicating cells during mitosis, leading to oncogenic cell death.

Recent evidence from a phase 3 trial showed that TTFields have a role in the treatment of newly diagnosed glioblastoma.[22] Patients from 83 centers were randomized to either receive TTFields plus temozolomide (n = 466) or temozolomide alone (n = 229). An planned interim analysis at a median follow-up of 38 months included 210 patients randomized to TTFields plus temozolomide and 105 randomized to temozolomide alone, and found that the median PFS (primary end point of the study) was improved from 4.0 to 7.1 months in the TTField group (HR, 0.62; 98.7% CI, 0.43–0.89; $P = .001$) (**Fig. 6.5**). The median overall survival was increased to 20.5 months for patients with TTFields and temozolomide versus 15.6 months for those with temozolomide alone (HR, 0.64; 99.4% CI, 0.42–0.98; $P = .004$). Median overall survival at 2 years was 48% in the group treated with TTFields versus 32% in patients treated with standard treatment alone.

Ongoing investigations are evaluating an antibody-drug conjugate against EGFR (ABT-414) in both recurrent and newly diagnosed GBM (NCT02343406, NCT02573324). A phase III trial with the EGFRviii targeting vaccine rindopepiumut was recently reported negative.[23]

REFERENCES

1. DeAngelis LM. Brain tumors. N Engl J Med 2001; 344:114–23.
2. Stupp R, Mason WP, van den Bent MJ, et al. Radiotherapy plus concomitant and adjuvant temozolomide for glioblastoma. N Engl J Med 2005;352: 987–96.
3. Gilbert MR, Dignam JJ, Armstrong TS, et al. A randomized trial of bevacizumab for newly diagnosed glioblastoma. N Engl J Med 2014;370: 699–708.
4. Stupp R, Hegi ME, Mason WP, et al. Effects of radiotherapy with concomitant and adjuvant temozolomide versus radiotherapy alone on survival in glioblastoma in a randomised phase III study: 5-year analysis of the EORTC-NCIC trial. Lancet Oncol 2009;10:459–66.
5. Jackson RJ, Fuller GN, Abi-Said D, et al. Limitations of stereotactic biopsy in the initial management of gliomas. Neuro Oncol 2001;3:193–200.
6. Woodworth G, McGirt MJ, Samdani A, et al. Accuracy of frameless and frame-based image-guided stereotactic brain biopsy in the diagnosis of glioma: comparison of biopsy and open resection specimen. Neurol Res 2005;27: 358–62.
7. Laws ER, Parney IF, Huang W, et al. Survival following surgery and prognostic factors for recently diagnosed malignant glioma: data from the Glioma Outcomes Project. J Neurosurg 2003; 99:467–73.
8. Sanai N, Polley MY, McDermott MW, et al. An extent of resection threshold for newly diagnosed glioblastomas. J Neurosurg 2011; 115:3–8.
9. Stummer W, Pichlmeier U, Meinel T, et al. Fluorescence-guided surgery with 5-aminolevulinic acid for resection of malignant glioma: a randomised controlled multicentre phase III trial. Lancet Oncol 2006;7:392–401.
10. Chowdhary SA, Ryken T, Newton HB. Survival outcomes and safety of carmustine wafers in the treatment of high-grade gliomas: a meta-analysis. J Neurooncol 2015;122:367–82.
11. Bregy A, Shah AH, Diaz MV, et al. The role of Gliadel wafers in the treatment of high-grade gliomas. Expert Rev Anticancer Ther 2013;13: 1453–61.
12. Hottinger AF, Stupp R, Homicsko K. Standards of care and novel approaches in the management of glioblastoma multiforme. Chin J Cancer 2014; 33:32–9.
13. Keime-Guibert F, Chinot O, Taillandier L, et al. Radiotherapy for glioblastoma in the elderly. N Engl J Med 2007;356:1527–35.
14. Malmström A, Gronberg BH, Marosi C, et al. Temozolomide versus standard 6-week radiotherapy versus hypofractionated radiotherapy in patients older than 60 years with glioblastoma: the Nordic randomised, phase 3 trial. Lancet Oncol 2012;13: 916–26.
15. Wick W, Platten M, Meisner C, et al. Temozolomide chemotherapy alone versus radiotherapy alone for malignant astrocytoma in the elderly: the NOA-08 randomised, phase 3 trial. Lancet Oncol 2012;13: 707–15.
16. Perry JR, Laperriere N, O'Callaghan CJ, et al. A phase III randomized controlled trial of short-course radiotherapy with or without concomitant and adjuvant temozolomide in elderly patients with glioblastoma (CCTG CE.6, EORTC 26062-22061, TROG

08.02, NCT00482677). J Clin Oncol 34, 2016 (suppl; abstr LBA2).

17. Stupp R, Hegi ME, Gorlia T, et al. Cilengitide combined with standard treatment for patients with newly diagnosed glioblastoma with methylated MGMT promoter (CENTRIC EORTC 26071-22072 study): a multicentre, randomised, open-label, phase 3 trial. Lancet Oncol 2014; 15:1100–8.

18. Batchelor TT, Mulholland P, Neyns B, et al. Phase III randomized trial comparing the efficacy of cediranib as monotherapy, and in combination with lomustine, versus lomustine alone in patients with recurrent glioblastoma. J Clin Oncol 2013;31:3212–8.

19. Chinot OL, Wick W, Mason W, et al. Bevacizumab plus radiotherapy-temozolomide for newly diagnosed glioblastoma. N Engl J Med 2014;370: 709–22.

20. Vredenburgh JJ, Desjardins A, Herndon JE 2nd, et al. Phase II trial of bevacizumab and irinotecan in recurrent malignant glioma. Clin Cancer Res 2007;13:1253–9.

21. Kreisl TN, Kim L, Moore K, et al. Phase II trial of single-agent bevacizumab followed by bevacizumab plus irinotecan at tumor progression in recurrent glioblastoma. J Clin Oncol 2009;27:740–5.

22. Stupp R, Taillibert S, Kanner AA, et al. Maintenance therapy with tumor-treating fields plus temozolomide vs temozolomide alone for glioblastoma: A randomized clinical trial. JAMA 2015;314:2535–43.

23. Weller M, Butowski NA, Tran DD, et al. ACT IV: An international, double-blind, phase 3 trial of rindopepimut in newly diagnosed, EGFRvIII-expressing glioblastoma. Proc Soc Neuro-Oncol 2016, in press.

CHAPTER 7

Radiographic Detection and Advanced Imaging of Glioblastoma

James Eric Schmitt, MD, PhD, Joel M. Stein, MD, PhD*

INTRODUCTION

Neuroimaging plays a critical role at each stage of glioblastoma (GBM) diagnosis and therapy. Imaging provides the first definitive evidence of GBM in most cases, facilitates maximal safe surgical resection of enhancing neoplasm, guides radiation therapy, characterizes residual or recurrent disease, determines progression or response to therapy, and identifies complications of tumor or treatment throughout the disease course. Thus, key features, techniques, and considerations in GBM imaging constitute essential knowledge for all members of the neuro-oncology team. The current chapter presents an overview of the practice and principles of neuroradiology in supporting the comprehensive management of patients with GBM by considering conventional imaging features, advanced imaging approaches, multifocal disease, GBM mimics, recurrent disease and treatment effects, and future directions in imaging.

CONVENTIONAL IMAGING FEATURES OF GLIOBLASTOMA

Although GBM can present with protean morphologies and locations, nearly all lesions have a constellation of typical imaging characteristics that mirror the pathophysiology of this tumor. Important imaging findings include aggressive infiltration, gyral expansion, hypercellularity, blood-brain barrier (BBB) disruption, and central necrosis.[1-3] The authors find it helpful to divide these key pathologic and radiologic features into 3 categories: infiltration, cellularity, and vascularity (Table 7.1). GBM has variably extensive infiltrative and cellular nonenhancing components, a property unique to glial tumors and shared by World Health Organization (WHO) grade II and III neoplasms. In addition, variable size and number of enhancing and hypervascular components are present, indicating inflammation with BBB breakdown and abnormal tumor vasculature. Irregular nonenhancing areas within cellular enhancing components indicate necrosis, which is a defining feature of GBM and differentiates this WHO grade IV neoplasm from grade III tumors. Although they may infiltrate widely, including across the corpus callosum, GBMs are usually centered in the white matter of the cerebral hemispheres, sometimes in the thalamus, rarely in the brainstem, and essentially never in the cerebellum in adults.

Important differential considerations include other primary glial neoplasms, metastases, lymphoma, subacute infarct, abscess, and tumefactive demyelination. However, knowledge of key radiologic features informed by clinical information makes initial diagnosis of GBM straightforward in most cases (Tables 7.2 and 7.3). The same principles apply when assessing for residual or recurrent disease, except that treatment-related changes complicate interpretation, and often treatment-related changes and tumor are intermixed. Although most GBM imaging focuses on MRI, computed tomography (CT) also deserves consideration as the initial imaging obtained in many patients. In our experience, diagnostic errors in these different modalities run in opposite directions; clinicians more readily attribute CT findings to other disorders and enhancing MRI lesions to GBM. Thus, this chapter emphasizes key differentiating features for both CT and MRI.

Division of Neuroradiology, Department of Radiology, Hospital of the University of Pennsylvania, 3400 Spruce Street, Philadelphia, PA 19104, USA
* Corresponding author.
E-mail address: joel.stein@uphs.upenn.edu

TABLE 7.1
Key properties of GBM with pathology-radiology correlates and relevant imaging sequences

Properties	Pathology	Radiology	Imaging
Infiltration	Ill-defined margins Widespread tumor cells	Nonenhancing signal abnormality Multifocal/multicentric pattern Cortical involvement Spread across corpus callosum	T2/FLAIR
Cellularity	Mitoses and cell density[a]	Increased tissue density	CT and T2
		Mild diffusion restriction	DWI
		Increased choline level	MRS
Vascularity	Microvascular proliferation Inflammation Necrosis[b]	Increased perfusion (rCBV, Vp)	DSC, DCE
		BBB breakdown	T1+C
		Necrosis	T1+C

Abbreviations: CT, computed tomography; DCE, dynamic contrast enhanced; DSC, dynamic susceptibility contrast; DWI, diffusion-weighted imaging; FLAIR, fluid attenuation inversion recovery; MRS, magnetic resonance spectroscopy; rCBV, relative cerebral blood volume; T1+C, contrast enhanced T1-weighted; Vp, plasma volume.

[a] Other related cellular features of anaplasia, atypia, and pleomorphism do not have specific radiology correlates.

[b] Necrosis is a symptom of cell proliferation with inadequate or abnormal vascular supply and so is also related to cellularity. Various factors in the tumor microenvironment may contribute, including ischemia, inflammation, and excitotoxicity.

Computed Tomography

CT is the most common neuroimaging modality in the acute setting and usually the first study performed on patients with symptoms of acute intracranial disorder. Depending on tumor location and presence or acuity of hemorrhage or mass effect, the clinical presentation of GBM can range from signs of increased intracranial pressure or herniation to focal neurologic deficits, seizures, functional decline, personality changes, or headaches. Note that the clinical history may be incomplete and should not dissuade the clinician from considering a primary brain tumor, particularly in the primary and secondary care settings, in which

TABLE 7.2
Typical imaging patterns of GBM and other intra-axial lesions

	Number of Lesions	Brain Region	Epicenter	Cortical Expansion	Crosses Midline
GBM	Often 1	Almost always supratentorial	WM	Common	Yes
Metastases	Sometimes 1	Supratentorial or infratentorial	GM-WM junction	No	No
Lymphoma (primary)	Variable	Classically periventricular	WM	Rare	Yes
Other glial neoplasms	Usually 1 unless gliomatosis or syndrome (NF1, VHL)	Supratentorial or infratentorial	WM	Common	Yes
Demyelination	Usually 1 when tumefactive	Usually supratentorial	WM	No	Yes
Abscess	Usually 1 unless hematogenous spread	Near routes of infection (frontal sinuses/temporal bones) unless hematogenous	WM	No	No
Infarct	Variable	Follows vascular territories	GM and/or WM	Common	No

Abbreviations: GM, gray matter; NF1, Neurofibromatosis type 1; VHL, von Hippel-Lindau disease.

TABLE 7.3
Conventional and advanced imaging features of GBM and other intra-axial lesions

	Enhancing Component (T1+C)	Nonenhancing Component (T2/FLAIR)	Hemorrhage (GRE/SWI)	Diffusion (DWI/ADC)	Perfusion (DSC, DCE, ASL)	Metabolism (MRS)
GBM	Solid, cystic, necrotic	Variable tumor and edema	Common	Variable	Increased	Neoplastic spectrum[a]
Metastases	Solid, cystic, necrotic	Marked edema	Often[b]	Variable	Increased	Neoplastic spectrum
Lymphoma	Solid[c]	Variable edema	Occasional	Uniform restricted	Mildly increased DSC overshoots	Neoplastic spectrum
Radiation necrosis	Solid, cystic, feathery, soap bubble	Variable edema	Absent	Variable	Decreased to mildly increased	Lipid/lactate
Demyelination	Partial ring, spares cortex	Chronic lesions	Absent	Peripheral restricted	Normal to decreased	Lipid/lactate
Pyogenic abscess	Ring	Marked edema	Typically absent	Central restricted	Increased peripheral	Lipid/lactate, amino acids
Subacute infarct	Gyriform	Cytotoxic edema	Variable	Variable	Decreased	Decreased metabolites

Abbreviations: ADC, apparent diffusion coefficient; ASL, arterial spin labeled; GRE, gradient echo; SWI, susceptibility-weighted.
[a] Characterized by increased choline/n-acetylaspartate and choline/creatine ratios. For GBM this is seen in enhancing components and adds specificity when present in nonenhancing components.
[b] Melanoma, renal cell carcinoma, choriocarcinoma, and thyroid cancer are known for hemorrhagic metastases. Lung and breast cancer produce more hemorrhagic metastases overall, because of increased prevalence.
[c] Peripheral enhancement may be seen with immune compromise, as in acquired immunodeficiency syndrome.

stroke, metastases, or hypertensive hemorrhage are typically higher on the differential diagnosis and may bias the provided history. In tertiary and quaternary care settings, patients may present with a known diagnosis of brain tumor on outside institution CT and MRI studies. In these cases, the CT should not be ignored because it provides complementary information that may help refine the differential diagnosis.

Although CT lacks the exquisite soft tissue resolution of MRI, significant diagnostic information can be obtained in most cases. A complete discussion of head CT physics and interpretation is beyond the scope of this chapter. Briefly, the CT scanner consists of 1 or more x-ray sources positioned across a ring from an array of detectors. As in conventional radiographs, high-energy photons are variably blocked (attenuated) as they travel through tissue. Passing the patient through the spinning ring enables attenuation to be calculated (reconstructed) at each point within the volume and a set of cross-sectional, quantitative, gray-scale images to be produced with brightness proportional to density. Reconstructions can emphasize different tissue types, such as soft tissue or bone, and the range and center (window level) of the gray-scale display values can be adjusted to bring out different features. Iodinated contrast increases density wherever it accumulates. Images can be reformatted in multiple planes and rendered to visualize bones, vessels, or other structures in 3 dimensions. CT excels relative to MRI in its spatial resolution, assessment of osseous structures, speed, and availability.

Consistent with its pathology, GBM typically appears as a peripherally isodense to slightly hyperdense, centrally hypodense intra-axial mass compared with normal gray matter[4] (**Fig. 7.1**). These imaging findings correlate with the pathologic findings of areas of dense cellularity and central regions of necrosis. Findings may be subtle and are usually better seen following careful windowing of CT images to maximize gray-white differentiation. Although regions of central necrosis generally appear hypoattenuating, superimposed hemorrhage can result in varied levels of attenuation.

Hypercellular and centrally necrotic areas are surrounded by a variable degree of hypoattenuation reflecting a combination of infiltrative tumor and superimposed edema. Expansion of adjacent

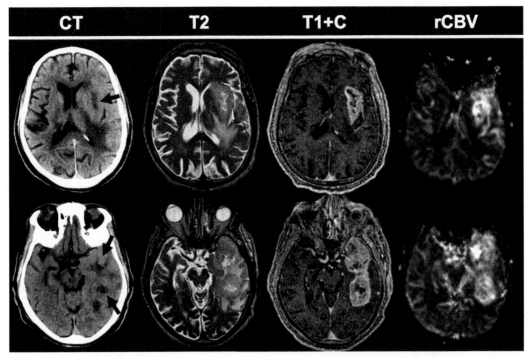

Fig. 7.1 Conventional imaging in an instructive case of GBM. The patient presented with cognitive decline and expressive aphasia. Unenhanced CT at the level of the insula (*top row*) and temporal lobe (*bottom*) shows areas of increased density in the white matter also extending into and expanding the cortex (*arrows*) reflecting infiltrative tumor. Central low density reflects necrosis with surrounding decreased density reflecting edema superimposed on neoplasm. T2-weighted and enhanced T1-weighted (T1+C) images show corresponding infiltrative tumor and edema with contiguous areas of solid peripheral enhancement and central necrosis. Relative cerebral blood volume (rCBV) is increased in the enhancing areas.

cortex may be present, indicating infiltrative tumor and increasing the likelihood of a primary neoplasm (see **Fig. 7.1**; **Fig. 7.2**). The presence or absence of calcium should be noted on CT, because parenchymal calcification in GBM is uncommon but is commonly seen with more slowly growing glial neoplasms, particularly oligodendroglioma and ganglioglioma.[5,6] Associated mass effect can manifest as asymmetric parenchymal expansion; variable effacement of ventricles, sulci, and cisterns; midline shift or herniation; and obstructive hydrocephalus or ventricular trapping. Intratumoral hemorrhage may also be present and is common in patients presenting with acute symptoms. Most important is to recognize when 1 or more signs of mass effect, edema, cellularity, or infiltration indicate that a scan is not showing a typical case of chronic small vessel ischemic disease and merits further evaluation with enhanced MRI.

Conventional MRI

Contrast-enhanced MRI remains the gold standard for imaging of brain tumors and is critical in assessing the full extent of neoplastic involvement, minimizing the risk of incorrect diagnosis,[2] and identifying potential complications of tumor or therapy. Technical principles of MRI are also beyond the scope of this chapter, although the general terminology of different pulse sequences is likely familiar to clinicians. Magnetic resonance (MR) images are created by measuring the current generated when spinning protons (typically hydrogen nuclei in water molecules) are induced by resonant radiofrequency pulses to flip out of and then return to alignment with a strong magnetic field. T1 and T2 are time constants describing different components of this relaxation and are influenced by the type of tissue in which the water molecules are located. Varying the strength of the magnetic field across the imaged area and the timing of pulses enables localization of signals in 3 dimensions and variable signal intensity according to tissue type. In T1-weighted images, white matter is bright and gray matter dark and the opposite is true for T2-weighted images. Cerebrospinal fluid (CSF), essentially water, is bright on T2-weighted images and dark on

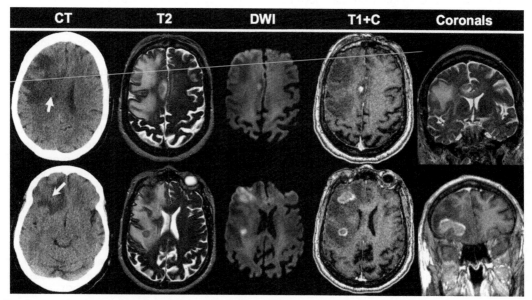

Fig. 7.2 Another instructive case of GBM. The patient presented with left facial droop and concern for metastases given a prior cancer history. Unenhanced CT more superiorly (*top row*) and inferiorly (*bottom*) shows a large region of right frontal lobe white matter hypodensity associated with sulcal effacement and midline shift. In addition, there is region of central hyperdensity (*long arrow*) and a subtle ring-shaped density (*short arrow*). Multiplicity and marked edema are good features for metastasis, but localization of numerous metastases exclusively to a single lobe is unusual. MRI is required for further characterization. T2-weighted MRI confirms the white matter signal abnormality and multiple isointense masses. Cortical involvement of the anterior frontal lesion and infiltration into the corpus callosum (far right top row of the coronal T2-weighted image) suggest glioma. Restricted diffusion on diffusion-weighted imaging (DWI) indicates cellularity of the multiple masses with corresponding enhancement, more intense peripherally. The dominant anterior enhancing mass follows rather than displaces the sulci (*arrows*, far right bottom row coronal enhanced T1-weighted image), suggestive of infiltration and preferential growth along white matter tracts. Considered in isolation, many features are compatible with metastases or lymphoma, but in combination these conventional imaging findings indicate high-grade glial neoplasm.

T1-weighted images. Typical gadolinium-based MRI contrast agents cause increased signal on T1-weighted images.

Routine brain imaging protocols include T2-weighted, fluid-attenuated inversion recovery (FLAIR; which is like T2 but suppresses signal from simple fluid), diffusion-weighted imaging (DWI), and multiplanar T1-weighted pregadolinium and postgadolinium contrast-enhanced sequences. Susceptibility-weighted or gradient echo sequences may be used to increase sensitivity for blood products and mineralization. Each sequence provides complementary information about the fundamental tissue properties of brain lesions and surrounding brain parenchyma (see **Figs. 7.1** and **7.2**). For glial tumors, both the enhancing potentially necrotic tumor components and surrounding nonenhancing components must be assessed. So-called advanced imaging techniques, which require additional postacquisition processing, can further characterize tumor tissue. These techniques include perfusion and permeability imaging as well as MR spectroscopy (MRS) and are discussed later. DWI could be considered advanced imaging but has become part of routine scans. High-resolution three-dimensional T1-weighted images are often added when the need for operative guidance is anticipated. Similarly, diffusion tensor imaging or functional MRI may be performed to aid surgery depending on tumor location. These topics are discussed in more detail in Chapter 14. Intraoperative MRI is only available at select centers and also discussed separately in Chapter 14.

Nonenhancing Components

Most primary glial tumors have a typical appearance on T2 and FLAIR imaging, with areas of hyperintense infiltrative signal abnormality following white matter tracts and variably associated with focal cortical or gyral expansion. White matter abnormalities are occasionally subtle but are usually readily identifiable when comparing affected regions with more typical-appearing white matter farther from the epicenter of the dominant lesion. FLAIR images generally increase the conspicuity of abnormal signal but the precise extent, especially of cortical involvement, may be better depicted on T2. Therefore, both sequences should be carefully scrutinized to identify the visible margins of the tumor, keeping in mind that tumor cells infiltrate much more widely. In our experience, cortical involvement, when present, is highly specific for glial neoplasm. This finding is in contrast with the increased signal caused by reactive vasogenic edema, which may compress the cortex because of mass effect but remains confined to the white

matter. In glial tumors there is usually a combination of infiltrative signal and vasogenic edema causing signal abnormality. Surrounding edema is generally less extensive relative to neoplastic burden than that seen with secondary neoplasms, but can be striking in some cases (as in **Fig. 7.2**).

DWI assesses the flow of water molecules within tissues, producing images that are brighter where diffusion is limited by the microenvironment. Because T2 weighting is inherent in this technique, vasogenic edema and overall increased water content also cause increased signal (T2 shine-through). To account for this, quantitative apparent diffusion coefficient (ADC) maps are calculated from DWI images, showing restricted diffusion as areas of decreased signal intensity. DWI images and ADC maps are interpreted in tandem, looking for areas of increased signal on DWI and corresponding low signal on ADC. For simplicity, some figures in this chapter may show DWI alone but restricted diffusion was confirmed on ADC maps.

Clinicians are most familiar with DWI from its striking sensitivity for acute cerebral infarcts, caused by increased intracellular water in areas where ischemia disrupts cell homeostasis. However, DWI has been used extensively to characterize GBM and other tumors, because the ratio of intracellular to extracellular water is also proportional to cell density and tumor grade. Areas of diffusion restriction usually correspond with enhancing regions, although the presence of restricted diffusion in regions of nonenhancing signal abnormality can help differentiate areas of glial neoplasm from vasogenic edema.[7] Diffusion restriction is also a well-known property of infected (and thus proteinaceous and viscous) fluid collections, including pyogenic cerebral abscess and empyema. The necrotic components of GBM can show restricted diffusion and are sometimes difficult to distinguish from abscess, but associated peripheral enhancement is usually thicker with GBM. In general, the degree of restricted diffusion is less in tumor tissue (less intense on DWI and less dark on ADC) compared with that seen in infarct or abscess.

DWI is affected by magnetic susceptibility, so apparent alterations in peritumoral signal may be caused by paramagnetic substances such as blood products, as seen in hemorrhagic tumors and postoperative studies. In the immediate postoperative period, small areas of restricted diffusion reflecting cytotoxic edema (infarct) can be expected at resection cavity margins, but should be distinguished from neoplasm and artifact from blood products. The purpose of identifying small areas of infarct induced by surgery is to recognize that these areas may enhance in the subacute phase when they might be confused for progressive neoplasm.

Blood products cause characteristic signal changes on T1-weighted and T2-weighted images depending on their age. More sensitive sequences tailored to assess for blood products are helpful and complementary in preoperative and postoperative assessment of GBM. Gradient echo and susceptibility-weighted imaging sequences exploit local magnetic field inhomogeneity produced by blood, mineralization, metal, and gas to better identify these materials. These substances show blooming; that is, conspicuous dark areas on the image extending beyond their physical boundaries, caused by perturbation of the local magnetic field. Note that gradient echo along with spin echo is a fundamental technique for acquiring MR images used in many different sequences, but in this case refers to a particular sequence attuned to hemorrhage.

Contrast Enhancement

Normal cerebral vessels possess specialized tight junctions between endothelial cells that form the BBB, excluding contrast and other molecules from the interstitium. Thus, contrast is particularly useful for brain MRI in general, because parenchymal accumulation highlights areas of BBB breakdown due to pathology, with low background signal. In GBM, contrast enhancement reflects a combination of inflammation causing disruption of the BBB and abnormal, leaky, tumoral vasculature. Contrast-enhancing areas may be solid, cystic with thin walls, or obviously necrotic. The presence of thick, irregular, nodular peripheral enhancement with central nonenhancement indicates necrosis[3] (see **Fig. 7.1**) and is a defining pathologic and radiologic feature of GBM compared with lower grade glial tumors. Regions of enhancement typically correspond with areas of hypercellularity (again seen as mildly restricted diffusion) and perfusional abnormalities on advanced imaging caused by the abnormal vasculature. Increasing patient age, tumor size, cellularity, necrosis, and perfusion are all predictive of higher grade.

Enhancing lesions in GBM can vary from 1 or more small foci, to a dominant lesion with satellite nodules, to a large lobar or transcallosal (butterfly) mass (**Fig. 7.3**). Although larger masses in general indicate more aggressive tumors, there is interplay between size and location causing symptomatic lesions that prompt imaging. Larger lesions with little nonenhancing signal abnormality are more typical of the mesenchymal GBM subtype.[8] Small enhancing lesions in a background of more extensive nonenhancing tumor may suggest secondary GBMs (proneural subtype) in younger patients. However, most lesions are primary GBMs in older patients and have variable-sized enhancing and nonenhancing components.

GBM may extend to the ventricular margin and show associated ependymal or subependymal enhancement. Sometimes tumoral enhancement is inseparable from choroid plexus, which precludes complete resection. More rarely, GBM shows extra-axial spread, leptomeningeal enhancement, involvement of adjacent vessels or dura, or dissemination in the CSF. Proximity to major vessels or evidence of vascular encasement or invasion should be noted preoperatively. Evidence of leptomeningeal spread or CSF dissemination usually mandates imaging of the spinal cord to assess for drop metastases.

ADVANCED IMAGING OF GLIOBLASTOMA

Advanced imaging techniques have become part of the standard evaluation of brain tumors at most academic centers and can be extremely valuable in patient management. The information gleaned from these methods complements conventional imaging in identifying and grading glial tumors, differentiating between other potential causes (**Table 7.4**),[9] and in general increases diagnostic confidence. In certain cases, advanced imaging findings can dramatically alter the interpretation of a study. Perhaps the best example of this is the use of perfusion imaging to diagnose pseudoprogression in patients treated with chemoradiation when conventional contrast-enhanced images suggest tumor recurrence[10] (see **Fig. 7.9**).

Again, note that advanced imaging techniques are reliant on additional postprocessing steps that must be performed before interpretation. Although all raw MRI data are heavily processed, each additional step allows the possible introduction of error or loss of information. Postprocessing may obscure artifacts inherent in the raw data. For example, colored overlays of perfusion data are often displayed on anatomic imaging. It is important to realize that these images depend on applying a threshold to the perfusion values. Good practice requires evaluating the source images for motion and susceptibility artifacts (discussed later) and viewing the derived perfusion maps without thresholding. Proper interpretation requires some familiarity with how various advanced imaging parameters are derived.

Dynamic Perfusion and Permeability Imaging

As tumors evolve, they induce alterations in the microvasculature within and surrounding them,

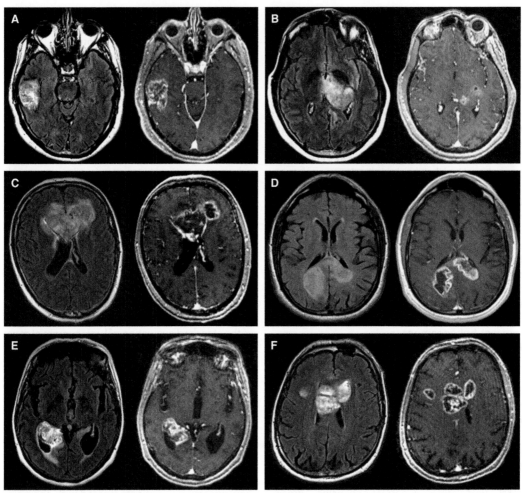

Fig. 7.3 Six patients with GBM. Representative postcontrast FLAIR (*left*) and T1-weighted images (*right*). (*A*) Right temporal lesion with cortical involvement. (*B*) Left thalamic multicentric GBM with multiple small rim-enhancing components and extension of nonenhancing neoplasm into the right thalamus through the massa intermedia. (*C*) Classic bifrontal butterfly GBM with extension through the anterior corpus callosum. (*D*) Posterior butterfly GBM extending through the splenium. (*E*) Partially intraventricular GBM protruding into the atrium of the right lateral ventricle. (*F*) Multifocal bifrontal GBM.

TABLE 7.4
Summary of Response Assessment in Neuro-Oncology response criteria

	Complete Response	Partial Response	Stable Disease	Progression
Enhancement	None	↓ by ≥50%	↓ <50% ↑ ≤25%	↑ >25%
T2/FLAIR	Stable or ↓	Stable or ↓	Stable or ↓	↑
New Lesion	None	None	None	+
Corticosteroids	None	Stable or ↓	Stable or ↓	—
Clinical Status	Stable or ↑	Stable or ↑	Stable or ↑	Decreased
Criteria Required	All	All	All	Any

Adapted from Wen PY, Macdonald DR, Reardon DA, et al. Updated response assessment criteria for high-grade gliomas: Response assessment in neuro-oncology working group. J Clin Oncol 2010;28(11):1970.

producing neoangiogenesis and disrupting the BBB.[11,12] A variety of imaging techniques have been developed to quantify alterations in microvasculature, including nuclear medicine techniques, arterial spin labeling, dynamic susceptibility contrast-enhanced (DSC), and dynamic contrast-enhancement (DCE) imaging; of these methods DSC and DCE are the most common methods in brain tumor imaging. These modalities may be of value both in predicting tumor grade[13,14] and in distinguishing neoplasm from treatment effects.[14]

Both DSC and DCE are similar in that they rapidly acquire multiple serial MRI data sets as a contrast bolus flows through the intracranial circulation. Dynamic imaging allows for mathematical modeling of microvascular kinetics based on the change in signal intensity over time. This approach differs from traditional contrast-enhanced images that are acquired several minutes following injection (when intravascular contrast has reached a steady state). DSC and DCE differ in how the presence of contrast affects the image. Similar to conventional imaging, gadolinium increases the signal of DCE images, whereas DSC exploits first-pass susceptibility effects of gadolinium on T2/T2* images to decrease image signal **(Fig. 7.4)**. As would be expected, other sources of magnetic susceptibility affect DSC images, including blood products and intracranial air commonly found after surgery.[11] Air-bone interfaces in the paranasal sinuses and temporal bones also cause susceptibility that may degrade imaging of frontal or temporal lesions. Significant underlying susceptibility can mask the DSC signal, resulting in apparently absent perfusion and potential false-negative results. Thus, DSC source images must be evaluated for underlying artifacts and DCE provides complimentary information in such cases.

Cerebral blood volume (CBV) is the most commonly calculated metric from DSC imaging for brain tumors[15] and provides an estimate of tissue microvascular density.[16] Increased CBV usually indicates higher tumor grade[13] and can be used to distinguish posttreatment effects from recurrent neoplasm. CBV measures are usually compared with the internal standard of contralateral white matter. As a general rule, the authors consider relative CBV (rCBV) 1.5 to 2 times contralateral white matter to be mild, 2 to 5 times to be intermediate, and greater than 5 times to be marked. Although mild increases may represent altered microvasculature from treatment, enhancing lesions with intermediate or marked increases in relative CBV should be considered suspicious for neoplasm, particularly if the appearance on conventional imaging supports that conclusion.

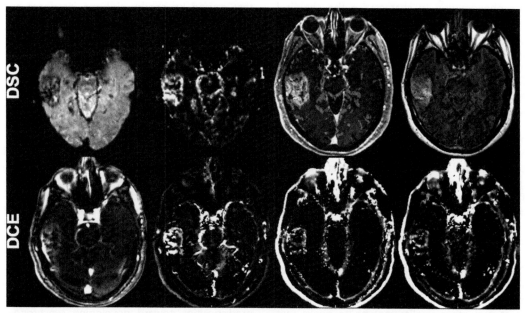

Fig. 7.4 DSC (*top*) and DCE (*bottom*) imaging of the right temporal GBM shown in Figure 7.3A. Panels on the left show the appearance of the raw data at the time the contrast bolus was passing through the mass; note the loss of signal on DSC and gain of signal on DCE. Subsequent DSC images represent processed rCBV data (the 2 panels on the right show rCBV in pseudocolor on anatomic images). Postprocessed DCE data provide examples of plasma volume, extracellular volume, and K^{trans} (volume transfer constant) (*left to right*). All metrics are suggestive of an aggressive neoplastic process.

For the evaluation of brain tumors, the information that DCE imaging provides is largely complementary to DSC.[17,18] Again, DCE has the advantage of being less prone to susceptibility artifacts compared with DSC. Calculated metrics include total plasma volume (Vp), extracellular volume (Ve), and K^{trans} (volume transfer constant, an estimate of capillary permeability). In our experience, Vp is the most useful of these metrics in the clinical setting; K^{trans} tends to mirror the appearance of conventional postcontrast images, which is not surprising given that both identify regions with disruptions to the BBB.

In most cases, abnormalities in perfusion metrics correspond with regions of tumoral enhancement on conventional images (although not all enhancing regions have abnormalities in perfusion). Perfusion values tend to be decreased in white matter areas with edema. In some cases, increased perfusion is evident in areas of nonenhancing signal abnormality, which again supports the diagnosis of glial neoplasm. For both DSC and DCE imaging, clinicians must be sure to recognize where increased perfusion is caused by normal vasculature, including cortical veins and choroidal vessels, to avoid false-positive interpretations.

Magnetic Resonance Spectroscopy

MRI traces its foundations to the discovery of nuclear MR (NMR) and subsequent exploitations of this phenomenon to characterize the chemical properties of matter.[19,20] NMR also allows the generation of exquisite chemical spectra (NMR spectroscopy), which are broadly used in chemistry. Although of diminished chemical resolution, the principles of NMR spectroscopy can be extended to analyze brain chemistry in vivo, where it has several applications in brain imaging.

A complete review of MRS is beyond the scope of this chapter. Briefly, any element with an odd number of nucleons (protons, neutrons, or both) can be imaged via MRS. ^1H MRS is most prevalent given the abundance of protons in organic matter. The MRS spectrum provides the relative abundance of different metabolites according to their chemical shift given in units of parts per million (ppm). Normal ^1H brain spectra have dominant characteristic peaks at 2 ppm (n-acetyl aspartate [NAA], a neuronal marker), at 3 ppm (creatine, an energy metabolite), and 3.2 ppm (choline, a measure of cellular membrane integrity), as well as several other smaller metabolite peaks that are poorly resolved on clinical imaging. The area under these peaks provides quantitative information on their relative concentrations.

GBM possesses a classic neoplastic spectrum with a reduced NAA peak and increases in the choline peak relative to NAA and creatine indicating cellular turnover[20] (Fig. 7.5). This spectrum should be sought in solid enhancing portions of the tumor, but is not specific for GBM. A neoplastic spectrum in regions of nonenhancing T2/FLAIR signal abnormality adds specificity, identifying regions of infiltrative nonenhancing neoplasm rather than merely edema. Useful thresholds are increases of the choline/NAA ratio greater than 2.2 in enhancing tissue and greater than 1 in regions of nonenhancing signal abnormality.[9] Increases in lipid/lactate concentration (1.3 ppm) may be seen and suggest necrosis. MRS may be helpful in differentiating lower grade primary glial neoplasms from GBM (GBM has been described as having lower NAA peak, more substantially increased choline peak, and increased likelihood of an increased lipid/lactate peak),[21] but the specificity of these findings is low. The utility of MRS continues to evolve as new applications and techniques become manifest. For example, advances in two-dimensional spectroscopy show promise in differentiating GBM from lower grade glial neoplasms as well as in predicting genetic subtypes.[22,23]

MRS data can be time consuming to acquire and therefore prone to motion artifacts. Because MRS differentiates substances via small differences in chemical shift, the technique is very sensitive to magnetic field inhomogeneity, such as that caused by nearby air-bone interfaces and blood products. MR spectra near the skull base, paranasal sinuses, or in proximity to intracranial hemorrhage and/or surgical sites are often of poor quality. In order to generate sufficient signal, MRS voxels are usually large and therefore spatial resolution is poor.

MULTIFOCAL LESIONS

Given their infiltrative nature, all aggressive glial neoplasms have the potential to involve multiple and distant brain structures. Several distinct patterns are traditionally defined. Multicentric glioblastoma (Fig. 7.6) connotes the presence of 2 or more distinct neoplasms, radiologically defined enhancing regions with an apparently normal intervening brain parenchyma.[24,25] It has been postulated that multicentric glioblastoma represents synchronous GBM.[26] Although it is conceivable that some patients possess a genetic predisposition toward developing synchronous GBM (akin to breast cancer in patients with BRCA1), it is also likely that many (if not most) multicentric tumors are part of the same primary neoplasm with infiltrative components below the level of resolution of standard clinical imaging. It

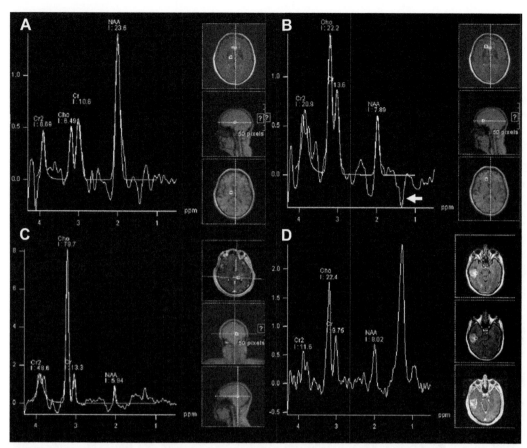

Fig. 7.5 Examples of MRS in assessment of brain tumors. (*A* and *B*) Spectra from a patient with pathology-proven butterfly GBM. A voxel sampled far from the visible lesion (*A*) has a fairly normal-appearing spectrum with dominant NAA peak and creatine (Cr) slightly greater than choline (Cho). In contrast, a voxel sampled from within the glioblastoma (*B*) shows neoplastic features with reversal of choline/creatine ratio, reductions in NAA peak, and a small lipid-lactate peak (*arrow*). (*C*) The intermediate TE (echo time) spectrum from a voxel placed within the left thalamic lesion from Figure 7.3B. The spectrum shows marked increases in choline and depression of NAA, again suggestive of high-grade glial neoplasm. (*D*) Short TE spectrum from within the right temporal lesion in Figure 7.3A shows aggressive neoplastic features with decreased (but present) NAA, reversed choline/creatine ratio, and an increased and broadened lipid-lactate peak centered at 1.3 ppm, findings suggestive of a necrotic glial neoplasm. Note that conventional imaging features should always be considered when interpreting spectroscopy data.

is important to keep in mind that GBM is highly aggressive and has numerous avenues for dissemination, including direct infiltration along axons, subarachnoid seeding, and even hematogenous dissemination.[25] Case reports have shown that some cases of radiographically multicentric disease have identical genetic profiles despite differences on pathology.[27] Further genomic analysis is likely to provide additional insights into the origins of multicentric tumors. Multifocal glioblastoma (see **Fig. 7.6**) indicates the presence of multiple discrete regions of enhancing tissue surrounded by a contiguous area of nonenhancing signal abnormality. In this case, different enhancing components are considered part of the same tumor. Again, careful genotyping within different parts of the same tumor or at different

time points following therapy can show divergent tumor lineages.[28–30] Gliomatosis cerebri represents an extensively infiltrative glial neoplasm that by definition involves 3 or more lobes in the cerebral hemispheres and may extend into the diencephalon and brainstem (**Fig. 7.7**). Gliomatosis cerebri can locally transform to GBM, with focal regions of enhancement most likely to include higher grade neoplasm.[31]

GLIOBLASTOMA MIMICS

Multiple other intracranial disorders may mimic glioblastoma, including metastases, lymphoma, radiation necrosis, lower grade gliomas, demyelination, abscess, and subacute to chronic infarcts. Differentiating between these causes on imaging

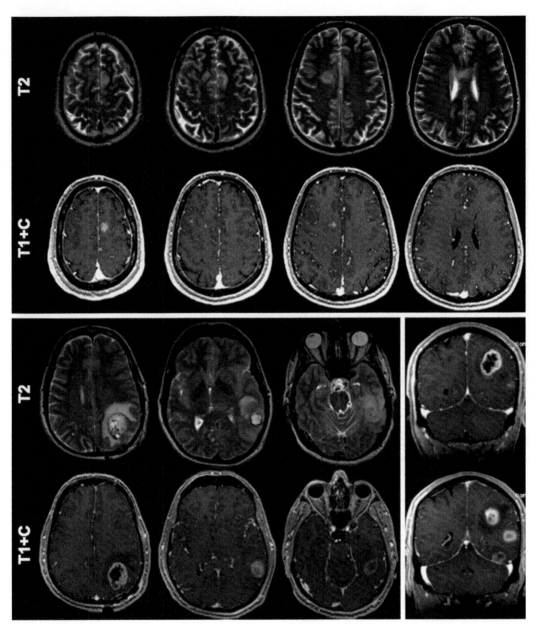

Fig. 7.6 Multicentric and multifocal GBM. (*A*) Bifrontal multicentric glioblastoma, by traditional definition. T2-weighted images (*top*) show numerous bilateral, discrete, hyperintense areas (including some with cortical infiltration as well as extension across the corpus callosum) and normal-appearing intervening brain parenchyma. Lesions partially enhance (*bottom*). (*B*) Multifocal glioma centered in the left parietal lobe with 3 thick and heterogeneous rim-enhancing masses (*bottom*) connected by nonenhancing infiltrative signal abnormality (*top*).

is critical to determining proper surgical management, or in some cases deferring surgery. A combination of conventional and advanced imaging findings (as presented in **Tables 7.2** and **7.3**, **Fig. 7.8**) is usually sufficient to make the correct diagnosis, but sometimes biopsy or follow-up imaging is indicated. Differentiating features of these alternative diagnoses are discussed below.

Radiation effects are described in the subsequent section on treatment changes.

Metastases

Solitary intracranial metastases occasionally mimic GBM. Approximately 50% of metastases are solitary at presentation, and large metastases often present as centrally necrotic rim-enhancing

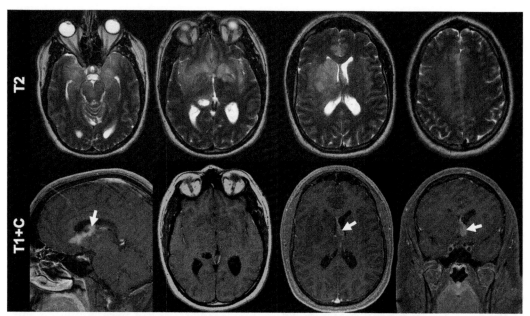

Fig. 7.7 T2-weighted images (*top*) show extensive gliomatosis involving both cerebral hemispheres, expanding the cortex at multiple locations, and within deep white matter, thalami, basal ganglia, and brainstem with a cystic region in the right thalamus (second from left images). Enhancing component near the left septum (indicated by the *arrows* on sagittal, axial, and coronal planes) was biopsied and was GBM by pathology.

lesions. In rare cases, multicentric GBM can be mistaken for metastases. Like GBM, the neoplastic tissue of a metastasis is usually hypercellular (ie, enhancing tissue with mild restricted diffusion) and is associated with solid, thick linear, and nodular enhancement. Further, like GBM, enhancing metastatic tissue usually has marked increases in perfusion and permeability metrics on advanced imaging.

Despite these superficial similarities, differentiating GBM from metastases on MRI is usually not a diagnostic challenge. In contrast with GBM, intra-axial metastases usually occur at the gray-white junction, are not infiltrative, do not extend into the cortex, and do not cross interhemispheric commissures. Metastases are commonly associated with disproportionately increased vasogenic edema relative to their size. Again, signal abnormality caused by vasogenic edema is restricted to white matter; any cortical involvement raises suspicion for a glial neoplasm. Infratentorial lesions are substantially more likely to be metastatic in adults. The presence of multiple, particularly widely separated, enhancing lesions also dramatically increases the likelihood that an intracranial mass represents a metastasis rather than GBM, as does a history of appropriate (eg, lung, breast, thyroid, testicular, melanoma) metastatic disease elsewhere in the body. In difficult cases, MRS

occasionally improves diagnostic accuracy, as noted earlier.

Lymphoma
Lymphoma can masquerade as multiple intracranial neoplastic and inflammatory processes, including GBM. Primary central nervous system (CNS) lymphoma often presents as a multicentric, hypercellular, infiltrative mass centered in the cerebral white matter. Note that secondary lymphoma has a different appearance, usually presenting as 1 or more dural-based masses that could be confused with meningiomas or solid organ metastases such as from breast cancer. Like GBM, primary CNS lymphoma often extends through interhemispheric white matter connections such as the corpus callosum. Lymphoma has a proclivity for the periventricular white matter and usually does not infiltrate the cortex. The key differentiating characteristic of lymphoma is its (usual) uniformity. Unlike GBM, lymphoma tends to enhance homogeneously and show uniform diffusion restriction.[32] An important exception to this rule is that lesions often show peripheral enhancement in immune-compromised patients, such as those with acquired immunodeficiency syndrome, who are also predisposed to developing lymphoma. Hemorrhage can also complicate lymphoma, affecting the pattern on

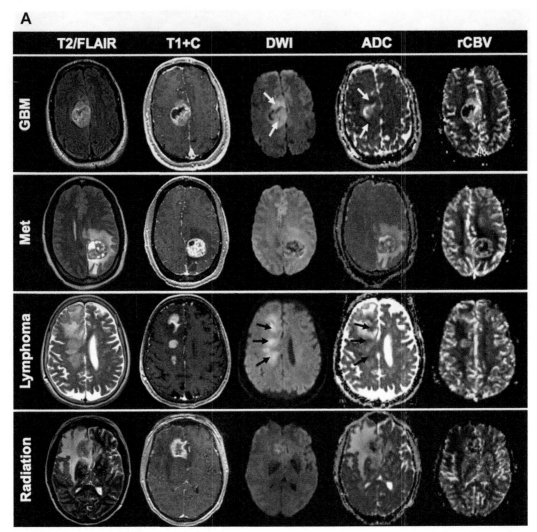

Fig. 7.8 MRI features of GBM and multiple potential mimicking lesions. (*A*) GBM: superior right frontal lesion shows cortical infiltration on FLAIR; solid, peripheral, and ill-defined enhancement with central necrosis; restricted diffusion (bright on DWI, dark on ADC; *arrows*) indicating cellularity as well as increased perfusion (rCBV) corresponding with the enhancing areas. Metastasis (Met): heterogeneously enhancing partially cystic high left parietal mass in a 45-year-old woman with 9 kg (20 pounds) of unintentional weight loss. The lesion is well circumscribed, surrounded by marked vasogenic edema, and near the gray-white junction. Increased perfusion is noted. *Lymphoma*: multiple periventricular homogeneously enhancing foci with corresponding restricted diffusion (*arrows*) with surrounding edema and involvement of the corpus callosum favor lymphoma. Mild associated increased perfusion. Radiation necrosis: right frontal heterogeneous, shaggy, peripherally enhancing lesion in a 63-year-old woman who previously received whole-brain and gamma knife radiotherapy for breast cancer metastases. Marked surrounding edema, which also involves the corpus callosum. Lack of significantly increased perfusion supports radiation necrosis.

postcontrast imaging and DWI. A variable amount of edema may be seen surrounding enhancing lesions in lymphoma.

In challenging situations, perfusion/permeability imaging may improve diagnostic accuracy.[33,34] rCBV is usually less increased than in GBM or metastasis. A characteristic finding on the DSC signal intensity curve is a return of signal above the baseline (overshoot) during the washout phase caused by leakage of contrast material into the interstitium.[34,35] In GBM, the signal intensity curve does not return to baseline.

Other Primary Glial Neoplasms

With good-quality MRI, experienced imagers can usually distinguish a primary brain tumor from other intracranial masses with high reliability. Distinguishing between different grades of glial

B

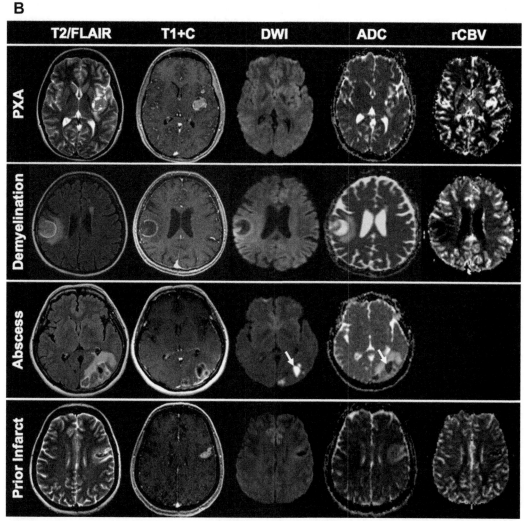

	T2/FLAIR	T1+C	DWI	ADC	rCBV
PXA					
Demyelination					
Abscess					
Prior Infarct					

Fig. 7.8 (continued). (B) Pleomorphic xanthoastrocytoma (PXA): solidly enhancing partially cystic mass in the left insula associated with infiltrative white matter signal abnormality. Increased perfusion. Low-grade glial neoplasms can show enhancement and increased perfusion. Most such lesions are seen in younger patients. *Tumefactive demyelination*: right lateral frontal lobe subcortical white matter lesion, hyperintense on FLAIR with a thin, incomplete peripheral rim of enhancement and diffusion restriction that spares the cortex. Surrounding vasogenic edema. Only mildly increased and predominantly decreased perfusion. *Abscess*: a 56-year-old woman with multiple clustered rim-enhancing masses in the left occipitotemporal cortex with prominent surrounding edema. Central restricted diffusion on DWI and ADC (arrows) confirm pyogenic abscess. Cultures grew *Streptococcus constellatus*, presumably from dental infection. Subacute to chronic prior infarct: left lateral frontal lesion shows evidence of prior cortical hemorrhage (low signal on T2-weighted, DWI, and rCBV images), residual edema, focal volume loss, and gyriform enhancement following the cortex. No increased perfusion.

neoplasms can be more challenging. Again, tumor size, growth rate, cellularity,[36] enhancement, perfusion, and particularly patient age are all associated with higher grade. Enhancement with necrosis indicates GBM but necrosis may not always be apparent at imaging. Pilocytic astrocytomas, pleomorphic xanthoastrocytomas, and gangliogliomas (mixed tumors) often do enhance and can mimic higher grade tumors. These tumors are usually found in younger

patients, the latter two most often with seizures. Grade II diffuse astrocytomas show infiltrative signal abnormality typically without enhancement. New enhancement in low grade tumors may indicate progression to higher grade. Grade II oligodendrogliomas are typically peripheral, wedge-shaped, and calcified with prominent gyral expansion. Enhancement and elevated rCBV may indicate anaplastic oligodendroglioma but oligodendrogliomas with 1p19q co-deletion can have these features and remain low grade.[37] Grade III anaplastic astrocytomas usually show areas of patchy enhancement and elevated rCBV without frank necrosis.

Tumefactive Demyelination

Demyelinating lesions can have a variety of appearances but typically appear as scattered regions of T2/FLAIR hyperintensity without significant mass effect. Regions of active demyelination may show enhancement or restricted diffusion at the periphery. In rare cases, active demyelinating lesions can produce significant mass effect and mimic neoplasm.[38] Enhancement of tumefactive demyelinating lesions tends to be smooth, peripheral, sometimes concentric, and may show a discontinuous lateral margin or open-ring sign, which has been reported to be approximately 90% specific for demyelination.[39,40] The open part of the ring reflects sparing of adjacent cortex. The presence of additional lesions in the brain or spinal cord that are more typical of a demyelinating process also may aid in diagnosis, although a tumefactive demyelinating lesion may be the only or first manifestation of disease.

Abscess

Like GBM, cerebral abscesses typically appear as rim-enhancing centrally debris-filled intra-axial masses. The pattern of rim enhancement tends to be smoother and thinner than that of GBM, with asymmetric thickness of the wall (thinner towards the white matter or ventricles) classically described.[39] Nevertheless, there is substantial overlap in the enhancement patterns between these entities. The most distinguishing imaging feature is on DWI[41]; abscesses tend to restrict centrally because of purulent material. Again, it is the hypercellular, peripherally enhancing tissue in GBM that restricts. The degree of restriction also differs substantially, because abscesses are usually lightbulb-bright on DWI.

Infarct

Arterial infarcts follow vascular territories and the mechanism and extent of vascular involvement dictate their appearance and multiplicity. Infarcts may be purely subcortical when caused by end-artery small vessel ischemia or watershed ischemia, cortical when caused by embolic disease, or wedge-shaped involving cortex and subcortical white matter when more proximal vessels are occluded by thromboembolic disease. Acute infarcts show restricted diffusion, hyperintensity on T2/FLAIR, and mass effect manifested by gyral swelling and sulcal effacement. In the subacute phase, DWI signal decreases, ADC values normalize because of the combined effects of cytotoxic and vasogenic edema, petechial cortical hemorrhage or frank hemorrhagic transformation may occur, and enhancement may be seen because of BBB disruption.

A subacute infarct with enhancement, persistent mass effect, edema, and possible hemorrhage may mimic GBM or other neoplasms if imaging in the acute phase is absent. However, enhancement is characteristically gyriform, following the cortex, rather than round and masslike. Sometimes coronal or sagittal images better depict this gyriform pattern. Note that venous infarcts follow different distributions, usually present with edema and hemorrhage rather than restricted diffusion, and may enhance. Appropriate evolution of imaging findings over time provides the best confirmation of infarct, with resolution of edema, hemorrhage, enhancement, and mass effect giving way to volume loss and gliosis (ie, encephalomalacia). Thus, follow-up imaging should be prescribed in uncertain cases.

RECURRENT DISEASE AND TREATMENT EFFECTS

Differentiating neoplasm from treatment effects represents one of the greatest challenges in brain tumor imaging, requiring experience, patience, and careful review of the extant clinical and imaging information. If available, pretreatment scans should be reviewed to understand the natural appearance of the tumor. Immediate postoperative scans also represent a critical time point. Knowledge of dates of surgery and radiation therapy, tumor pathology, other interventions (eg, chemotherapy, steroids), and the patient's clinical trajectory are of great value.

In the immediate postoperative setting, the surgical cavity is expected to contain heterogeneous blood products and gas and may be lined with regions of ischemia. Although expected, the heterogeneous appearance of the surgical bed can complicate interpretation. Of particular importance is the varied appearance of blood products on MRI, which may appear bright or dark on multiple sequences based on oxygenation, oxidation, and location of hemoglobin. Subacute blood usually appears hyperintense on T1-weighted images and can be confused with enhancement. Conversely, hyperintense background signal from blood products may obscure residual enhancing tumor. Thus, when evaluating for residual enhancing neoplasm, it is critical to examine precontrast and postcontrast T1-weighted images in parallel.

Within 24 to 48 hours of surgery, enhancement at the resection site represents residual neoplasm. Over time, granulation tissue forms, which usually appears as thin linear enhancement surrounding the resection cavity and of the overlying dura. Subacute regions of ischemia may also enhance.[42] Development of nodular or thick enhancement in the surgical cavity should raise concern for recurrence. The surgical bed is expected to evolve over time, with decreases in the size of the resection cavity, improvement in mass effect, continued evolution of blood products, and resolution of pneumocephalus.

Variations from the expected postoperative time course should raise concerns for recurrence or superimposed infection. For example, fluid in the surgical cavity does not suppress initially because of the presence of blood products but signal should approach that of CSF over time. However, new incomplete FLAIR suppression in a cavity that previously suppressed suggests tumor progression.[43] Similarly, surgical cavities and overlying fluid collections may have persistent, heterogeneously increased signal on DWI caused by blood products. However, new homogeneous areas of diffusion restriction confirmed on ADC maps prompt concern for infection, which should be correlated with clinical findings.

Nearly all patients with high-grade glial neoplasms also receive chemoradiation as standard of care. Radiation has the potential to produce numerous effects, including favorable tumor response, pseudoprogression, and radiation necrosis, all superimposed on the tumor's natural proclivity for continued growth. The conventional imaging appearances of these effects overlap substantially. Pseudoprogression is thought to represent a combination of radiation effects on the tumor and increased permeability of the BBB, typically beginning within the first 12 weeks of completing therapy and resolving by 6 months.[44,45] In contrast, radiation necrosis is thought to represent primarily brain parenchymal injury, usually occurs months to years following completion of therapy, and potentially results in widespread geographic edema and enhancement within the radiation field.[46]

In contrast to the typical thick and localized enhancement of GBM recurrence, radiation effects are classically described as feathery or bubbly.[10] Nevertheless, there is substantial overlap between progression and treatment effects on conventional imaging[47] and perfusion/permeability imaging may be required to distinguish radiation effects from recurrence with confidence (**Fig. 7.9**). A discriminatory rCBV threshold of 1.8 times normal white matter has been described

as having a 94% sensitivity and 92% specify for recurrent tumor, with each unit increase in relative CBV conveying a 254-fold increase in the odds of tumor.[48] MRS may also be of value, because the spectrum of radiation necrosis has been described to have a reduced choline peak relative to neoplasm.[46,49] However, there is overlap in the perfusion values seen with neoplasm and treatment change. In addition, in many cases there is a combination of enhancing tumor and treatment effects.

New enhancing lesions are often small and below the resolution level of DSC/DCE imaging or spectroscopy and must simply be followed over time. Such small enhancing foci are common along ventricular margins in the radiation port, attributed to particular sensitivity of periventricular white matter caused by radiation-induced vasculopathy.[46] Such small enhancing foci are common along ventricular margins in the radiation port; this finding is attributed to the particular sensitivity of periventricular white matter to radiation-induced vasculopathy. Even larger areas of radiation necrosis may extend up to and around the ventricular margin or into the corpus callosum.

Clinical information can be integrated into imaging interpretation as further detailed below in the context of response criteria. Either recurrent tumor or treatment effects with edema may cause worsening symptoms, but increasing enhancement with stable symptoms and no change in steroid therapy usually results in continued follow-up imaging rather than a change in treatment course. Note that O6-methylguanine-DNA-methyltransferase (MGMT)-promotor methylation is associated with greater incidence of pseudoprogression (and better outcome overall)[50] so increasing enhancement and signal abnormality in the early postradiation period can be more readily attributed to treatment in patients with this modification.

Addition of the anti–vascular endothelial growth factor monoclonal antibody bevacizumab (Avastin) to GBM treatment regimens has further complicated the radiographic differentiation of treatment effects from tumor.[45] The principles and evolving evidence behind antiangiogenic therapy are described in detail elsewhere. Bevacizumab typically produces dramatic reductions in enhancement within neoplastic tissue[51] (**Fig. 7.10**); however, underlying neoplasm may remain stable, increase, or even adopt a more infiltrative phenotype.[52] Thus, contrast enhancement becomes less reliable as a marker of progression. DSC and DCE parameters also provided limited information in the setting of bevacizumab.

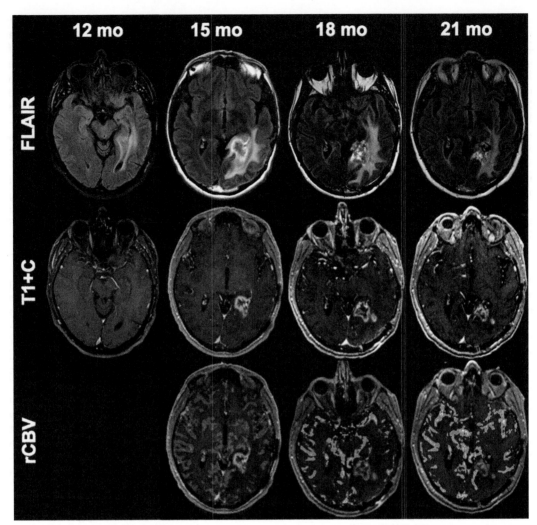

Fig. 7.9 Pseudoprogression (radiation necrosis) in a patient with resected GBM additionally treated with chemoradiation. Initial images on the left performed 12 months after radiotherapy completion show FLAIR hyperintensity along the margins of the occipital and temporal horns of the lateral ventricle and no abnormal enhancement. This hyperintensity is in the radiation field near the patient's lateral parietotemporal resection cavity (not shown) and consistent with treatment changes. Imaging at 15 months shows a new heterogeneous, peripherally enhancing lesion with increased surrounding nonenhancing signal and mass effect but no apparent increased perfusion. Follow-up imaging at 18 and 20 months showed decreasing enhancement and edema. Contiguous component of the lesion was resected before the 18-month scan with pathology showing predominantly treatment effects (not shown).

Eventually, clear progression with enhancement may be seen despite antiangiogenic therapy, but, in the absence of enhancement, careful attention must be paid to increasing infiltrative nonenhancing components over time. Here again, evidence of cellularity, expansion, or cortical infiltration should be sought. Diffusion restriction indicates cellular tumor in some cases.[53] However, bevacizumab can also induce atypical necrosis in radiated brains (see **Fig. 7.10**), particularly in the periventricular white matter, characterized by areas of persistent striking restricted diffusion.[54–56] These areas tend to have lower ADC values than expected for viable tissue. Extent of atypical necrosis and associated edema and mass effect may increase initially but often stabilize, and development of atypical necrosis may be associated with improved outcomes.[56]

In order to standardize reporting of response to therapy, several guidelines that include imaging data have been published.[45,57,58] The Macdonald Criteria have traditionally been the most commonly used metric, combining postcontrast imaging data with clinical information and corticosteroid use to defines disease progression. In 2010, the Response Assessment in Neuro-Oncology (RANO) group

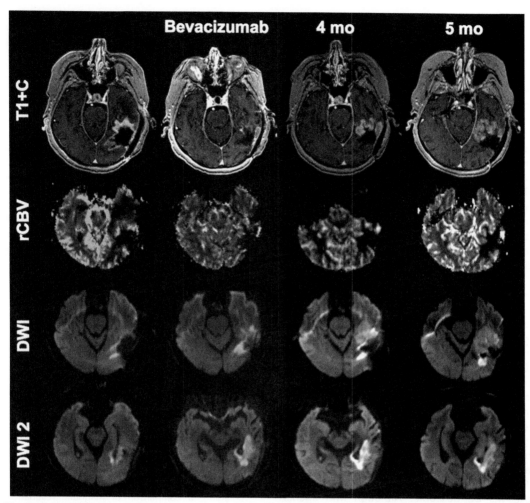

Fig. 7.10 Pseudoresponse and progression on bevacizumab. Initial images on the left show heterogeneous nodular enhancement with increased perfusion along the margins of a left temporo-occipital resection cavity in a 65-year-old woman with GBM after multiple resections and chemoradiation. She was subsequently started on bevacizumab with corresponding marked reduction in enhancement as well as perfusion at the cavity margins. However, over the next 4 to 5 months, scans show recurrent and increased nodular enhancement and increased perfusion at the cavity margin reflecting progression of neoplasm. A dural-based enhancing nodule at the superficial cavity margin showed fairly persistent enhancement throughout. Two bottom rows of images show the pattern on DWI at the same level and a little more superiorly (DWI 2). Note the increase in intermediate signal on DWI at the anterior margin of the cavity corresponding with the increasing enhancement and consistent with cellular tumor. In addition, a more pronounced area of diffusion restriction developed along the posterior and lateral ventricular margin immediately after bevacizumab therapy, remained fairly stable over the following 4 to 5 months, and never enhanced. This finding may represent atypical necrosis, possibly superimposed on underlying tumor.

modified the Macdonald Criteria in order to increase the precision of imaging measurements, as well as to account for the imaging effects of chemoradiation and antiangiogenic therapy.[45] The modified Macdonald Criteria require more convincing evidence of progression on scans performed less than 12 weeks following the completion of chemoradiation, given the common occurrence of pseudoprogression during this time period. In addition, in patients on antiangiogenic therapy on stable or decreasing doses of corticosteroids, the revised criteria include increases in nonenhancing signal abnormalities as evidence of neoplastic progression.

FUTURE DIRECTIONS IN IMAGING
As the most common and deadly adult primary brain tumor and one of the most aggressive neoplasms overall, GBM remains a subject of considerable imaging research. As in other areas of brain imaging and radiology more generally, improving

scanner technology and higher resolution imaging along with ever-increasing computing power has enabled more quantitative approaches to tumor characterization. Volumetric measurements of enhancing and nonenhancing tumor components can be derived automatically or semiautomatically and may aid tumor follow-up and response assessment. Applying such techniques to institutional and publically available brain tumor databases that include preoperative imaging and tumor genotypes permits combined analyses (radiogenomics) that are revealing the imaging phenotypes of glioblastoma subtypes and imaging features that may predict response to therapy and other outcomes.[8,59,60] Computer algorithms can also be trained on such data, including conventional and advanced imaging features, to predict tumor subtypes and overall survival.[61]

Nuclear medicine techniques are likely to take on a greater role in glioblastoma imaging. PET using 18F-fluorodeoxyglucose (FDG) is now widely used for staging and restaging of extracranial malignancies. Signal to background is poor for intracranial malignancy because of the high uptake of FDG within normal brain tissue, although GBM does show greater uptake and this can be used to distinguish recurrent tumor from treatment changes. As clinicians learn more about GBM genetics and the tumor microenvironment, other agents designed to evaluate hypoxia or tumor markers may be useful. With increasing use of targeted T-cell therapy (discussed in Chapter 19), means to measure cell distribution and uptake will be desirable. Although MRI agents have been used for cell tracking in preclinical models, nuclear medicine techniques are both quantitative and more sensitive, and therefore may be advantageous for cell tracking.

Numerous nanoparticle agents have been developed for diagnostic and/or therapeutic purposes for GBM and tested in preclinical models. Nanoparticles can target tumors passively, relying on long circulation time, BBB disruption, and enhanced permeability and retention properties of tumor tissues. In addition, particles may be modified to bind to cell surface markers by conjugating various peptides, receptors, antibodies, or antibody fragments. The BBB remains a significant barrier to targeting infiltrative and nonenhancing tumor components. Nanoparticles have been developed as single or multimodal contrast agents to guide resection,[62,63] delivery vehicles for chemotherapy,[64] and sensitizer agents to enhance radiation therapy and thermal ablation.[65,66] Translation of these technologies to clinical use remains a challenge.

SUMMARY

Neuroimaging will continue to play a critical role in the management of patients with GBM. Successful interpretation of imaging data requires understanding the principles of image generation, pathophysiology of disease, and effects of treatment. Imaging must be assessed within the context of each patient's history, demographics, current symptoms, and prior or ongoing therapies. Imaging features of infiltration, cellularity, and abnormal vascularity mirror the pathologic findings in GBM. Conventional enhanced MRI is the primary modality for GBM evaluation. Advanced imaging techniques provide important adjunct information during initial diagnosis and follow-up evaluation. Imaging will continue to support, adapt to, and in some cases drive emerging brain tumor therapies.

REFERENCES

1. Yamashita K, Hiwatashi A, Togao O, et al. MR imaging–based analysis of glioblastoma multiforme: estimation of IDH1 mutation status. AJNR Am J Neuroradiol 2016;37:58–65.
2. Dean BL, Drayer BP, Bird CR, et al. Gliomas: classification with MR imaging. Radiology 1990;174(2):411–5.
3. Claussen C, Laniado M, Schorner W, et al. Gadolinium-DTPA in MR imaging of glioblastomas and intracranial metastases. AJNR Am J Neuroradiol 1985;6(5):669–74.
4. Brant-Zawadzki M, Badami J, Mills C, et al. Tumor imaging: a comparison of magnetic resonance and CT. Radiology 1984;150(2):435–40.
5. Keogh BP, Henson JW. Clinical manifestations and diagnostic imaging of brain tumors. Hematol Oncol Clin North Am 2012;26(4):733–55.
6. Berberat J, Grobholz R, Boxheimer L, et al. Differentiation between calcification and hemorrhage in brain tumors using susceptibility-weighted imaging: a pilot study. Am J Roentgenol 2014;202(4):847–50.
7. Provenzale JM, McGraw P, Mhatre P, et al. Peritumoral brain regions in gliomas and meningiomas: investigation with isotropic diffusion-weighted MR imaging and diffusion-tensor MR imaging. Radiology 2004;232(2):451–60.
8. Naeini KM, Pope WB, Cloughesy TF, et al. Identifying the mesenchymal molecular subtype of glioblastoma using quantitative volumetric analysis of anatomic magnetic resonance images. Neuro Oncol 2013;15(5):626–34.
9. Al-Okaili RN, Krejza J, Wang S, et al. Advanced MR imaging techniques in the diagnosis of intraaxial brain tumors in adults. Radiographics 2006;26(Suppl 1):173–90.

10. Kumar AJ, Leeds NE, Fuller GN, et al. Malignant gliomas: MR imaging spectrum of radiation therapy- and chemotherapy-induced necrosis of the brain after treatment. Radiology 2000;217(2):377–84.

11. Lacerda S, Law M. Magnetic resonance perfusion and permeability imaging in brain tumors. Neuroimaging Clin N Am 2009;19(4):527–57.

12. Shweiki D, Neeman M, Itin A, et al. Induction of vascular endothelial growth factor expression by hypoxia and by glucose deficiency in multicell spheroids: implications for tumor angiogenesis. Proc Natl Acad Sci U S A 1995;92(3):768–72.

13. Knopp EA, Cha S, Johnson G, et al. Glial neoplasms: dynamic contrast-enhanced T2*-weighted MR imaging. Radiology 1999;211(3):791–8.

14. Law M, Yang S, Wang H, et al. Glioma grading: sensitivity, specificity, and predictive values of perfusion MR imaging and proton MR spectroscopic imaging compared with conventional MR imaging. AJNR Am J Neuroradiol 2003;24(10): 1989–98.

15. Cha S, Knopp EA, Johnson G, et al. Intracranial mass lesions: dynamic contrast-enhanced susceptibility-weighted echo-planar perfusion MR imaging. Radiology 2002;223(1):11–29.

16. Hu LS, Baxter LC, Smith KA, et al. Relative cerebral blood volume values to differentiate high-grade glioma recurrence from posttreatment radiation effect: Direct correlation between image-guided tissue histopathology and localized dynamic susceptibility-weighted contrast-enhanced perfusion MR imaging measurements. AJNR Am J Neuroradiol 2009;30(3):552–8.

17. Buckley DL. Uncertainty in the analysis of tracer kinetics using dynamic contrast-enhanced T1-weighted MRI. Magn Reson Med 2002;47(3):601–6.

18. Haroon HA, Patankar TF, Zhu XP, et al. Comparison of cerebral blood volume maps generated from T2* and T1 weighted MRI data in intra-axial cerebral tumours. Br J Radiol 2007;80(951):161–8.

19. Bulik M, Jancalek R, Vanicek J, et al. Potential of MR spectroscopy for assessment of glioma grading. Clin Neurol Neurosurg 2013;115(2):146–53.

20. Ott M, Henning J, Ernst T. Human brain tumors: assessment with in vivo proton MR spectroscopy. Radiology 1993;186(3):745–52.

21. Stadlbauer A, Gruber S, Nimsky C, et al. Preoperative grading of gliomas by using metabolite quantification with high-spatial-resolution proton MR spectroscopic imaging. Radiology 2006;238(3): 958–69.

22. Yang F, Shan ZY. Mapping developmental precentral and postcentral gyral changes in children on magnetic resonance images. J Magn Reson Imaging 2011;33(1):62–70.

23. Andronesi OC, Kim GS, Gerstner E, et al. Detection of 2-hydroxyglutarate in IDH-mutated glioma patients by in vivo spectral-editing and 2D correlation magnetic resonance spectroscopy. Sci Transl Med 2012;4(116):116ra4.

24. Kyritsis AP, Levin VA, Yung WK, et al. Imaging patterns of multifocal gliomas. Eur J Radiol 1993; 16(3):163–70.

25. Showalter TN, Andrel J, Andrews DW, et al. Multifocal glioblastoma multiforme: prognostic factors and patterns of progression. Int J Radiat Oncol Biol Phys 2007;69(3):820–4.

26. Parsa AT, Wachhorst S, Lamborn KR, et al. Prognostic significance of intracranial dissemination of glioblastoma multiforme in adults. J Neurosurg 2005;102(4):622–8.

27. Akimoto J, Sasaki H, Haraoka R, et al. A case of radiologically multicentric but genetically identical multiple glioblastomas. Brain Tumor Pathol 2014; 31(2):113–7.

28. Diehn M, Nardini C, Wang DS, et al. Identification of noninvasive imaging surrogates for brain tumor gene-expression modules. Proc Natl Acad Sci U S A 2008;105(13):5213–8.

29. Pope WB, Mirsadraei L, Lai A, et al. Differential gene expression in glioblastoma defined by ADC histogram analysis: relationship to extracellular matrix molecules and survival. AJNR Am J Neuroradiol 2012;33(6):1059–64.

30. Rutman AM, Kuo MD. Radiogenomics: creating a link between molecular diagnostics and diagnostic imaging. Eur J Radiol 2009;70(2):232–41.

31. Kannuki S, Hirose T, Horiguchi H, et al. Gliomatosis cerebri with secondary glioblastoma formation: report of two cases. Brain Tumor Pathol 1998; 15(2):111–6.

32. Yamashita K, Yoshiura T, Hiwatashi A, et al. Differentiating primary CNS lymphoma from glioblastoma multiforme: assessment using arterial spin labeling, diffusion-weighted imaging, and ^{18}F-fluorodeoxyglucose positron emission tomography. Neuroradiology 2013;55(2):135–43.

33. Kickingereder P, Sahm F, Wiestler B, et al. Evaluation of microvascular permeability with dynamic contrast-enhanced MRI for the differentiation of primary CNS lymphoma and glioblastoma: radiologic-pathologic correlation. AJNR Am J Neuroradiol 2014;35(8):1503–8.

34. Mangla R, Kolar B, Zhu T, et al. Percentage signal recovery derived from MR dynamic susceptibility contrast imaging is useful to differentiate common enhancing malignant lesions of the brain. AJNR Am J Neuroradiol 2011;32(6):1004–10.

35. Wang LL, Leach JL, Breneman JC, et al. Critical role of imaging in the neurosurgical and radiotherapeutic management of brain tumors. Radiographics 2014;34(3):702–21.

36. Higano S, Yun X, Kumabe T, et al. Malignant astrocytic tumors: clinical importance of apparent

diffusion coefficient in prediction of grade and prognosis. Radiology 2006;241(3):839–46.

37. Whitmore RG, Krejza J, Kapoor GS, et al. Prediction of oligodendroglial tumor subtype and grade using perfusion weighted magnetic resonance imaging. J Neurosurg 2007;107(3):600–9.

38. Tsui EYK, Leung WH, Chan JH, et al. Tumefactive demyelinating lesions by combined perfusion-weighted and diffusion weighted imaging. Comput Med Imaging Graph 2002;26(5):343–6.

39. Smirniotopoulos JG, Murphy FM, Rushing EJ, et al. Patterns of contrast enhancement in the brain and meninges. Radiographics 2007;27:525–51.

40. Masdeu J, Quinto C, Olivera C, et al. Open-ring imaging sign: highly specific for atypical brain demyelination. Neurology 2000;54(7):1427–33.

41. Kim Y, Chang KH, Song IC, et al. Brain abscess and necrotic or cystic brain tumor: discrimination with signal intensity on diffusion weighted MR imaging. Am J Roentgenol 1998;171(6):1487–90.

42. Ulmer S, Braga TA, Barker FG 2nd, et al. Clinical and radiographic features of peritumoral infarction following resection of glioblastoma. Neurology 2006;67:1668–70.

43. Winterstein M, Münter MW, Burkholder I. Partially resected gliomas: diagnostic performance of fluid-attenuated inversion recovery MR imaging for detection of progression. Radiology 2010;254(3):907–16.

44. de Wit MCY, de Bruin HG, Eijkenboom W, et al. Immediate post-radiotherapy changes in malignant glioma can mimic tumor progression. Neurology 2004;63(3):535–7.

45. Wen PY, Macdonald DR, Reardon DA, et al. Updated response assessment criteria for high-grade gliomas: response assessment in neuro-oncology working group. J Clin Oncol 2010;28(11):1963–72.

46. Shah R, Vattoth S, Jacob R, et al. Radiation necrosis in the brain: imaging features and differentiation from tumor recurrence. Radiographics 2012;32(5):1343–59.

47. Young RJ, Gupta A, Shah AD, et al. Potential utility of conventional MRI signs in diagnosing pseudo-progression in glioblastoma. Neurology 2011;76(22):1918–24.

48. Gasparetto EL, Pawlak MA, Patel SH, et al. Post-treatment recurrence of malignant brain neoplasm: accuracy of relative cerebral blood volume fraction in discriminating low from high malignant histologic volume fraction. Radiology 2009;250(3):887–96.

49. Siu A, Wind JJ, Iorgulescu JB, et al. Radiation necrosis following treatment of high grade glioma–a review of the literature and current understanding. Acta Neurochir 2012;154(2):191–201.

50. Brandes AA, Franceschi E, Tosoni A, et al. MGMT promoter methylation status can predict the incidence and outcome of pseudoprogression after concomitant radiochemotherapy in newly diagnosed glioblastoma patients. J Clin Oncol 2008;26(13):2192–7.

51. Pope W, Lai A, Nghiemphu P, et al. MRI in patients with high-grade gliomas treated with bevacizumab and chemotherapy. Neurology 2006;66(8):2089–91.

52. De Groot JF, Fuller G, Kumar AJ, et al. Tumor invasion after treatment of glioblastoma with bevacizumab: radiographic and pathologic correlation in humans and mice. Neuro Oncol 2010;12(3):233–42.

53. Gerstner E, Frosch M, Batchelor T. Diffusion magnetic resonance imaging detects pathologically confirmed, nonenhancing tumor progression in a patient with recurrent glioblastoma receiving bevacizumab. J Clin Oncol 2010;28(6):e91–3.

54. Rieger J, Bähr O, Muller K, et al. Bevacizumab-induced diffusion-restricted lesions in malignant glioma patients. J Neurooncol 2010;99(1):49–56.

55. Rieger J, Bähr O, Ronellenfitsch MW, et al. Bevacizumab-induced diffusion restriction in patients with glioma: Tumor progression or surrogate marker of hypoxia? J Clin Oncol 2010;28(27):2016.

56. Mong S, Ellingson BM, Nghiemphu PL, et al. Persistent diffusion-restricted lesions in bevacizumab-treated malignant gliomas are associated with improved survival compared with matched controls. AJNR Am J Neuroradiol 2012;33(9):1763–70.

57. Macdonald DR, Cascino TL, Schold SCJ, et al. Response criteria for phase II studies of supratentorial malignant glioma. J Clin Oncol 1990;8(7):1277–80.

58. Therasse P, Arbuck S, Eisenhauer E, et al. New guidelines to evaluate the response to treatment in solid tumors. J Natl Cancer Inst 2000;87(12):881–6.

59. Ellingson BM, Lai A, Harris RJ, et al. Probabilistic radiographic atlas of glioblastoma phenotypes. AJNR Am J Neuroradiol 2013;34(3):533–40.

60. Gevaert O, Mitchell LA, Achrol AS, et al. Glioblastoma multiforme: exploratory radiogenomic analysis by using quantitative image features. Radiology 2014;273(1):131731.

61. Macyszyn L, Akbari H, Pisapia JM, et al. Imaging patterns predict patient survival and molecular subtype in glioblastoma via machine learning techniques. Neuro Oncol 2016;18(3):417–25.

62. Kircher MF, Mahmood U, King RS, et al. A multimodal nanoparticle for preoperative magnetic resonance imaging and intraoperative optical brain tumor delineation. Cancer Res 2003;63:8122–5.

63. Kircher MF, de la Zerda A, Jokerst JV, et al. A brain tumor molecular imaging strategy using a new triple-modality MRI-photoacoustic-Raman nanoparticle. Nat Med 2012;18(5):829–34.

64. Cho K, Wang X, Nie S, et al. Therapeutic nanoparticles for drug delivery in cancer. Clin Cancer Res 2008;14(5):1310–6.

65. Joh DY, Sun L, Stangl M, et al. Selective targeting of brain tumors with gold nanoparticle-induced radiosensitization. PLoS One 2013;8(4): e62425.

66. Schwartz JA, Shetty AM, Price RE, et al. Feasibility study of particle-assisted laser ablation of brain tumors in orthotopic canine model. Cancer Res 2009;69(4):1659–67.

ACKNOWLEDGMENTS

The authors would like to acknowledge our colleagues and teachers in neuroradiology at the University of Pennsylvania for their insights on brain tumor imaging, particularly Drs Ronald Wolf, Linda Bagley, Suyash Mohan, and John Woo.

CHAPTER 8

Principles and Tenets of Radiation Treatment in Glioblastoma

Edward W. Jung, MD[a], John Choi, MEd[b],
Samuel T. Chao, MD[c], Erin S. Murphy, MD[c],
John H. Suh, MD[c],*

STANDARD-OF-CARE RADIATION REGIMENS

Historical Context of Radiation Therapy and Dose

Historically, standard treatment for glioblastoma (GBM) was surgical resection alone. The first randomized trial to show a survival benefit with adjuvant radiation therapy (RT) was the Brain Tumor Study Group trial published in 1978, which showed a median survival of 37.5 weeks for RT alone, 25 weeks for adjuvant carmustine [1,3-bis(2-chloroethyl)-1-nitrosourea (BCNU)] chemotherapy alone, and 17 weeks for supportive care without adjuvant treatment; combination of RT plus (+) BCNU yielded a survival of 40.5 weeks.[1] In this study, whole-brain radiation therapy (WBRT) was delivered with parallel opposed fields to a dose of 50 to 60 Gy. The same group also conducted a dose-response analysis from less than 45 to 60 Gy and found improvement in median survival for doses of 50 to 60 Gy.[2] A combined Eastern Cooperative Oncology Group (ECOG)/Radiation Therapy Oncology Group (RTOG) study in 1983 compared standard 60 Gy WBRT with 3 other arms: 60 Gy WBRT + 10 Gy partial-brain RT boost, 60 Gy WBRT + BCNU, and 60 Gy WBRT + lomustine and dacarbazine.[3] This study showed no survival benefit with the 10 Gy boost and 60 Gy became the standard treatment dose with external beam RT (EBRT) for GBM.

Interstitial brachytherapy is a form of internal radiation that involves intraoperative placement of small radioactive sources into a tumor or resection cavity. Brachytherapy allows the delivery of high doses of radiation with significant dose fall-off at a short (brachy) distance to minimize damage to surrounding tissues. Early attempts at dose escalation were investigated using interstitial brachytherapy with iodine 125 (I-125) in 2 prospective randomized trials. The first randomized trial from Princess Margaret Hospital compared EBRT to 50 Gy in 2 Gy fractions versus (vs) EBRT 50 Gy + I-125 brachytherapy implant delivering an additional 60 Gy to the tumor or resection cavity.[4] This study showed no survival benefit with the brachytherapy implant, yielding a median survival of 13.2 months in the standard arm vs 13.8 months in the brachytherapy arm ($P = .49$). The Brain Tumor Cooperative Group went on to conduct the largest prospective randomized study with brachytherapy for malignant gliomas with 270 patients enrolled.[5] Patients were assigned to either EBRT (60.2 Gy in 35 fractions) + BCNU or EBRT + BCNU + I-125 implant (60 Gy). Median survival was 68.1 weeks with I-125 compared with 58.8 weeks without I-125 ($P = .101$). The lack of a statistically significant survival benefit despite large boost doses of brachytherapy, along with the logistical complexity, time factor, and operator dependence of the procedure, tempered the impetus for further investigation with

Disclosures: Varian Medical Systems (consultant), Elekta (Travel and Lodging) (J.H. Suh); Varian Medical Systems (Honorarium) (S.T. Chao).

[a] Therapeutic Radiology Associates, Hagerstown, MD, USA; [b] Johns Hopkins University School of Medicine, Baltimore, MD, USA; [c] Department of Radiation Oncology, Rose Ella Burkhardt Brain Tumor and Neuro-oncology Center, Cleveland Clinic Foundation, 9500 Euclid Avenue, Cleveland, OH 44195, USA
* Corresponding author. Department of Radiation Oncology, Rose Ella Burkhardt Brain Tumor and Neuro-oncology Center, Cleveland Clinic Foundation, T28, 9500 Euclid Avenue, Cleveland, OH 44195.
E-mail address: suhj@ccf.org

brachytherapy. Enthusiasm for brachytherapy has further waned with advances in EBRT for dose escalation, including stereotactic radiosurgery as described later in this chapter as well as heavy particle RT such as proton therapy and carbon ion therapy.

With the advent of three-dimensional (3D) conformal RT (3DCRT), the dose could be further escalated to the tumor volume with EBRT. A study from the University of Michigan examined dose escalation up to 80 Gy without dose-limiting toxicity.[6] Despite higher doses, 89% of patients developed an in-field recurrence. RTOG 8302 was a prospective phase I/II trial comparing dose escalation with hyperfractionation or accelerated hyperfractionation with BCNU. Hyperfractionation dosing included 64.8 Gy, 72 Gy, 76.8 Gy, and 81.6 Gy delivered twice daily in 1.2 Gy fractions, whereas accelerated hyperfractionation included 48 Gy and 54.4 Gy in 1.6 Gy twice-daily treatments. A preliminary report from this trial showed best survival in the 72 Gy hyperfractionation arm.[7] Subsequently, a phase III study (RTOG 9006) examined 72 Gy hyperfractionation vs 60 Gy conventional fractionation; however, there was no survival benefit to hyperfractionation.[8] Therefore, 60 Gy in 2 Gy daily fractions remains the standard of care with EBRT.

Current Standard of Care

The current standard of care for management of GBM is maximal surgical resection followed by concurrent chemoradiation therapy (chemoRT) with daily temozolomide (TMZ) to a radiation dose of 60 Gy, followed by further adjuvant TMZ. This regimen is based on level I evidence from the landmark European Organisation for Research and Treatment of Cancer (EORTC)–National Cancer Institute of Canada (NCIC) study published in 2005 by Stupp and colleagues,[9] which showed a survival benefit to chemoRT with TMZ vs adjuvant RT alone. Before this study, adjuvant RT + BCNU was considered standard of care, but no randomized phase III trial had shown a statistically significant survival benefit with RT + BCNU compared with adjuvant RT alone for GBM. RT in the EORTC-NCIC study was delivered with 3DCRT to a dose of 60 Gy in 2 Gy fractions 5 days per week with a 2-cm to 3-cm margin around the gross tumor volume. For the chemoRT arm, TMZ was administered 7 days per week at a dose of 75 mg/m² from the first day until the last day of RT. After a 4-week break, adjuvant TMZ dosed at 150 to 200 mg/m² for 5 days was administered every 28 days for 6 cycles. Because TMZ can lead to lymphocytopenia, patients were administered prophylaxis against *Pneumocystis*

carinii pneumonia with either pentamidine or trimethoprim-sulfamethoxazole. Median survival was 14.6 months with RT + TMZ and 12.1 months with RT alone, which translates to a 37% relative reduction in risk of death (P<.001). Survival at 2 years was 26.5% for RT + TMZ and 10.4% with RT alone. Tumor progression was defined as an increase in tumor size by 25%, the appearance of a new lesion, or an increased need for corticosteroids. Median progression-free survival (PFS) was 6.9 months for RT + TMZ vs 5 months for RT alone (P<.001). Only 8% of patients discontinued adjuvant TMZ because of toxic effects, and grade 3 or 4 toxicity was seen in 7% of patients in the RT + TMZ arm.

An update of the EORTC-NCIC trial reported that the long-term survival advantage with TMZ persists at 5 years follow-up.[10] Overall survival (OS) comparing RT + TMZ vs RT alone was 16% vs 4.4% at 3 years, 12.1% vs 3% at 4 years, and 9.8% vs 1.9% at 5 years, respectively (hazard ratio, 0.56; 95% confidence interval [CI], 0.47–0.66; P<.0001). Patients who had gross total resection survived longer than those with subtotal resection. The worst outcome was in patients with unresectable tumors who had undergone biopsy only. Promotor methylation of O6-methylguanine-DNA methyltransferase (MGMT) was the strongest prognostic factor and predictor for survival with TMZ, as discussed in further detail later in this chapter.

Immobilization

To minimize daily setup errors and intrafractional patient movement, creating a reproducible immobilization device is paramount to delivering an accurate RT plan. Patients should be simulated supine on a head cup or pad, with a thermoplastic mask that conforms to the patient's face for immobilization (Fig. 8.1). This position confers a daily setup error of 3 mm, which is the current standard for clinical target volume (CTV) to planning target volume (PTV) expansion when creating RT volumes. Newer technologies include an open-faced mask that uses an optical surface tracking system via camera pods to capture facial features for tracking to ensure correct patient setup. The benefit of this newer system is that it circumvents daily x-ray radiation exposure for patient alignment and potentially mitigates patient discomfort and claustrophobia compared with a standard thermoplastic mask. This technology also allows radiation oncologists to track intrafractional movement with the ability to halt RT via real-time feedback if the patient moves past a threshold (eg, 3 mm) during treatment.[11] Once the patient is immobilized, a computed tomography (CT)

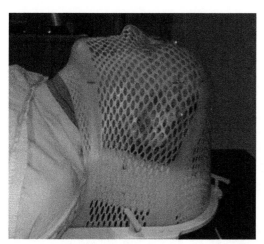

Fig. 8.1 Aquaplast mask immobilization for fractionated radiation therapy. The thermoplastic mask material conforms to the patient's face and skull, with pegs or screws that fasten to a board that is indexed on the table of the computed tomography (CT) simulator and treatment machine. The patient is immobilized daily in the same position to ensure treatment accuracy.

simulation scan is performed using 1-mm to 3-mm slice thickness from vertex to below the skull base for treatment planning.

Target Volumes

A postoperative MRI scan including T1-weighted postcontrast (T1C+) MRI and T2-weighted fluid-attenuated inversion recovery (FLAIR) MRI should be fused with the CT simulation scan to generate target volumes for radiation treatment planning. A postoperative MRI within 72 hours after surgery allows for the best assessment of the extent of residual tumor before blood and postoperative edema cloud the clinical picture. MRI performed <2 weeks before RT is ideal because further edema may cause midline shift.[12] There is also the potential for tumor regrowth from the time of surgery to RT. Although functional imaging modalities such as magnetic resonance spectroscopy (MRS) and dynamic contrast-enhanced MRI may potentially add information regarding target volume contouring and treatment planning, these modalities have not been validated and are still considered investigational. There are some differences in target volume delineation between the EORTC and the RTOG, as detailed in (Table 8.1). The main difference is that the RTOG treats the FLAIR signal hyperintensity with a margin to account for peritumoral spread from edema followed by a cone-down boost to the T1C+ MRI enhancement, whereas the EORTC treats only the T1C+ MRI volume without a boost. Regardless, both the RTOG and EORTC advocate a 2-cm volumetric 3D expansion around the gross tumor volume (GTV) visualized on T1C+ MRI to create the CTV, with a reduction in margins to respect anatomic barriers, including the skull, ventricles, falx cerebri, tentorium cerebelli, optic chiasm/nerve, and brainstem. The CTV margins are based on historical studies showing that approximately 80% of recurrences are within a 2-cm margin of the enhancement seen on T1C+

TABLE 8.1 EORTC and RTOG Target Volume Definitions	
EORTC Treatment Volumes (EORTC 22981/ 22961, 26071/22072 [Centric], 26981–22981, and AVAglio Trials)	**RTOG Treatment Volumes (RTOG 0525, 0825, 0913, and AVAglio Trials)**
Phase 1 (to 60 Gy in 30 fractions) GTV = surgical resection cavity + any residual enhancing tumor (postcontrast T1-weighted MRI scans) CTV = GTV + a margin of 2 cm[a] PTV = CTV + a margin of 3–5 mm	**Phase 1 (to 46 Gy in 23 fractions)** GTV1 = surgical resection cavity + any residual enhancing tumor (postcontrast T1-weighted MRI scans) + surrounding edema (hyperintensity on T2 or FLAIR MRI scans) CTV1 = GTV1 + a margin of 2 cm (if no surrounding edema is present, the CTV is the contrast enhancing tumor + 2.5 cm) PTV1 = CTV1 + a margin of 3–5 mm **Phase 2 (14 Gy boost in 7 fractions)** GTV2 = surgical resection cavity + any residual enhancing tumor (postcontrast T1-weighted MRI scans) CTV2 = GTV2 + a margin of 2 cm PTV2 = CTV2 + a margin of 3–5 mm

Abbreviations: CTV, clinical target volume; GTV, gross tumor volume; PTV, planning target volume.
[a] Margins up to 3 cm were allowed in 22981/22961 trial, and 1.5 cm in 26981–22981 trial.
From Niyazi M, Brada M, Chalmers AJ, et al. ESTRO-ACROP guideline "target delineation of glioblastomas". Radiother Oncol 2016;118(1):37; with permission.

MRI scans.[13–18] An additional 3-mm to 5-mm margin is added to the CTV to account for daily setup error to create the PTV. An example of target volume contouring based on RTOG guidelines is shown in **Fig. 8.2**. RTOG 0525 and CENTRIC clinical trials allowed for contouring based on either guideline and showed no difference in PFS or OS when comparing the 2

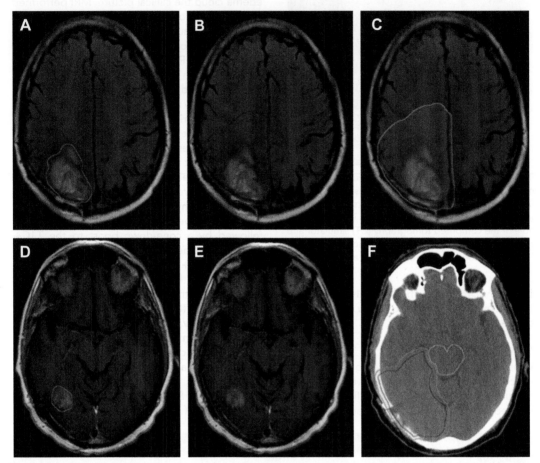

Fig. 8.2 Target volume delineation for a patient with GBM following subtotal resection. (*A*) Axial postoperative FLAIR MRI is fused with the CT simulation scan to contour the initial GTV (*red*), which is treated to 46 Gy (GTV 46). Areas of FLAIR changes are included in the GTV. (*B*) A 2-cm volumetric expansion around the GTV is used to create the CTV 46 (*blue*) to account for microscopic disease. Margins are reduced to respect anatomic barriers of tumor infiltration. In this example, the CTV does not extend to the left hemisphere, because the falx cerebri is a barrier to contralateral tumor spread. (*C*) The PTV is a 3-mm volumetric margin around the CTV to account for daily setup error. Note that the PTV 46 (*orange shaded*) extends to the contralateral hemisphere because it is not modified by barriers of tumor spread. (*D*) Postoperative T1 postcontrast MRI is fused with CT simulation scan to create the GTV boost volume (*red*), which is treated to 60 Gy (GTV 60). Area of enhancement is included in the GTV. This patient is the same as in *A–C*, but shown at a more inferior (caudal) extent of the tumor. (*E*) A 2-cm expansion around the GTV 60 is used to create the CTV 60 (*blue*), with reduced margins to respect anatomic boundaries. CTV margin is shaved off areas that extend into or are in close proximity to critical OARs. In this example, note how the CTV is shaved off the superior aspect of the right cerebellar hemisphere, because the tentorium cerebelli is a barrier to anatomic spread. As well, the CTV is shaved off the brainstem because the perimesencephalic cistern is an anatomic barrier to tumor spread. (*F*) PTV 60 (*orange shaded*) expansion for the 60 Gy boost volume shown on the CT simulation scan. The GTV 60 (*red*) and CTV 60 (*blue*) are also outlined. The brainstem is contoured (*light green*). Normally, the PTV should not be modified. However, in this situation, the PTV is shaved off the brainstem, which must be kept at less than 60 Gy point maximum dose. For institutions that incorporate a planning risk volume (PRV), there is an even greater separation between the brainstem and the juxtaposed PTV. Note that the PTV is not shaved off the right cerebellar hemisphere because it is not an OAR. In addition, note that the 3-mm CTV → PTV expansion does not appear uniform on this single CT axial slice; the reason for this is that the 3-mm expansion is a volumetric 3D expansion, as opposed to a 3-mm two-dimensional expansion on each axial slice. Hence, the CTV volumes on the superior and inferior axial CT slices contribute to the PTV volume seen on this axial CT slice.

guidelines for target volumes.[19,20] Retrospective studies comparing the EORTC and RTOG contouring guidelines also showed no difference in tumor recurrence.[14,21] In the United States, most radiation oncologists follow the RTOG guidelines, although the EORTC margins may lead to reduced toxicity with no proven disadvantage in local control or survival.

Organs at Risk

Organs at risk (OARs) to be contoured along with tolerance doses and toxicity are summarized in **Table 8.2**. Doses to OARs should be evaluated by a dose-volume histogram (DVH). Sometimes the dosimetric goals of the OARs may not be achievable because of the location and size of the PTV. In these scenarios, the radiation oncologist must make a clinical decision regarding the risks of reducing PTV coverage against the benefits of avoiding potential radiation damage to OARs. The most critical organs to avoid exceeding the tolerance dose are the brainstem, optic chiasm, and optic nerves, because of the potentially severe consequences of radiation-induced injury to these structures. Some radiation oncologists incorporate a planning risk volume (PRV) around the OARs, which is congruous to the CTV → PTV expansion, to also account for variability in daily setup for the OARs during fractionated RT.

Treatment Planning and Delivery

In the past, 3DCRT was used for partial-brain treatment planning for GBM. However, with modern treatment techniques such as intensity-modulated RT (IMRT) and volumetric intensity-modulated arc therapy (VMAT), which are now available at most radiation centers, a more conformal treatment plan can be created to deliver the prescribed treatment dose while minimizing dose to OARs. Ideally, the treatment planning goals should be the following: 95% of the PTV should receive 100% of the prescription dose (D95 = 100%) and 100% of the CTV and GTV should receive 100% of the prescription dose. Maximum plan dose (hot spots) should be ≤115% of the prescription dose. Daily image-guided RT with cone-beam CT should be aligned to the skull to maintain treatment accuracy. A treatment plan with isodose lines and DVH for a patient with GBM is shown in **Fig. 8.3**.

Prognosis

MGMT repairs DNA damage induced by alkylating agents. The MGMT gene can be silenced by methylation of its promoter, thereby preventing DNA damage repair and increasing the effectiveness of TMZ. MGMT promoter methylation is prognostic (meaning that it affects survival regardless of treatment) and also predictive for improved survival with TMZ in patients with GBM.[10,22] In the updated results of the EORTC-NCIC trial, MGMT methylation was the strongest prognostic factor for survival.[10] Methylation status of the MGMT gene promoter was determined retrospectively by methylation-specific polymerase chain reaction analysis. The 2-year OS for patients treated with RT + TMZ was 48.9% for MGMT-methylated and 14.8% for unmethylated tumors. MGMT methylation is present in approximately 45% of patients with GBM.[22]

Loss of heterozygosity on chromosome arms 1p and 19q are frequently found in oligodendrogliomas. Codeletion of 1p/19q has been associated with improved PCV (procarbazine,

---

TABLE 8.2
OARs for fractionated RT

OAR	Dose Parameter (Gy)	Toxicity
Brainstem	D_{max} <54; D1-10 cc ≤59	Permanent cranial neuropathy or necrosis
Optic nerves/chiasm	D_{max} <55	Optic neuropathy, blindness
Retina	D_{max} <45	Radiation retinopathy, decreased visual acuity
Cochlea	Mean dose ≤45	Sensory neural hearing loss
Lens	D_{max} <10	Cataract formation
Pituitary	D_{max} <50	Hypopituitarism
Lacrimal gland	D_{max} ≤40	Dry eyes
Spinal cord	D_{max} ≤50	Myelopathy

Abbreviation: D_{max}, maximum dose.
Adapted from Marks LB, Yorke ED, Jackson A, et al. Use of normal tissue complication probability models in the clinic. Int J Radiat Oncol Biol Phys 2010;76(Suppl 3):S15.

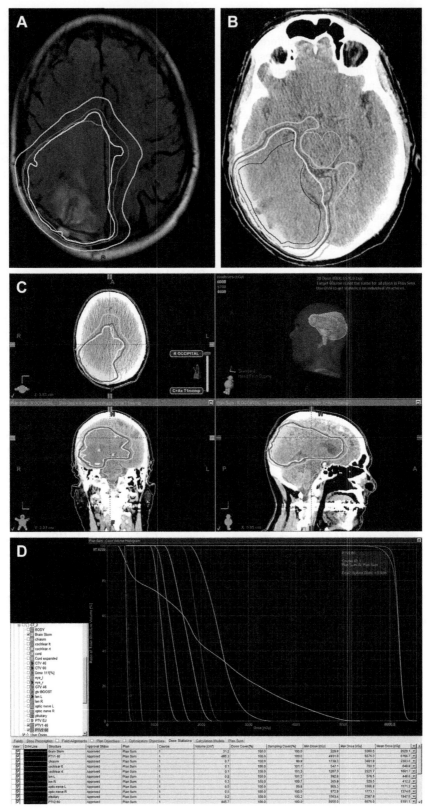

Fig. 8.3 Treatment plan and DVH. VMAT treatment plan with isodose lines and DVH for the patient shown in **Fig. 8.2.** (A) PTV 46 *(orange shaded)* with isodose lines shown. Isodose lines: light blue, 46 Gy; red, 54 Gy; yellow,

lomustine, and vincristine) chemosensitivity in grade III gliomas with a trend for improved PFS and OS.[23,24] However, codeletion of 1p/19q is rare in GBM, presenting in approximately 5% of cases.[25] An oligodendroglioma-like component (GBM-O) was seen in 15% of 339 patients with GBM, but was not found to have prognostic significance.[26]

Recursive partitioning analysis (RPA) classification for malignant gliomas was developed to categorize patients based on factors that could affect survival and prognosis. The EORTC and RTOG have both developed RPA classifications, as detailed in **Table 8.3**.[27,28] Of note, the RTOG classification also includes anaplastic astrocytomas, whereas the EORTC RPA only includes GBM. There are also some differences in performance status and neurologic functioning assessment. Survival data by RPA class from the phase II and phase III EORTC trials along with the RTOG database are compared in **Table 8.4**. The EORTC RPA classification retains prognostic significance in patients receiving RT + TMZ and patients treated with RT alone for GBM. RPA is predictive of survival with TMZ in class III ($P = .006$) and class IV ($P = .0001$) patients, with a trend for survival prediction in class V patients ($P = .054$).[28] In summary, RPA classification is an important tool for assessing survival outcomes and should be used as a guide to discuss prognosis for patients with GBM.

Management of Elderly Patients

In patients more than 70 years old with good performance status and in otherwise good overall health, standard of care remains maximal surgical resection followed by concurrent chemoRT and adjuvant TMZ. In the landmark EORTC-NCIC study, median OS was similar (10.9 vs 11.8 months) when comparing RT + TMZ vs RT alone for patients 60 to 70 years old. However, there was a statistically significant advantage in OS with TMZ when comparing OS at 2 years (21.8% vs 5.7%) and 5 years (6.6% vs 0%). Note that older patients who are not in good health or with poor Karnofsky performance status (KPS) may not be able to tolerate RT + TMZ, and the risks of toxicity in these patients should be weighed against the

potential for improved survival. For these patients, alternative treatments include hypofractionated RT with concurrent chemotherapy, RT alone, or chemotherapy alone. This section will focus specifically on radiation therapy and modifications in dosing and fractionation for elderly patients who may not be able to tolerate the standard regimen.

A phase II trial of 71 patients with age ≥ 70 years and KPS $\geq$ to 60 was designed to evaluate the efficacy and safety of concurrent and adjuvant TMZ with short-course RT (40 Gy in 2.66 Gy fractions).[29] Median and 1-year OS were 12.4 months and 58%, respectively. Median and 1-year PFS were 6 months and 20%, respectively. All patients completed RT. TMZ was discontinued because of toxicity in 6 patients (8%). Health-related quality of life was maintained until the time of disease progression in most patients.[30] Subsequently, the same group retrospectively reviewed patients with age ≥ 65 years and KPS ≥ 60 who received concurrent and adjuvant TMZ with standard RT (60 Gy) vs short-course RT (40 Gy).[31] CTV was defined as a 2-cm expansion around the T1C+ MRI enhancement while respecting anatomic boundaries, with a 3-mm to 4-mm margin for PTV. Standard RT was administered in 1.8 Gy to 2 Gy fractions to a dose of 59.4 to 60 Gy without a cone-down boost, and short course was treated at 2.66 Gy for 15 fractions to a dose of 40 Gy. Median OS and PFS were similar: 12 months and 5.6 months for standard RT vs 12.5 months and 6.7 months for short-course RT, respectively. MGMT methylation was the most favorable prognostic factor ($P = .0001$). Standard RT was associated with higher rates of grade 2 and 3 neurotoxicity ($P = .01$), worsening KPS after treatment ($P = .01$), and higher doses of corticosteroids ($P = .02$). The investigators concluded that short-course RT is an effective alternative in older patients that yields similar survival and reduced toxicity compared with conventional RT for GBM. Standard RT vs short-course RT with TMZ is currently being investigated prospectively in a phase III trial (NCT00482677).

RT alone is an effective alternative in older patients with poor performance status and may be preferable to TMZ alone, especially for

---

60 Gy. (B) PTV 60 (*orange shaded*). Sometimes the PTV needs to be undercovered to protect a critical OAR, such as the brainstem in this case. (C) PTV 60 with isodose lines on multiple CT simulation scan views. Clockwise from upper left image: axial, 3D reconstruction, sagittal, and coronal views. (D) DVH. X-axis: dose in centigray (cGy). Y-axis: percent volume. The DVH is used to evaluate dose delivered to the GTV, CTV, PTV, and OARs. The GTV and CTV should receive 100% of the prescription dose. At least 95% of the PTV should receive 100% of the prescription dose. As shown in this example, with crosshairs placed on 6000 cGy (60 Gy), more than 95% of the PTV 60 is covered by 100% of the prescription dose (60 Gy).

TABLE 8.3
RTOG and EORTC RPA classification

	RTOG (Original)	EORTC (Adapted)
RPA Class III		
Age (y)	<50	<50
Tumor Type	Anaplastic astrocytomas	GBM
Mental Status	Abnormal	—
Performance Status	—	WHO PS 0
Or		
Age (y)	<50	—
Tumor Type	GBM	—
Performance Status	KPS 90–100	—
RPA Class IV		
Age (y)	<50	<50
Tumor Type	GBM	GBM
Performance Status	KPS <90	WHO PS 1–2
Or		
Age (y)	≥50	≥50
Tumor Type	Anaplastic astrocytomas	GBM
Performance Status	KPS 70–100	—
Treatment Status	≤3 from time of first symptom to start of treatment	Complete/partial surgery
Mental Status	—	MMSE ≥27
Or		
Age (y)	≥50	—
Tumor Type	GBM	—
Mental Status	Good neurologic function	—
Treatment Status	Surgical resection	—
RPA Class V		
Age (y)	≥50	≥50
Tumor Type	GBM	GBM
Performance Status	KPS 70–100	—
Mental Status	Neurologic function that inhibits the ability to work	MMSE <27
Treatment Status	Surgical resection or biopsy only followed by at least 54.4 Gy radiotherapy	Biopsy only
Or		
Age (y)	≥50	—
Tumor Type	GBM	—
Performance Status	KPS <70	—
Mental Status	Normal	—

Abbreviations: KPS, Karnofsky performance status; MMSE, Mini-Mental Status Examination; PS, performance status.
From Mirimanoff RO, Gorlia T, Mason W, et al. Radiotherapy and temozolomide for newly diagnosed glioblastoma: recursive partitioning analysis of the EORTC 26981/22981-NCIC CE3 phase III randomized trial. J Clin Oncol 2006;24(16):2564; with permission.

TABLE 8.4
Comparison of survival data by RPA class from the RTOG database and 2 EORTC trials with TMZ

RPA Class	Phase II Survival with RT/TMZ[15]		Phase III Survival[a,18]		RTOG Database[4,5]	
	Median (months)	2-y (%)	Median (months)	2-y (%)	Median (months)	2-y (%)
III	24+	51	21.4	43.4	17.9	35
IV	13.8	32	16.3	27.9	11.1	15
V	9.2	0	10.3	16.5	8.9	6

[a] EORTC 26981/22981-NCIC CE3 study, RT/TMZ arm.
From Mirimanoff RO, Gorlia T, Mason W, et al. Radiotherapy and temozolomide for newly diagnosed glioblastoma: recursive partitioning analysis of the EORTC 26981/22981-NCIC CE3 phase III randomized trial. J Clin Oncol 2006;24(16):2568; with permission.

MGMT-unmethylated tumors. A retrospective study comparing hypofractionated RT with or without concurrent and adjuvant TMZ for age >70 years was conducted and showed no survival benefit with the addition of TMZ.[32] Median OS was actually higher in the RT-alone patients (9.3 vs 6.9 months), although it was not statistically significant (P = .351). On subgroup analysis of the RT-alone group, patients salvaged with TMZ for disease progression had increased OS of 13.3 months compared with 5.7 months with no further treatment (P = .012). This study suggests that concurrent TMZ does not confer survival benefit in patients >70 years of age and that a sequential approach of hypofractionated RT alone followed by TMZ for salvage may be a more effective strategy.

A prospective trial of 81 elderly patients randomly assigned to receive RT alone vs supportive care alone after undergoing surgery showed median survival of 29.1 weeks and 16.9 weeks, respectively.[33] Biopsy alone was performed in half (42 of 81) of the patients. Median PFS was 14.9 weeks with RT vs 5.4 weeks with supportive care. Fractionated RT was delivered at 1.8 Gy per fraction to a total dose of 50.4 Gy. CTV was defined as a 2-cm margin around the enhancement seen on T1C+ MRI. There was no impairment of quality of life or cognitive function with RT.

A prospective randomized comparison of hypofractionated RT vs standard RT alone in 100 patients ≥60 years old showed no difference in OS (5.6 vs 5.1 months; P = .57).[34] However, more patients receiving standard RT required a post-treatment increase in dexamethasone dose (49%) vs hypofractionated RT patients (23%), (P = .02). Recognizing the reduced treatment time and lower dexamethasone requirement with hypofractionated RT in the setting of equivalent OS, the investigators advocate hypofractionated RT in older patients with GBM who are not

good candidates for combined treatment with TMZ. In a subsequent prospective randomized trial by the same group, an even more hypofractionated course of RT (25 Gy in 5 fractions) was compared with 40 Gy in 15 fractions.[35] The study included elderly (≥65 years old) and frail patients (age ≥50 years and KPS 50–70). The 25 Gy short-course arm was non-inferior to the 40 Gy arm with median OS of 7.9 vs 6.4 months (P = .988). There was no difference in quality of life between the two arms. As such, this study supports an even shorter hypofractionated course for elderly patients with poor KPS.

There are 2 major randomized prospective trials that examined the efficacy of RT alone compared with TMZ alone for older patients: the Methusalem (NOA-8) trial and the Nordic Clinical Brain Tumor Study Group trial.[36,37] The NOA-8 trial compared TMZ alone vs standard fractionation RT alone to 60 Gy with a 2-cm margin around the GTV with no boost.[36] There was no difference in OS between the two groups (8.6 months for TMZ vs 9.6 months for RT). Event-free survival was longer in patients with MGMT methylation who received TMZ than in those who underwent RT alone (8.4 months [95% CI, 5.5–11.7] vs 4.6 months [95% CI, 4.2–5.0]), whereas the opposite was true for patients with unmethylated MGMT (3.3 months [95% CI, 3.0–3.5] with TMZ vs 4.6 months with RT [95% CI, 3.7–6.3]). This study suggests that MGMT methylation status may help with clinical decision making in patients undergoing single-modality therapy for GBM when deciding between chemotherapy vs RT alone. Notably, MGMT methylation was associated with longer survival regardless of treatment, and TMZ was associated with more grade 3 or 4 hematologic toxicity compared with RT alone.

The Nordic trial randomly assigned patients with median age 70 years to 3 arms: TMZ alone, standard RT (60 Gy), and hypofractionated RT

(34 Gy in 10 fractions).[37] This study found that although TMZ resulted in significantly improved median OS compared with standard RT (8.3 vs 6 months; $P = .01$), TMZ showed no survival advantage compared with hypofractionated RT (7.5 months; $P = .24$). MGMT methylation was associated with improved survival for patients receiving TMZ (9.7 vs 6.8 months; $P = .02$), but MGMT methylation status did not affect survival in patients receiving RT in either arm. The results of these two trials are conflicting, and further study using a more common hypofractionated regimen (40 Gy in 15 fractions) compared with standard TMZ dosing is warranted to further investigate the efficacy of single-modality treatment in elderly patients.

Patients with GBM older than 65 years have worse prognosis compared with younger patients.[38,39] RPA classification of more than 700 patients with GBM ≥70 years of age demonstrated 4 prognostic groups (Table 8.5).[40] MGMT methylation is present in approximately 58% of patients with GBM over 70 years of age, and the prognostic and predictive values have been reported in elderly patients.[41–43] Acknowledging that single-modality therapy is better tolerated than chemoRT, MGMT methylation status may guide selection between TMZ vs RT alone for older patients.

Stereotactic Radiosurgery

Stereotactic radiosurgery (SRS) is an RT technique that is available at many radiation oncology facilities and allows physicians to administer large doses of RT in one or a few treatments with high conformity and steep dose fall-off outside the target to spare normal tissues. Treatment platforms include Gamma Knife radiosurgery (GKRS) and linear accelerator (LINAC)–based radiosurgery. GKRS consists of 192 or 201 cobalt-60 sources with a helmet over a fixed frame with 4 screws attached to the patient's skull for immobilization. The latest Leksell GKRS unit (Icon) now allows for a thermoplastic mask–based system without screws. LINAC-based radiosurgery uses a standard RT linear accelerator that generates photon beams to deliver conformal SRS. LINAC SRS can involve a rigid head frame or a mask that conforms to the patient's skull and face. Several newer immobilization technologies have emerged for LINAC SRS, including infrared sensors that can be attached either to the surface of the mask or a bite block, as well as frameless immobilization that uses a series of cameras to detect facial structures to verify patient positioning before and during treatment.

RTOG 9305 is the only level I study to assess the efficacy of SRS for GBM. Patients were randomly assigned to chemoRT with BCNU to 60 Gy vs SRS boost (15–24 Gy) followed by chemoRT with BCNU to 60 Gy.[44] Patients who had gross total resection (GTR) were not eligible for the trial. This trial turned out to be a negative study because there was no difference in median survival between the two groups (13.6 months with no SRS vs 13.5 months with SRS) and no difference in 2-year or 3-year survival rates. Quality of life and cognitive decline were comparable. RTOG 0023 was a phase II trial of 76 patients treated with fractionated RT to 50 Gy with weekly fractionated stereotactic radiotherapy boost (5 or 7 Gy for 4 treatments) to a total cumulative dose of 70 to 78 Gy.[45] BCNU chemotherapy was given adjuvantly after RT. Median survival was 12.5 months and no survival benefit was seen compared with the historical RTOG database. One patient developed radionecrosis and 11 patients experienced grade 3 neurologic toxicity. There was a trend for improved survival in patients who had GTR and underwent stereotactic boost compared with historical RTOG controls.

There have been several single-institution and retrospective SRS studies (some of which include TMZ) that showed promising survival rates after treatment. These studies are summarized in Table 8.6.[44–56] Although the 2 major RTOG trials for SRS in GBM failed to show benefit, examination of SRS boost with TMZ in a prospective trial may be warranted. Other areas of potential investigation include a rethinking of the tumor volume treated with SRS for GBM. Leading-edge SRS treats a volume of predictive likelihood of relapse along with the T1C+ MRI enhancement, which can be aided with multiparametric MRI and other

TABLE 8.5
RPA classification for patients with GBM ≥70 years old

RPA Subgroup	Surgery	Age (y)	KPS	Median OS (mo)
I	GTR or STR	<75.5	Any	8.5
II	GTR or STR	≥75.5	Any	7.7
III	Biopsy	Any	≥70	4.3
IV	Biopsy	Any	<70	3.1

Abbreviations: GTR, gross total resection; STR, subtotal resection.
Data from Scott JG, Bauchet L, Fraum TJ, et al. Recursive partitioning analysis of prognostic factors for glioblastoma patients aged 70 years or older. Cancer 2012;118(22): 5595–600.

TABLE 8.6
SRS for treatment of newly diagnosed GBM

Author	N	SRS Modality	Radiation Dose (Range)	Surgical Resection Extent	Survival Rate	Median OS (mo)	Toxicity
Souhami et al,[44] 2004	89	GKRS or LINAC	15–24 Gy SRS + 60 Gy RT + BCNU	GTR not eligible	2-y OS, 21%; 3-y OS, 9%	13.5	Neurologic grade 1, 3 patients; grade 2, 6 patients; grade 3, 3 patients
Cardinale et al,[45] 2006	76	LINAC	50 Gy RT + (5–7 Gy × 4 FSRS) + BCNU	Biopsy (24%), STR (35%), GTR (41%)	22 mo OS, 17%	12.5	1 patient (1%) developed radionecrosis; 11 patients (14%) with grade 3 neurologic toxicity
Sarkaria et al,[46] 1995	115	LINAC	54–60 Gy RT + 12 Gy (6–20) SRS	Biopsy (44%), STR (53%), GTR (3%)	2-y OS, 45%; 2-y OS for KPS ≥70, 51%; 2-y OS for KPS <70, 0%	NR	19 out of 115 (16%) patients experienced complications from radiosurgery: 17 patients with radiation necrosis, 1 patient with hemiparesis, 1 patient with double vision and hydrocephalus requiring ventricular shunt. 47% of patients required prolonged steroid use
Gannett et al,[47] 1995	30	LINAC	44–62 Gy RT + 10 Gy (0.5–18) SRS	Biopsy (10%), STR (60%), GTR (30%)	1-y DSS, 57%; 2-y DSS, 25%	13.9	No significant acute or late toxicity; no documented occurrence of symptomatic radiation necrosis. All patients were managed with oral steroids for prophylaxis
Masciopinto et al,[48] 1995	31	LINAC	50–66 Gy RT + 10–20 Gy SRS	Biopsy (11%), tumor debulking (65%)	1-y OS, 37%	9.5	NR
Mehta et al,[49] 1994	31	LINAC	54 Gy RT + 12 Gy (10–20) SRS	Biopsy (39%), STR (55%), near-total resection (6%)	1-y OS, 38%; 2-y OS, 28%	10.5	NR
Nwokedi et al,[50] 2002	33 RT alone; 31 RT + SRS	GKRS	59.7 Gy (28–80) RT + 17.1 Gy (10–28) SRS	Biopsy (30%), maximal safe resection (70%)	For all patients: 1-y OS, 67%; 2-y OS, 40%; 3 y OS, 26%	RT alone, 13; RT + SRS, 25	No patients experienced acute grade 3–4 toxicity that could be attributed to radiotherapy alone; of the patients who received RT + SRS, 2 patients (7%) developed radiation necrosis

(continued on next page)

TABLE 8.6 (continued)

Author	N	SRS Modality	Radiation Dose (Range)	Surgical Resection Extent	Survival Rate	Median OS (mo)	Toxicity
Balducci et al,[51] 2010	41 (36 GBM, 5 AA)	LINAC	59.4 Gy or 50.4 Gy RT + 10 or 19 Gy SRS + TMZ	STR (68%), GTR (32%)	2-y OS, 63%	All patients, 30; GBM, 28	12% of patients experienced G1–2 neurologic acute toxicity such as headache, confusion and seizures. G3 toxicity was observed in 1 patient. Hematologic acute toxicity G1–2 was observed in 2% of patients. During adjuvant chemotherapy, 10% of patients experienced G2 hematologic toxicity and G3 toxicity was seen in 7% of patients. Late neurologic toxicity included 2 cases (4.8%) of radionecrosis
Cardinale et al,[52] 1998	12 (9 GBM, 3 AA)	LINAC	44 Gy RT + 36 Gy SRS	Biopsy (17%), STR (83%)	NR	GBM, 16; AA, 33	1 patient required an increase in steroid dose because of headache and neurologic progression. 1 patient with a history of seizures had a seizure 5 wk after completion of radiation with significant edema that was then managed with steroid therapy. Another patient developed new seizures 6 mo after treatment. 4 patients (33%) were diagnosed with radionecrosis
Shrieve et al,[53] 1999	78	LINAC	12 Gy (6–24) SRS	Stereotactic biopsy (27%), STR (64%), GTR (9%)	1-y OS, 88.5%; 2-y OS, 35.9%	19.9	Acute toxicity following SRS showed exacerbation of existing symptoms (eg, seizure activity, aphasia, or paresis). 50% had reoperation for symptomatic necrosis or recurrent tumor. Rate of reoperation at 24 mo after SRS was 54.8%

Study	n	Technique	Dose	Resection	Survival		Toxicity
Floyd et al,[54] 2012	20	CyberKnife	40 Gy RT + SRS (lesions <2 cm, 22 Gy; 2.1–3.0 cm, 18 Gy; 3.1–4.1 cm, 15 Gy; >4.1 cm, 8 Gy) + TMZ	Biopsy (35%), STR (15%), GTR (50%)	NR	13	All patients experienced fatigue and skin reactions (erythema and alopecia) without requiring further treatment (grade I). 4 patients required prolonged dexamethasone for symptomatic cerebral edema, which eventually resolved in all but 2 patients (20% grade II toxicity). Overall, 4 patients (20%) experienced grade III toxicity
Landy et al,[55] 2004	23	GKRS	Estramustine + SRS (tumor maximum diameter ≤20 mm, 21 Gy; 21–30 mm, 18 Gy; 31–40 mm, 15 Gy) + 72 Gy RT for new tumors	NR	2-y OS, 38%	16	7 patients (30%) experienced moderate nausea, with emesis in 4 of these patients (17%). 4 other patients (17%) developed DVT and 1 patient experienced vaginal bleeding
Omuro et al,[56] 2014	40	LINAC	6 Gy × 6 or 4 Gy × 6 FSRS + TMZ + bevacizumab	STR or biopsy (75%), GTR (25%)	1-y OS, 93%	19	1 patient (2.5%) developed grade 4 surgical wound infection without dehiscence; 2 patients (5%) had grade 4 pulmonary embolisms and 1 experienced a late ischemic stroke. 1 patient (2.5%) had a history of difficult to control seizures and died suddenly during sleep while on treatment. 2 patients (5%) had CNS bleeding, both grade 1 and asymptomatic

Abbreviations: AA, anaplastic astrocytoma; CNS, central nervous system; DSS, disease-specific survival; DVT, deep vein thrombosis; FSRS, fractionated stereotactic radiosurgery; RT, radiation therapy.

Adapted from Redmond KJ, Mehta M. Stereotactic Radiosurgery for Glioblastoma. Cureus 2015;7(12):e413.

imaging modalities such as PET.[57] It would also be interesting to evaluate the benefit of SRS boost specifically for unresectable (biopsy alone) cases. Dose escalation with SRS boost for patients with unresectable GBM may provide improved tumor control compared with fractionated RT, analogous to how lung SBRT (stereotactic body radiation therapy) has now become the standard of care for early-stage unresectable lung tumors.

REIRRADIATION FOR RECURRENT GLIOMAS

Because of the aggressiveness of the disease, GBM has high rates of recurrence and disease progression. Historical data suggest median PFS of 6.9 months after treatment with current standard of care.[9] Because of this, there is ongoing multidisciplinary investigation to improve outcomes in the setting of disease recurrence or tumor progression. This chapter focuses specifically on current developments in radiation oncology. Innovative treatment strategies such as gene therapy, vaccines, low-intensity alternating electric fields (Novocure), and novel chemosensitizers are discussed in other chapters.

Stereotactic Radiosurgery for Recurrent Glioblastoma

SRS for treatment of recurrent GBM has been evaluated in small prospective and retrospective studies, as outlined in **Table 8.7**.[58–77] A phase II trial on border zone SRS with bevacizumab (Avastin) for recurrent GBM is underway.[78] Border zone SRS is defined as treating a 2-cm margin around the T2 FLAIR signal intensity to cover potential areas of tumor spread with SRS.

Pulsed Reduced-Dose-Rate Radiation Therapy

Pulsed reduced-dose-rate RT (PRDR) is a radiation treatment method that has been developed for reirradiation settings. In PRDR, fractionated RT is still administered daily at 2 Gy, but in a series of ten 0.2 Gy pulses separated by 3-minute time intervals; this creates an apparent dose rate of 0.0667 Gy/min.[79] In contrast, 2 Gy of conventional RT is delivered at a dose rate of 4 to 6 Gy/min. Thus, PRDR can increase daily treatment times up to 45 minutes compared with conventional fractionated RT, which is typically around 10 minutes daily using IMRT. PRDR improves the therapeutic ratio by reducing toxic effects and increasing therapeutic effects of radiation. By lengthening the time of delivery of daily radiation, PRDR can reduce normal tissue toxicity compared with standard dose rates by allowing normal cell repair to be active during RT. PRDR can improve tumor cell kill via the inverse dose-rate effect, which is a paradoxic increase in cell kill at a low dose rate by radiating tumor cells in radiosensitive phases of the cell cycle. This inverse dose-rate effect on human GBM cell lines has been shown at 37 cGy/h, which is thought to be related to the blockade of cycling cells in G2M.[80] RT kills tumor cells by inducing double-stranded breaks in the DNA. Cells in the G2M phase are more sensitive to DNA damage than in G1 or S phase, which allows increased tumor cell death during ongoing continuous low-dose-rate irradiation.

The efficacy of PRDR on GBM has been studied in murine models. A comparison of standard dose rate vs PRDR at Beaumont Hospital (Royal Oak, MI) was performed in nude mice with GBM tumor implantation.[81] Animals received WBRT with either daily 2 Gy fractions delivered continuously over 8 minutes or with PRDR in a series of ten 0.2 Gy pulses separated by 3-minute intervals over a total of 38 minutes. A significant difference ($P = .049$) in median survival was observed when comparing the standard dose rate (29 ± 1.8 days) vs PRDR (34.2 ± 1.9 days) in mice treated to a total dose of 30 Gy with WBRT. Compared with the standard dose rate, PRDR resulted in a 53% reduction in normalized tumor volume ($P = .01$) and a 70% reduction in tumor growth rate ($P<.01$) as assessed with micro-PET/CT imaging. When comparing the effects on normal tissue, the standard dose rate resulted in a 28% increase ($P = .05$) in neuron degeneration in the surrounding normal brain parenchyma, thus highlighting the significant benefit in normal tissue toxicity with PRDR. Note that the standard dose rate resulted in 40% ($P = .05$) reduction in tumor vascular density compared with PRDR, with no difference in vascular density between PRDR and untreated mice. Preserving tumor vasculature may enhance the ionizing effects of irradiation by increasing the amount of substrate for free radical formation. Moreover, preserved tumor vasculature after PRDR suggests that antivascular agents such as bevacizumab may provide greater benefit if given adjuvantly after PRDR.

Most of the clinical investigation with PRDR for recurrent GBM in humans has been performed at the University of Wisconsin. A study of 103 patients with recurrent gliomas, 86 of which were grade 4 at the time of recurrence, demonstrated the safety and efficacy of PRDR for salvage treatment.[82] All patients had been previously treated with the standard dose rate to 59.4 Gy. Median interval from initial treatment to salvage PRDR therapy was 18.2 months (range, 2–227.6 months). Median PRDR retreatment dose was 50 Gy, with a goal of 54 Gy once the investigators' experience

TABLE 8.7
SRS for recurrent GBM

Author	N	Modality	SRS Dose (Range)	Median OS (mo)	Toxicity
Shrieve et al,[58] 1995	118 (86 SRS alone, 32 brachytherapy alone)	LINAC	13 Gy (6–20) SRS	10.2 (SRS)	1 patient (1%) developed *P carinii* pneumonia 1 mo after SRS, most likely from steroid treatment. 3 patients (3%) with a history of seizures experienced seizures within 24 h of treatment. 1 patient (1%) had acute herniation secondary to edema and died. 1 patient (1%) developed hydrocephalus and required a ventricular shunt. 2 patients (2%) had transient aphasia. 2 patients (2%) developed transient motor deficits
Vordermark et al,[59] 2005	19 (14 GBM, 5 AA)	LINAC	45–61 Gy RT + 30 Gy (20–30) SRS	9.3	No acute neurotoxicity or deterioration in general health status
Lederman et al,[60] 1997	23 (9 SRS alone, 14 SRS + Taxol)	LINAC	60 Gy RT + (SRS alone, 20 Gy [9–25]; SRS + Taxol, 6 Gy [4.5–9.0])	SRS alone, 6.3; SRS + Taxol, 14.2	Minimal toxicity without neuropathy, nausea, vomiting, diarrhea, stomatitis, myalgia, arthralgia, or seizures. 1 patient (7%) developed a pruritic eruption. In 3 patients (21%), resected tissue revealed radionecrosis. In 1 patient (7%), both radiation necrosis and tumor were present
Combs et al,[61] 2005	32	LINAC	54 Gy (40–64) RT + 15 Gy (10–20) SRS	10	27 patients (84%) presented with neurologic symptoms, including headache, seizures, nausea, vomiting, and motor and sensory deficits
Fogh et al,[62] 2010	147	LINAC	60 Gy RT + 35 Gy (28–80) SRS	11	1 late grade 3 CNS toxicity 4 mo after hypofractionated SRS
Maranzano et al,[63] 2011	22	LINAC	17 Gy SRS or 30 Gy FSRS	11	No acute toxicity of more than grade II. 4 patients (18%) experienced headache and nausea/vomiting. Only FSRS patients presented with skin erythema and alopecia, all of which were self-limiting. 3 of 13 patients (23%) with SRS developed brain radionecrosis
Greenspoon et al,[64] 2014	31	LINAC	25–30 Gy or 30–35 Gy FSRS depending on size of PTV + TMZ	9	Acute grade 3 CNS necrosis was seen in 3 patients (10%). 1 patient (3%) experienced an acute grade 4 CNS necrosis

(continued on next page)

TABLE 8.7
(continued)

Author	N	Modality	SRS Dose (Range)	Median OS (mo)	Toxicity
Hudes et al,[65] 1999	20 (19 GBM, 1 AA)	LINAC	5 lesions, 24 Gy/3 Gy fractions SRS; 10 lesions, 30 Gy/3 Gy fractions SRS; 9 lesions, 35 Gy/3.5 Gy fractions SRS; 1 lesion, 21 Gy/3 Gy fractions SRS	20	Grade 2 toxicities: 2 patients experienced headaches (10%) and 1 patient (5%) tinnitus/hearing loss. Transient increase of steroids was required in these 2 patients. These toxicities occurred within 8 wk after treatment
Lederman et al,[66] 2000	88	LINAC	Paclitaxel + 6 Gy (4.5–9) SRS weekly	7	2 patients (2%) experienced a pruritic rash and another 2 patients (2%) experienced both radiation necrosis and tumor
Cuneo et al,[67] 2012	63 (WHO grade 3, 14; WHO grade 4, 49)	LINAC	15 Gy (12.5–25) SRS + bevacizumab	WHO grade 4 glioma, 5.2	32% of patients experienced acute grade 2 toxicity, whereas 11% of patients experienced grade 3 toxicity. 1 patient died 2 wk after salvage SRS. 25% of all patients treated reported worsening of preexisting neurologic symptoms; these side effects were managed with dexamethasone. 21% of patients had increased seizure frequency within 3 mo of receiving SRS, although there were no new onsets of seizures. Radionecrosis was found in 10% of patients who received salvage SRS
Minniti et al,[68] 2013	54	LINAC	30 Gy SRS + TMZ	12.4	4 patients (7%) experienced grade 3 neurologic deterioration. Hematologic toxicities during continuous dose-intense TMZ were observed in 14 patients (26%), with 10 patients (19%) experiencing grade 3 or 4 lymphopenia, 2 patients (4%) experiencing grade 3 thrombocytopenia, and 2 patients (4%) experiencing grade 3 leukopenia. 11 patients (20%) experienced grade 2 or 3 fatigue, 2 patients (4%) experienced headache, and nausea/vomiting occurred in 4 patients (8%)
Skeie et al,[69] 2012	77 (51 SRS, 26 reoperation only)	GKRS	39–60 Gy RT + 12.2 Gy (8–20) SRS	SRS, 12; reoperation only, 6	5 patients (10%) had increasing edema. 1 of 7 patients (14%) with a second GKRS treatment had a transient worsening of neurologic function

Study	No. of patients	Modality	Dose	Survival (mo)	Toxicity/outcomes
Park et al,[70] 2012	55 (11 SRS + bevacizumab, 44 SRS alone)	GKRS	16 Gy (13–18) SRS	SRS + bevacizumab, 17.9; SRS alone, 12.2	4 patients (37%) developed mild (grade I or II) toxicity. 2 patients (18%) developed diarrhea (grade I and II, respectively), 2 patients (18%) developed a grade II hypertension, and 1 (9%) showed grade II lymphocytopenia. All of these toxicities were transient. 1 patient (9%) experienced grade III toxicity after treatment, including fatigue and lymphopenia. Another patient (9%) developed new neurologic symptoms, including hemiparesis and regional edema
Koga et al,[71] 2012	18 (9 conventional SRS, 9 extended-field SRS)	GKRS	20 Gy conventional SRS; 20 Gy extended-field SRS	Conventional SRS, 10.5; extended-field SRS, 9	Radiation necrosis was observed in 4 lesions in 4 patients (29%). 5 patients (28%) experienced steroid-related toxicities
Elliott et al,[72] 2011	26	GKRS	15 Gy (10–18) SRS	13	4 patients (25%) had fixed hemiparesis (mild in 2 and moderate in 2) after resection. 2 patients (12%) had fixed homonymous hemianopia and 1 patient (6%) had mild expressive aphasia. One patient (6%) had moderate hemiparesis, homonymous hemianopsia and mild receptive aphasia
Pouratian et al,[73] 2009	48	GKRS	6 Gy (3–15) SRS	9.4	No significant acute toxicities or recorded radiation necrosis attributed to GKRS therapy
Kida et al,[74] 2009	172 astrocytoma cases (25 GI, 52 GII, 41 GIII, 54 GIV)	GKRS	GII to GIV tumors treated with 15 Gy SRS	14	Perifocal edema and neurologic deterioration
Kong et al,[75] 2008	114	GKRS	16 Gy (12–50) SRS	13	22 patients (24%) experienced radiation necrosis induced by SRS
Kohshi et al,[76] 2008	25 (11 GBM, 14 AA)	GKRS	22 Gy (18–27) SRS	11	After FSRS treatment, 7 patients (27%) had signs of radionecrosis or tumor progression
Hsieh et al,[77] 2005	51	GKRS	12 Gy SRS	10	16 patients (62%) experienced radionecrosis. 1 patient (4%) had a sarcoma associated with radiation changes

Abbreviations: AA, anaplastic astrocytoma; FSRS, fractionated stereotactic radiosurgery; GI, grade I; GII, grade II; GIII, grade III; GIV, grade IV; Gy, gray; RT, radiation therapy.
Adapted from Redmond KJ, Mehta M. Stereotactic radiosurgery for glioblastoma. Cureus 2015;7(12):e413.

with PRDR increased. Tumor volumes were contoured with a 2-cm margin around T2 FLAIR or T2-weighted MRI signal intensity to create the PTV. In the absence of T2-weighted imaging, a 2.5-cm margin around the T1C+ MRI enhancement was used. Dose constraints were determined from the PRDR plan only, irrespective of the initial RT plan. The lens and cervical spine were shielded from the direct beam at all times. OAR dose limits were as follows: the retreatment dose to the optic chiasm <54 Gy, the retina of at least one eye <50 Gy, and the brainstem <54 Gy. No patient discontinued treatment because of radiation toxicity, and no patient became blind from treatment. A total of 15 patients underwent autopsy of the brain, and 4 had notable necrosis. One patient had also been treated previously with SRS to 12 Gy. Three patients underwent post-PRDR subtotal resection for progressive disease with the pathologic findings revealing progressive disease without treatment-related necrosis. The 6-month and 1-year actuarial survival rate was 34.8% and 4.4% respectively for patients with grade 4 tumors, with median survival of 5.1 months (range, 1–48.4 months). KPS at initiation of PRDR was an important factor for survival, because patients with KPS ≥70 had better survival compared with patients with KPS <70 (2.4 vs 6 months; P<.0001).

A more recent study published in 2014 reviewed 23 patients treated with PRDR for disease progression during bevacizumab therapy for recurrent GBM.[83] All patients had undergone maximal safe resection followed by chemoRT with TMZ to a dose of 59.4 to 60 Gy followed by adjuvant TMZ as per the EORTC-NCIC trial. At the time of recurrence, patients were administered bevacizumab 10 mg/kg every 2 weeks until disease progression. Patients were treated with PRDR within 14 days after progression on bevacizumab. During reirradiation, bevacizumab (10 mg/kg) was given every 4 weeks for 2 cycles to minimize edema and radiation necrosis. There were no grade 3 or 4 toxicities. Median survival was 6.9 months, which was an improvement compared with the investigators' literature review of 16 phase II trials with median survival of 3.8 months after bevacizumab failure. Although further investigation is needed, PRDR may play an important role as salvage therapy after bevacizumab failure with the potential to prolong survival.

In conclusion, PRDR is a promising salvage treatment technique for recurrent or progressive GBM. In particular, it may be the reirradiation method of choice for large-volume recurrences not amenable to SRS. Of note,

PRDR should be administered at radiation oncology centers with strong physics support. For instance, when using a TomoTherapy (Sunnyvale, CA) unit, reducing the dose per fraction to <0.6 Gy/fraction results in a clinically unacceptable plan with a dramatic decrease in PTV dose homogeneity because TomoTherapy uses a fixed-dose-rate output and modulates the beam using a binary multileaf collimator. To counteract this problem, physicists at the University of Wisconsin developed a virtual grid-style blocking scheme, in which half of the beam angles are directionally blocked using 15 equally spaced segments surrounding the center of the image set to create an acceptable homogeneity index.[84] Extra care should also be taken during weekly on-treatment-evaluations of patients treated with PRDR for recurrent GBM.

FUTURE DIRECTIONS IN RADIOTHERAPY FOR GLIOBLASTOMA
Proton Therapy
Proton therapy is currently being used and studied for treatment of many central nervous system (CNS) diseases. The advantage of this technology lies in the physical properties of proton particles. Protons exhibit a Bragg peak phenomenon, which allows these particles to deposit a large dose of radiation at a specific depth, followed by a sharp dose fall-off. Therefore, high doses of radiation can be delivered with proton therapy to tumors in close proximity to critical structures. There has been a recent proliferation of proton centers in the United States with piqued interest to expand utilization in the field of radiation oncology. Currently the data on protons for treatment of GBM is limited. The first published phase II proton study for GBM from Massachusetts General Hospital enrolled 23 patients treated with twice-daily accelerated fractionation with conformal photon (x-ray) and proton radiotherapy to 90 Gy equivalent (GyE). Of note, chemotherapy was not administered in these patients. Median survival was 20 months, and actuarial 2-year survival was 34%. However, this dose escalation with protons led to high rates of surgical re-resection and necrosis, with 13 of 23 patients (57%) undergoing reoperation and 10 patients (43%) exhibiting radiation necrosis.

A study from Japan examined 20 patients with supratentorial GBM treated with concomitant x-ray radiotherapy with proton boost.[85] Three CTVs were generated: CTV1 included the entire surgical bed and T1C+ MRI enhancement areas, CTV2 was defined as the area of T1C+ MRI enhancement + a 1-cm margin, and CTV3 was defined as T2 FLAIR signal abnormality. A 5-mm expansion was used to create the PTVs. Conventional x-ray radiotherapy with 6 or 10 MV (50.4 Gy in 28 fractions) was delivered to PTV3. Concomitant proton boost (23.1 GyE in 14 fractions) was delivered to PTV2 more than 6 hours after x-ray radiotherapy and subsequent proton boost (23.1 GyE in 14 fractions) was delivered to PTV1. Total doses were 96.6 GyE in 56 fractions for PTV1, 73.5 GyE in 42 fractions for PTV2, and 50.4 Gy in 28 fractions for PTV3. Nimustine hydrochloride (ACNU) was administered intravenously for 1 day during weeks 1 and 4 of RT. Median OS was 21.6 months, with 1-year and 2-year OS of 71.1% and 45.3%, respectively. PFS at 1 and 2 years was 45% and 15.5%, respectively. A mixture of tumor recurrence and radionecrosis was seen in 6 patients who underwent surgical re-resection. A follow-up study by the same group examined 23 patients treated in the same manner as the prior study, except for 2 patients who received TMZ instead of ACNU.[86] Survival rates were similar to the prior study, because almost all of the same patients were included. There were 6 patients who developed radionecrosis with a reduction in KPS by an increment of 10 to 30 at last follow-up.

In conclusion, concomitant proton therapy could potentially improve outcomes by allowing higher dose escalation in GBM. Initial results with regard to survival are promising and superior to historical rates, but further clinical data are needed, including studies that administer concurrent TMZ. NRG-BN001 is a 3-arm prospective randomized phase II trial that is currently enrolling patients to evaluate dose escalation with either x-ray IMRT or proton therapy with TMZ compared with the current standard-of-care regimen. The standard arm consists of x-ray radiotherapy using 3DCRT or IMRT to an initial 46 Gy, followed by a boost to 60 Gy using RTOG treatment volume guidelines. The 2 dose escalation arms (x-ray IMRT or protons) incorporate a simultaneous integrated boost. Using a standard 2-cm CTV margin, 50 Gy is delivered at 1.67 Gy in 30 fractions to the T2 FLAIR abnormality; simultaneously, 75 Gy at 2.5 Gy in 30 fractions is delivered to the T1C+ MRI enhancement, but at a reduced CTV margin of 5 mm. The x-ray experimental arm only allows for IMRT planning. The proton experimental arm is delivered with either passive scattered, uniform scanning beam, pencil beam scanning, or intensity-modulated proton therapy techniques. TMZ is administered identically in all 3 arms with standard dosing as per the EORTC-NCIC trial.[9]

Carbon Ion Therapy

Heavy particle carbon ion therapy has been used for certain disease sites and tumors as a method for delivering high linear energy transfer radiation, which confers a greater relative biological effectiveness than fractionated x-ray or proton therapy. Carbon ions are less dependent on the oxygen enhancement ratio compared with x-rays and may be more effective in treating hypoxic GBM cells.

The first and only published clinical trial using carbon ion therapy for patients with high-grade glioma was a phase I/II study from Japan.[87] A total of 48 patients were enrolled (16 anaplastic astrocytoma and 32 GBM). RT consisted of 2 x-ray fields (opposed lateral or wedge pair) to a CTV defined as a 5-mm margin around the T2 FLAIR signal intensity to a dose of 50 Gy in 2 Gy fractions. ACNU chemotherapy was delivered concurrently with RT. Afterward, carbon ion radiotherapy was administered 4 days/week for a total of 8 fractions. The total carbon ion boost dose was escalated from 16.8 GyE to 24.8 GyE in 10% increments. The CTV for carbon ion boost was a 5-mm margin around the T1C+ MRI enhancement. Median survival for patients with GBM was 17 months. Median PFS and OS in patients with GBM by carbon ion boost dose were the following: low-dose group (16.8 GyE), 4 and 7 months respectively; middle-dose group (18.4–22.4 GyE), 7 and 19 months; and high-dose group (24.8 GyE), 14 and 26 months. There were no grade 3 CNS toxicities and 4 grade 2 (moderate headache, significant lethargy) toxicities. A following collaborative retrospective analysis compared 3 groups: the same carbon ion–treated patients vs patients treated with x-ray RT alone vs patients receiving RT + TMZ.[88] OS at 1 and 2 years were the following: carbon ion therapy, 72% and 34%; RT alone, 26% and 4%; RT + TMZ, 66% and 26%, respectively. There was a statistically significant improvement in survival comparing carbon ion boost vs RT alone ($P = .0003$), and a trend difference in survival comparing carbon ion boost vs RT + TMZ ($P = .09$). There was also a statistically significant difference in PFS comparing carbon ion boost (8 months) vs RT + TMZ (6 months) and RT alone (5 months).

Carbon ion boost is currently being investigated in prospective trials. CLEOPATRA is a randomized phase II study evaluating carbon ion boost vs proton boost with RT + TMZ for GBM and is currently enrolling patients.[89] The CINDERELLA trial is a randomized phase I/II study evaluating carbon ion monotherapy alone vs fractionated stereotactic radiotherapy for salvage of recurrent or progressive gliomas.[90]

study): a multicentre, randomised, open-label, phase 3 trial. Lancet Oncol 2014;15(10):1100–8.

21. Minniti G, Amelio D, Amichetti M, et al. Patterns of failure and comparison of different target volume delineations in patients with glioblastoma treated with conformal radiotherapy plus concomitant and adjuvant temozolomide. Radiother Oncol 2010; 97(3):377–81.

22. Hegi ME, Diserens AC, Gorlia T, et al. MGMT gene silencing and benefit from temozolomide in glioblastoma. N Engl J Med 2005;352(10): 997–1003.

23. van den Bent MJ, Brandes AA, Taphoorn MJ, et al. Adjuvant procarbazine, lomustine, and vincristine chemotherapy in newly diagnosed anaplastic oligodendroglioma: long-term follow-up of EORTC brain tumor group study 26951. J Clin Oncol 2013;31(3):344–50.

24. Cairncross G, Wang M, Shaw E, et al. Phase III trial of chemoradiotherapy for anaplastic oligodendroglioma: long-term results of RTOG 9402. J Clin Oncol 2013;31(3):337–43.

25. Tabatabai G, Stupp R, van den Bent MJ, et al. Molecular diagnostics of gliomas: the clinical perspective. Acta Neuropathol 2010;120(5):585–92.

26. Hegi ME, Janzer RC, Lambiv WL, et al. Presence of an oligodendroglioma-like component in newly diagnosed glioblastoma identifies a pathogenetically heterogeneous subgroup and lacks prognostic value: central pathology review of the EORTC_26981/NCIC_CE.3 trial. Acta Neuropathol 2012;123(6):841–52.

27. Curran WJ, Scott CB, Horton J, et al. Recursive partitioning analysis of prognostic factors in three Radiation Therapy Oncology Group malignant glioma trials. J Natl Cancer Inst 1993;85(9): 704–10.

28. Mirimanoff RO, Gorlia T, Mason W, et al. Radiotherapy and temozolomide for newly diagnosed glioblastoma: recursive partitioning analysis of the EORTC 26981/22981-NCIC CE3 phase III randomized trial. J Clin Oncol 2006;24(16):2563–9.

29. Minniti G, Lanzetta G, Scaringi C, et al. Phase II study of short-course radiotherapy plus concomitant and adjuvant temozolomide in elderly patients with glioblastoma. Int J Radiat Oncol Biol Phys 2012;83(1):93–9.

30. Minniti G, Scaringi C, Baldoni A, et al. Health-related quality of life in elderly patients with newly diagnosed glioblastoma treated with short-course radiation therapy plus concomitant and adjuvant temozolomide. Int J Radiat Oncol Biol Phys 2013; 86(2):285–91.

31. Minniti G, Scaringi C, Lanzetta G, et al. Standard (60 Gy) or short-course (40 Gy) irradiation plus concomitant and adjuvant temozolomide for elderly patients with glioblastoma: a propensity-matched analysis. Int J Radiat Oncol Biol Phys 2015;91(1):109–15.

32. Cao JQ, Fisher BJ, Bauman GS, et al. Hypofractionated radiotherapy with or without concurrent temozolomide in elderly patients with glioblastoma multiforme: a review of ten-year single institutional experience. J Neurooncol 2012;107(2): 395–405.

33. Keime-Guibert F, Chinot O, Taillandier L, et al. Radiotherapy for glioblastoma in the elderly. N Engl J Med 2007;356(15):1527–35.

34. Roa W, Brasher PM, Bauman G, et al. Abbreviated course of radiation therapy in older patients with glioblastoma multiforme: a prospective randomized clinical trial. J Clin Oncol 2004;22(9):1583–8.

35. Roa W, Kepka L, Kumar N, et al. International Atomic Energy Agency randomized phase III study of radiation therapy in elderly and/or frail patients with newly diagnosed glioblastoma multiforme. J Clin Oncol 2015;33(35):4145–50.

36. Wick W, Platten M, Meisner C, et al. Temozolomide chemotherapy alone versus radiotherapy alone for malignant astrocytoma in the elderly: the NOA-08 randomised, phase 3 trial. Lancet Oncol 2012;13(7):707–15.

37. Malmström A, Grønberg BH, Marosi C, et al. Temozolomide versus standard 6-week radiotherapy versus hypofractionated radiotherapy in patients older than 60 years with glioblastoma: the Nordic randomised, phase 3 trial. Lancet Oncol 2012;13(9):916–26.

38. Paszat L, Laperriere N, Groome P, et al. A population-based study of glioblastoma multiforme. Int J Radiat Oncol Biol Phys 2001;51(1): 100–7.

39. Kita D, Ciernik IF, Vaccarella S, et al. Age as a predictive factor in glioblastomas: population-based study. Neuroepidemiology 2009;33(1):17–22.

40. Scott JG, Bauchet L, Fraum TJ, et al. Recursive partitioning analysis of prognostic factors for glioblastoma patients aged 70 years or older. Cancer 2012;118(22):5595–600.

41. Gerstner ER, Yip S, Wang DL, et al. Mgmt methylation is a prognostic biomarker in elderly patients with newly diagnosed glioblastoma. Neurology 2009;73(18):1509–10.

42. Brandes AA, Franceschi E, Tosoni A, et al. Temozolomide concomitant and adjuvant to radiotherapy in elderly patients with glioblastoma: correlation with MGMT promoter methylation status. Cancer 2009;115(15):3512–8.

43. Reifenberger G, Hentschel B, Felsberg J, et al. Predictive impact of MGMT promoter methylation in glioblastoma of the elderly. Int J Cancer 2012; 131(6):1342–50.

44. Souhami L, Seiferheld W, Brachman D, et al. Randomized comparison of stereotactic radiosurgery

followed by conventional radiotherapy with car-mustine to conventional radiotherapy with carmus-tine for patients with glioblastoma multiforme: report of Radiation Therapy Oncology Group 93-05 protocol. Int J Radiat Oncol Biol Phys 2004; 60(3):853–60.

45. Cardinale R, Won M, Choucair A, et al. A phase II trial of accelerated radiotherapy using weekly ste-reotactic conformal boost for supratentorial glio-blastoma multiforme: RTOG 0023. Int J Radiat Oncol Biol Phys 2006;65(5):1422–8.

46. Sarkaria JN, Mehta MP, Loeffler JS, et al. Radiosur-gery in the initial management of malignant gli-omas: survival comparison with the RTOG recursive partitioning analysis. Radiation Therapy Oncology Group. Int J Radiat Oncol Biol Phys 1995;32(4):931–41.

47. Gannett D, Stea B, Lulu B, et al. Stereotactic radio-surgery as an adjunct to surgery and external beam radiotherapy in the treatment of patients with malignant gliomas. Int J Radiat Oncol Biol Phys 1995;33(2):461–8.

48. Masciopinto JE, Levin AB, Mehta MP, et al. Stereo-tactic radiosurgery for glioblastoma: a final report of 31 patients. J Neurosurg 1995;82(4):530–5.

49. Mehta MP, Masciopinto J, Rozental J, et al. Ste-reotactic radiosurgery for glioblastoma multi-forme: report of a prospective study evaluating prognostic factors and analyzing long-term sur-vival advantage. Int J Radiat Oncol Biol Phys 1994;30(3):541–9.

50. Nwokedi EC, DiBiase SJ, Jabbour S, et al. Gamma knife stereotactic radiosurgery for patients with glioblastoma multiforme. Neurosurgery 2002; 50(1):41–6 [discussion: 6–7].

51. Balducci M, Apicella G, Manfrida S, et al. Single-arm phase II study of conformal radiation therapy and temozolomide plus fractionated stereotactic conformal boost in high-grade gliomas: final report. Strahlenther Onkol 2010;186(10):558–64.

52. Cardinale RM, Schmidt-Ullrich RK, Benedict SH, et al. Accelerated radiotherapy regimen for malig-nant gliomas using stereotactic concomitant boosts for dose escalation. Radiat Oncol Investig 1998;6(4):175–81.

53. Shrieve DC, Alexander E 3rd, Black PM, et al. Treatment of patients with primary glioblastoma multiforme with standard postoperative radio-therapy and radiosurgical boost: prognostic fac-tors and long-term outcome. J Neurosurg 1999; 90(1):72–7.

54. Floyd SR, Kasper EM, Uhlmann EJ, et al. Hypofrac-tionated radiotherapy and stereotactic boost with concurrent and adjuvant temozolamide for glio-blastoma in good performance status elderly pa-tients - early results of a phase II trial. Front Oncol 2012;2:122.

55. Landy H, Markoe A, Potter P, et al. Pilot study of estramustine added to radiosurgery and radio-therapy for treatment of high grade glioma. J Neurooncol 2004;67(1–2):215–20.

56. Omuro A, Beal K, Gutin P, et al. Phase II study of bev-acizumab, temozolomide, and hypofractionated stereotactic radiotherapy for newly diagnosed glio-blastoma. Clin Cancer Res 2014;20(19):5023–31.

57. Redmond KJ, Mehta M. Stereotactic radiosurgery for glioblastoma. Cureus 2015;7(12):e413.

58. Shrieve DC, Alexander E 3rd, Wen PY, et al. Comparison of stereotactic radiosurgery and brachytherapy in the treatment of recurrent glio-blastoma multiforme. Neurosurgery 1995;36(2): 275–82 [discussion: 82–4].

59. Vordermark D, Kolbl O, Ruprecht K, et al. Hypo-fractionated stereotactic re-irradiation: treatment option in recurrent malignant glioma. BMC Cancer 2005;5:55.

60. Lederman G, Arbit E, Odaimi M, et al. Recurrent glioblastoma multiforme: potential benefits using fractionated stereotactic radiotherapy and con-current taxol. Stereotact Funct Neurosurg 1997; 69(1–4 Pt 2):162–74.

61. Combs SE, Widmer V, Thilmann C, et al. Stereo-tactic radiosurgery (SRS): treatment option for recurrent glioblastoma multiforme (GBM). Cancer 2005;104(10):2168–73.

62. Fogh SE, Andrews DW, Glass J, et al. Hypofractio-nated stereotactic radiation therapy: an effective therapy for recurrent high-grade gliomas. J Clin Oncol 2010;28(18):3048–53.

63. Maranzano E, Anselmo P, Casale M, et al. Treat-ment of recurrent glioblastoma with stereotactic radiotherapy: long-term results of a mono-institutional trial. Tumori 2011;97(1):56–61.

64. Greenspoon JN, Sharieff W, Hirte H, et al. Frac-tionated stereotactic radiosurgery with concurrent temozolomide chemotherapy for locally recurrent glioblastoma multiforme: a prospective cohort study. Onco Targets Ther 2014;7:485–90.

65. Hudes RS, Corn BW, Werner-Wasik M, et al. A phase I dose escalation study of hypofractio-nated stereotactic radiotherapy as salvage therapy for persistent or recurrent malignant glioma. Int J Radiat Oncol Biol Phys 1999;43(2):293–8.

66. Lederman G, Wronski M, Arbit E, et al. Treatment of recurrent glioblastoma multiforme using frac-tionated stereotactic radiosurgery and concurrent paclitaxel. Am J Clin Oncol 2000;23(2):155–9.

67. Cuneo KC, Vredenburgh JJ, Sampson JH, et al. Safety and efficacy of stereotactic radiosurgery and adjuvant bevacizumab in patients with recur-rent malignant gliomas. Int J Radiat Oncol Biol Phys 2012;82(5):2018–24.

68. Minniti G, Scaringi C, De Sanctis V, et al. Hypofrac-tionated stereotactic radiotherapy and continuous

low-dose temozolomide in patients with recurrent or progressive malignant gliomas. J Neurooncol 2013;111(2):187–94.

69. Skeie BS, Enger PO, Brogger J, et al. gamma knife surgery versus reoperation for recurrent glioblastoma multiforme. World Neurosurg 2012;78(6): 658–69.

70. Park KJ, Kano H, Iyer A, et al. Salvage gamma knife stereotactic radiosurgery followed by bevacizumab for recurrent glioblastoma multiforme: a case-control study. J Neurooncol 2012;107(2): 323–33.

71. Koga T, Maruyama K, Tanaka M, et al. Extended field stereotactic radiosurgery for recurrent glioblastoma. Cancer 2012;118(17):4193–200.

72. Elliott RE, Parker EC, Rush SC, et al. Efficacy of gamma knife radiosurgery for small-volume recurrent malignant gliomas after initial radical resection. World Neurosurg 2011;76(1–2):128–40 [discussion: 61–2].

73. Pouratian N, Crowley RW, Sherman JH, et al. Gamma Knife radiosurgery after radiation therapy as an adjunctive treatment for glioblastoma. J Neurooncol 2009;94(3):409–18.

74. Kida Y, Yoshimoto M, Hasegawa T. Radiosurgery for intracranial gliomas. Prog Neurol Surg 2009; 22:122–8.

75. Kong DS, Lee JI, Park K, et al. Efficacy of stereotactic radiosurgery as a salvage treatment for recurrent malignant gliomas. Cancer 2008;112(9):2046–51.

76. Kohshi K, Yamamoto H, Nakahara A, et al. Fractionated stereotactic radiotherapy using gamma unit after hyperbaric oxygenation on recurrent high-grade gliomas. J Neurooncol 2007;82(3): 297–303.

77. Hsieh PC, Chandler JP, Bhangoo S, et al. Adjuvant gamma knife stereotactic radiosurgery at the time of tumor progression potentially improves survival for patients with glioblastoma multiforme. Neurosurgery 2005;57(4):684–92 [discussion: 92].

78. Multicenter phase II study of border zone stereotactic radiosurgery with bevacizumab in patients with recurrent or progressive glioblastoma multiforme. 2014. Available at: http://clinicaltrials feeds.org/clinical-trials/show/NCT02120287.

79. Tomé WA, Howard SP. On the possible increase in local tumour control probability for gliomas exhibiting low dose hyper-radiosensitivity using a pulsed schedule. Br J Radiol 2007;80(949):32–7.

80. Schultz CJ, Geard CR. Radioresponse of human astrocytic tumors across grade as a function of acute and chronic irradiation. Int J Radiat Oncol Biol Phys 1990;19(6):1397–403.

81. Dilworth JT, Krueger SA, Dabjan M, et al. Pulsed low-dose irradiation of orthotopic glioblastoma multiforme (GBM) in a pre-clinical model: effects on vascularization and tumor control. Radiother Oncol 2013;108(1):149–54.

82. Adkison JB, Tomé W, Seo S, et al. Reirradiation of large-volume recurrent glioma with pulsed reduced-dose-rate radiotherapy. Int J Radiat Oncol Biol Phys 2011;79(3):835–41.

83. Magnuson W, Ian Robins H, Mohindra P, et al. Large volume reirradiation as salvage therapy for glioblastoma after progression on bevacizumab. J Neurooncol 2014;117(1):133–9.

84. Rasmussen KH, Hardcastle N, Howard S, et al. Reirradiation of glioblastoma through the use of a reduced dose rate on a tomotherapy unit. Technol Cancer Res Treat 2010;9(4):399–406.

85. Mizumoto M, Tsuboi K, Igaki H, et al. Phase I/II trial of hyperfractionated concomitant boost proton radiotherapy for supratentorial glioblastoma multiforme. Int J Radiat Oncol Biol Phys 2010;77(1): 98–105.

86. Mizumoto M, Yamamoto T, Takano S, et al. Long-term survival after treatment of glioblastoma multiforme with hyperfractionated concomitant boost proton beam therapy. Pract Radiat Oncol 2015; 5(1):e9–16.

87. Mizoe JE, Tsujii H, Hasegawa A, et al. Phase I/II clinical trial of carbon ion radiotherapy for malignant gliomas: combined X-ray radiotherapy, chemotherapy, and carbon ion radiotherapy. Int J Radiat Oncol Biol Phys 2007;69(2):390–6.

88. Combs SE, Bruckner T, Mizoe JE, et al. Comparison of carbon ion radiotherapy to photon radiation alone or in combination with temozolomide in patients with high-grade gliomas: explorative hypothesis-generating retrospective analysis. Radiother Oncol 2013;108(1):132–5.

89. Combs SE, Kieser M, Rieken S, et al. Randomized phase II study evaluating a carbon ion boost applied after combined radiochemotherapy with temozolomide versus a proton boost after radiochemotherapy with temozolomide in patients with primary glioblastoma: the CLEOPATRA trial. BMC Cancer 2010;10:478.

90. Combs SE, Burkholder I, Edler L, et al. Randomised phase I/II study to evaluate carbon ion radiotherapy versus fractionated stereotactic radiotherapy in patients with recurrent or progressive gliomas: the CINDERELLA trial. BMC Cancer 2010;10:533.

91. Goitein M, Jermann M. The relative costs of proton and X-ray radiation therapy. Clin Oncol (R Coll Radiol) 2003;15(1):S37–50.

92. Peeters A, Grutters JP, Pijls-Johannesma M, et al. How costly is particle therapy? Cost analysis of external beam radiotherapy with carbon-ions, protons and photons. Radiother Oncol 2010; 95(1):45–53.

93. Brandsma D, Stalpers L, Taal W, et al. Clinical features, mechanisms, and management of pseudoprogression in malignant gliomas. Lancet Oncol 2008;9(5):453–61.

94. Hygino da Cruz LC, Rodriguez I, Domingues RC, et al. Pseudoprogression and pseudoresponse: imaging challenges in the assessment of post-treatment glioma. AJNR Am J Neuroradiol 2011; 32(11):1978–85.

95. Brandes AA, Franceschi E, Tosoni A, et al. MGMT promoter methylation status can predict the incidence and outcome of pseudoprogression after concomitant radiochemotherapy in newly diagnosed glioblastoma patients. J Clin Oncol 2008; 26(13):2192–7.

96. Fink J, Born D, Chamberlain MC. Radiation necrosis: relevance with respect to treatment of primary and secondary brain tumors. Curr Neurol Neurosci Rep 2012;12(3):276–85.

97. Dequesada IM, Quisling RG, Yachnis A, et al. Can standard magnetic resonance imaging reliably distinguish recurrent tumor from radiation necrosis after radiosurgery for brain metastases? A radiographic-pathological study. Neurosurgery 2008;63(5):898–903 [discussion: 4].

98. Stockham AL, Tievsky AL, Koyfman SA, et al. Conventional MRI does not reliably distinguish radiation necrosis from tumor recurrence after stereotactic radiosurgery. J Neurooncol 2012; 109(1):149–58.

99. Larsen VA, Simonsen HJ, Law I, et al. Evaluation of dynamic contrast-enhanced T1-weighted perfusion MRI in the differentiation of tumor recurrence from radiation necrosis. Neuroradiology 2013;55(3):361–9.

100. Thomas AA, Arevalo-Perez J, Kaley T, et al. Dynamic contrast enhanced T1 MRI perfusion differentiates pseudoprogression from recurrent glioblastoma. J Neurooncol 2015;125(1):183–90.

101. Bulik M, Kazda T, Slampa P, et al. The diagnostic ability of follow-up imaging biomarkers after treatment of glioblastoma in the temozolomide era: implications from proton MR spectroscopy and apparent diffusion coefficient mapping. Biomed Res Int 2015;2015:641023.

102. Di Costanzo A, Scarabino T, Trojsi F, et al. Recurrent glioblastoma multiforme versus radiation injury: a multiparametric 3-T MR approach. Radiol Med 2014;119(8):616–24.

103. Pirzkall A, McKnight TR, Graves EE, et al. MR-spectroscopy guided target delineation for high-grade gliomas. Int J Radiat Oncol Biol Phys 2001;50(4): 915–28.

104. Pirzkall A, Li X, Oh J, et al. 3D MRSI for resected high-grade gliomas before RT: tumor extent according to metabolic activity in relation to MRI. Int J Radiat Oncol Biol Phys 2004;59(1):126–37.

105. Niyazi M, Geisler J, Siefert A, et al. FET-PET for malignant glioma treatment planning. Radiother Oncol 2011;99(1):44–8.

106. Rieken S, Habermehl D, Giesel FL, et al. Analysis of FET-PET imaging for target volume definition in patients with gliomas treated with conformal radiotherapy. Radiother Oncol 2013;109(3): 487–92.

107. Terakawa Y, Tsuyuguchi N, Iwai Y, et al. Diagnostic accuracy of 11C-methionine PET for differentiation of recurrent brain tumors from radiation necrosis after radiotherapy. J Nucl Med 2008;49(5):694–9.

108. Parvez K, Parvez A, Zadeh G. The diagnosis and treatment of pseudoprogression, radiation necrosis and brain tumor recurrence. Int J Mol Sci 2014; 15(7):11832–46.

109. Li YQ, Ballinger JR, Nordal RA, et al. Hypoxia in radiation-induced blood-spinal cord barrier breakdown. Cancer Res 2001;61(8):3348–54.

110. Rahman M, Hoh BL. Avastin in the treatment for radiation necrosis: exciting results from a recent randomized trial. World Neurosurg 2011;75(1):4–5.

111. Levin VA, Bidaut L, Hou P, et al. Randomized double-blind placebo-controlled trial of bevacizumab therapy for radiation necrosis of the central nervous system. Int J Radiat Oncol Biol Phys 2011;79(5):1487–95.

112. Glantz MJ, Burger PC, Friedman AH, et al. Treatment of radiation-induced nervous system injury with heparin and warfarin. Neurology 1994;44(11): 2020–7.

113. Leber KA, Eder HG, Kovac H, et al. Treatment of cerebral radionecrosis by hyperbaric oxygen therapy. Stereotact Funct Neurosurg 1998;70(Suppl 1): 229–36.

114. Rahmathulla G, Recinos PF, Valerio JE, et al. Laser interstitial thermal therapy for focal cerebral radiation necrosis: a case report and literature review. Stereotact Funct Neurosurg 2012;90(3):192–200.

115. Ballesteros-Zebadúa P, Chavarria A, Celis MA, et al. Radiation-induced neuroinflammation and radiation somnolence syndrome. CNS Neurol Disord Drug Targets 2012;11(7):937–49.

116. Ryan J. Radiation somnolence syndrome. J Pediatr Oncol Nurs 2000;17(1):50–3.

117. Uzal D, Ozyar E, Hayran M, et al. Reduced incidence of the somnolence syndrome after prophylactic cranial irradiation in children with acute lymphoblastic leukemia. Radiother Oncol 1998;48(1):29–32.

118. Brown PD, Jensen AW, Felten SJ, et al. Detrimental effects of tumor progression on cognitive function of patients with high-grade glioma. J Clin Oncol 2006;24(34):5427–33.

119. Bosma I, Vos MJ, Heimans JJ, et al. The course of neurocognitive functioning in high-grade glioma patients. Neuro Oncol 2007;9(1):53–62.

120. Hilverda K, Bosma I, Heimans JJ, et al. Cognitive functioning in glioblastoma patients during radiotherapy and temozolomide treatment: initial findings. J Neurooncol 2010; 97(1):89–94.

121. Brown PD, Pugh S, Laack NN, et al. Memantine for the prevention of cognitive dysfunction in patients receiving whole-brain radiotherapy: a randomized, double-blind, placebo-controlled trial. Neuro Oncol 2013;15(10):1429–37.

CHAPTER 9

Chemotherapeutics and Their Efficacy

H. Westley Phillips, MD[a], Andrew S. Chi, MD, PhD[a,b,c,*]

INTRODUCTION

Glioblastoma (GBM), the most common primary brain malignancy, carries a poor prognosis and has therefore been the subject of numerous studies attempting to improve outcomes. Although a plethora of investigative studies and clinical trials have focused on this patient population, the median overall survival from time of diagnosis has remained largely unchanged over many decades, with a current range of 15 to 17 months and a median time to recurrence of approximately 7 months.[1]

Traditional therapy was predicated on surgical resection or biopsy, if amenable; however, the highly infiltrative nature of these tumors renders complete resection nearly impossible. Accordingly, effective treatment relies on neoadjuvant and adjuvant therapy. Subsequent therapies have consisted of a combination of radiation with concurrent and adjuvant chemotherapeutics after surgical debulking with the current gold standard chemotherapeutic agent for newly diagnosed disease being temozolomide (TMZ), which is used concomitantly with radiotherapy.[2–4]

Over the past decade, TMZ-based chemoradiotherapy has emerged worldwide as the standard therapy for newly diagnosed GBM. Although TMZ represents a landmark achievement in the treatment landscape of GBM because it remains the only chemotherapy agent that has definitively improved survival in a randomized controlled phase III trial in GBM, the absolute survival improvement is modest (**Table 9.1**). Numerous novel therapeutic strategies for GBM are being developed. In this chapter, the historical context and rationale for chemotherapy in GBM are highlighted and the current gold standard are highlighted and the current gold standard

reviewed. In addition, recent attempts to improve on the current standard are discussed with a focus on randomized controlled clinical trials given the plethora of early-stage clinical trials that have been conducted in GBM over the last several decades.

CONTEXT OF CURRENT GOLD STANDARD

In the past, the mainstay of GBM treatment solely consisted of surgical resection of the lesion. However, in 1978, Walker and colleagues[5] showed a statistically significant increased overall survival in patients with anaplastic gliomas receiving either radiotherapy or 1,3-bis(2-chloroethyl)-l-nitrosourea (BCNU, or carmustine), a nitrosourea DNA-alkylating chemotherapy that penetrates the blood-brain barrier (BBB), compared with supportive care alone. This controlled, prospective trial randomized patients into 1 of 4 arms: BCNU, given as 80 $mg/m^2/d$ on 3 consecutive days every 6 to 8 weeks; radiotherapy alone (5000–6000 rad to the whole brain); BCNU plus radiotherapy; and best supportive care. In the analysis of 222 patients who received any amount of therapy, there was a statistically significant improvement in overall survival with each of the 3 treatment arms compared with supportive care alone. However, the increases in median overall survival were small (18.5 weeks, 35 weeks, and 34.5 weeks for BCNU, radiotherapy, and BCNU plus radiotherapy, respectively, compared with 14 weeks for supportive care only), and the overall outcomes remained bleak. However, this study showed that both radiotherapy and BCNU had some efficacy in anaplastic gliomas, and, as a result, adjuvant radiotherapy in addition to surgical debulking of

a Department of Neurosurgery, NYU Langone Medical Center, NYU School of Medicine, 462 1st Avenue, 7th Floor, New York, NY 10016, USA; b Department of Neurology, Laura and Isaac Perlmutter Cancer Center, NYU Langone Medical Center, NYU School of Medicine, 240 East 38th Street, Floor 19, New York, NY 10016, USA; c Department of Medicine, Laura and Isaac Perlmutter Cancer Center, NYU Langone Medical Center, NYU School of Medicine, 240 East 38th Street, Floor 19, New York, NY 10016, USA
* Corresponding author. 240 East 38th Street, Floor 19, New York, NY 10016.
E-mail address: chia01@nyumc.org

TABLE 9.1
Median overall survival (OS) outcomes in phase III GBM trials

| | Survival of GBM in 2016 | |
Trial (Year Published)	Median OS (mo)	95% Confidence Interval
Walker (BCNU) (1978)[5]	8.75	NA
EORTC-NCIC (2005)[4]	14.6	13.2–16.8
RTOG 0525 (control) (2013)[29]	16.6	14.9–18.0
RTOG 0525 (dose-dense TMZ) (2013)[29]	14.9	13.7–16.5
RTOG 0825 (control) (2014)[31]	16.1	14.8–16.8
RTOG 0825 (bevacizumab) (2014)[31]	15.7	14.2–16.8
EORTC 26071–2072 (cilengitide) (2014)[36]	26.3	23.8–28.8
TTFields (2015)[37]	20.5	16.7–25.0

Abbreviations: BCNU, 1,3-bis(2-chloroethyl)-l- nitrosourea; EORTC, European Organization for Research and Treatment of Cancer; NA, not available; NCIC, National Cancer Institute of Canada; RTOG, Radiation Therapy Oncology Group; TTFields, tumor-treating fields.

the lesion became standard therapy in these patients for decades to follow. Another finding of this study that would be a subject of further investigation was that the patients on the combined radiotherapy plus chemotherapy arm did not live significantly longer than patients treated with radiotherapy alone.[5]

Later, chemotherapy agents used for other solid tumors were trialed in patients with GBM. In 1999, Friedman and colleagues[6] published a single-arm study on the pharmacokinetics and preliminary efficacy of irinotecan, an alkaloid derivative of camptothecin and inhibitor of topoisomerase I originally marketed for colon cancer, in patients with recurrent or progressive malignant glioma. Preclinical studies of irinotecan showed promising results against a broad array of central nervous system neoplasms, prompting a phase II trial to further investigate its role in malignant glioma. The study enrolled 60 patients with recurrent malignant glioma treated with intravenous irinotecan at a starting dose of 125 mg/m^2 given weekly for a 4-week cycle followed by a 2-week rest period. There were 15% confirmed partial responses and the 1-year median overall survival was 43 weeks, indicating moderate preliminary efficacy. By the early 2000s many other cytotoxic agents used for other cancers were studied in trials for malignant glioma, mostly using nitrosoureas such as carmustine or lomustine (CCNU) because these agents are lipid soluble and penetrate the BBB. However, most studies were inconclusive, and the median survival times for newly diagnosed GBM continued to be less than 1 year.[7]

Eventually, a meta-analysis of patients from randomized trials comparing patients treated with radiotherapy alone versus radiotherapy plus nitrosourea-based chemotherapy was conducted,

which suggested a small but statistically significant improvement in survival with the addition of chemotherapy to radiotherapy.[8] Chemotherapy resulted in an apparent increase in median survival time of approximately 2 months compared with radiotherapy alone, with an increase in the 1-year survival rate of 6% (40% vs 46%). Although the effect of chemotherapy seemed modest at best, this analysis encouraged further study of chemotherapy in malignant glioma, with the focus on the imidazotetrazinone class of chemotherapeutic agents that crossed the BBB, such as dacarbazine and TMZ.[8]

TMZ was developed in the 1980s at Aston University with support from the UK Cancer Research Campaign. Like earlier imidazotetrazinone derivatives, such as dacarbazine, TMZ converts to an active metabolite, 5-(3-methyl)1-triazen-1-yl-imidazole-4-carboxamide (MTIC). Advantageously, it spontaneously converted to the active agent after oral administration at physiologic pH without hepatic metabolism. MTIC is an unstable compound that quickly degrades into a methyldiazonium ion, which is a potent methylating agent. MTIC is readily available throughout the body, has excellent bioavailability, and, like nitrosourea compounds, has excellent penetration through the BBB.[9] The drug acts as a major groove-directed DNA-alkylating agent methylating DNA at the N^7 and O^6 on guanine and the O^3 atom on adenine, with guanine O^6 and N^7 methylation being the main cytotoxic factors leading to apoptosis. In preclinical studies, TMZ showed antitumor activity in a wide variety of both intracranial and extracranial malignancies (reviewed by Friedman and colleagues[10]).

Yung and colleagues[11] ultimately showed that TMZ had promising efficacy in a randomized phase II trial of patients with GBM at first relapse. This study showed that the 6-month progression-free survival rate (PFS6), which is the now-standard efficacy measure for recurrent GBM phase II trials, was improved with TMZ versus procarbazine (21% vs 8%). TMZ was given orally at 150 or 200 mg/m^2 for 5 consecutive days on days 1 to 5 of each 28-day cycle. Although the study showed that TMZ had some activity against GBM, the median progression-free survival (PFS) rates remained modest (12 weeks) and the objective radiographic response rate was low (5.4%). In 1999, TMZ received US Food and Drug Administration (FDA) approval for second-line treatment of refractory anaplastic astrocytoma and GBM.[7]

Later, combined radiotherapy and TMZ strategies were explored. Preclinical studies showed that concurrent TMZ and radiation resulted in at least additive cytotoxicity against several GBM cell lines in vitro.[12–14] In 2002, Stupp and colleagues[2] conducted a single-arm phase II trial of 64 newly diagnosed patients with GBM investigating concurrent daily fractionated radiotherapy with a continuous schedule of low-dose TMZ. The continuous TMZ schedule was originally designed as an attempt to mitigate a TMZ resistance mechanism mediated through the O^6 methylguanine-DNA methyltransferase (MGMT) enzyme, a DNA repair protein that rapidly reverses DNA alkylation at the O^6 position of guanine.[15,16] Continuous TMZ exposure to TMZ resulted in depletion of MGMT in vitro, and this schedule was found to be safe in patients.[17] Stupp and colleagues'[2] study exploited this schedule, providing patients with concurrent 75 mg/m^2/d TMZ in addition to fractionated radiotherapy (total dose of 60 Gy given in 2-Gy fractions 5 times per week) for 6 weeks. Following this period, TMZ was given as monotherapy at a standard dose of 200 mg/m^2 during days 1 to 5 of 28-day cycles for 6 cycles. The regimen was found to be safe and reported promising 1-year and 2-year survival rates of 58% and 31% with a median survival of 16 months.

The promising results of the phase II trial prompted a multi-institutional randomized phase III trial by the European Organization for Research and Treatment of Cancer (EORTC) and National Cancer Institute of Canada (NCIC) Clinical Trials Group in patients newly diagnosed with GBM. Patients were randomized to receive either standard radiotherapy or concurrent radiotherapy with TMZ followed by 6 cycles of adjuvant TMZ in dosing described in the previous phase II study. A total of 573 patients were enrolled at 85 centers and overall survival was the primary end point. The median survival was 14.6 months with radiotherapy plus TMZ and 12.1 months with radiotherapy alone, and notably there was a significant improvement in the 2-year survival rate (26.5% for combined therapy vs 10.4% for radiotherapy alone).[3] At 5-year follow-up, the survival results were sustained, with a significantly increased fraction of long-term survivors in the combination therapy group (5-year survival rate of 9.8% vs 1.9% in the radiotherapy-alone group). As a result of this study, the FDA approved TMZ for patients with newly diagnosed GBM in 2005 and this combined regimen of TMZ chemoradiotherapy became the standard of care.[3,4]

In a companion molecular correlative study to the EORTC-NCIC phase III trial, Hegi and colleagues[18] confirmed the positive prognostic impact of MGMT promoter DNA methylation. Methylation of the promoter silences expression of the MGMT gene, rendering cancer cells no longer able to produce MGMT protein, presumably limiting repair of DNA methylation induced by TMZ. Esteller and colleagues[19] had earlier reported in a retrospective cohort of 47 patients with malignant glioma that MGMT promoter methylation was independently associated with response to nitrosourea therapy and increased overall survival. Using the same methylation-specific polymerase chain reaction assay, Hegi and colleagues[18] found that, in the entire group of patients with GBM with evaluable MGMT status (206 patients), approximately half (44.7%) had MGMT promoter methylation, and this was also independently associated with significantly longer median overall survival (18.2 months for methylated vs 12.2 months for unmethylated MGMT promoter). Notably, Hegi and colleagues[18] suggested that MGMT promoter methylation could predict response to TMZ. Within the subgroup of patients with methylated MGMT promoter, patients who received TMZ chemoradiotherapy lived significantly longer than patients who received radiotherapy alone (median overall survival, 21.7 months vs 15.3 months; $P = .007$). In patients without MGMT methylation, there was a small and marginally statistically significant improvement in overall survival for TMZ chemoradiotherapy compared with radiation alone (median overall survival, 12.7 months vs 11.8 months; $P = .06$).

TMZ has first-degree pharmacokinetics and excretion is predominantly renal, but dosing recommendations remain the same regardless of kidney function. Individual absorption is variable and the maximum plasma concentration occurs 30 to 90 minutes after ingestion, with an average volume of distribution of 171/m^2 and cerebrospinal fluid concentrations 30% to 40% of plasma concentrations.[20] The drug is more effective in the

TMZ dosing schedules. The trial was terminated in the planned interim analysis because of a benefit observed in PFS in the intent-to-treat population, which was the primary end point of the study. The overall survival, a secondary end point, was also increased when the study was halted (20.5 months for TTFields vs 15.6 months for standard therapy; $P = .004$).[36] Although this study was the first phase III trial in a decade since the pivotal TMZ chemoradiotherapy study to show improved survival, there remain some debate about TTFields therapy. The study was neither blinded nor placebo controlled because a sham treatment was considered inappropriate, and it remains to be seen whether the favorable overall survival results reported in the interim analysis will be sustained in the final study report. Furthermore, the FDA had previously granted approval for TTFields therapy as a device for monotherapy in recurrent GBM based on a phase III trial that randomized patients to receive either the TTFields therapy or a physician's choice of chemotherapy and this study showed that, although the TTFields therapy was clearly less toxic than chemotherapy, it was not superior to standard chemotherapy with regard to overall survival or PFS.[37] Based on these factors, questions remain regarding the efficacy of this therapy in GBM.

CHEMOTHERAPY IN RECURRENT GLIOBLASTOMA IN THE ERA OF TEMOZOLOMIDE CHEMORADIOTHERAPY

Although TMZ chemoradiotherapy is modestly effective in improving survival of patients with newly diagnosed GBM, the tumors invariably recur and GBM remains a uniformly fatal disease with overall dismal outcomes. A plethora of experimental therapeutic strategies have been and are currently being used and have thus far had varying degrees of success in preclinical or early-stage clinical studies. The array of strategies, which are beyond the scope of this chapter, include antiangiogenic therapy, molecularly targeted therapy, stem cell–targeted therapy, epigenetic therapy, locoregional therapy, and immunotherapy. Early-phase clinical studies of many of these strategies have been largely disappointing, with the possible exception of bevacizumab, which was granted accelerated FDA approved for monotherapy in progressive GBM. However, a recently reported multi-institutional randomized (2:1) phase III trial of 437 patients with GBM at first recurrence testing the combination of bevacizumab (10 mg/kg every 2 weeks) plus lomustine (90 mg/m^2 every 6 weeks) versus lomustine monotherapy (110 mg/m^2 every

6 weeks) failed to show improved survival in the combination therapy arm compared with lomustine monotherapy.[38] Although subgroup analyses are ongoing, this result failed to resolve the uncertainty regarding the impact of bevacizumab on the survival of patients with GBM.

Although a substantial number of single-arm phase I and II trials for recurrent GBM after progression on standard TMZ chemoradiotherapy have been conducted, there has been a paucity of randomized controlled trials in this setting. However, the few that have been performed have more clearly delineated the efficacy and role of cytotoxic chemotherapy in the recurrent setting after TMZ chemoradiotherapy because single-agent chemotherapy was used as a control arm in these studies. Lomustine has been used in the control arm in several recently reported randomized controlled phase III trials in recurrent GBM, including trials of bevacizumab,[38] enzastaurin,[39] and cediranib.[40] Aggregate data from these studies indicate that lomustine results in a median PFS of approximately 1.5 to 4 months, a PFS6 rate of approximately 20% to 25%, and a median overall survival ranging between 7 and 10 months.[38–40] Carboplatin was also studied in a large, multi-institutional, randomized controlled, phase II trial in recurrent GBM comparing carboplatin monotherapy (AUC 5 every 4 weeks) versus carboplatin plus bevacizumab (10 mg/kg every 2 weeks).[41] The study did not find a difference in PFS or overall survival between the two treatment groups, and the median PFS, PFS6, and median overall survival rates with carboplatin monotherapy (3.5 months, 18%, 7.5 months, respectively) were comparable with those observed with lomustine.[41] In the TTFields randomized phase III trial in recurrent GBM, the control arm of investigator's choice chemotherapy included a mix of chemotherapies, including nitrosoureas, irinotecan, carboplatin, TMZ, and other therapies with or without bevacizumab. The median PFS, PFS6, and median overall survival rates (2.1 months, 15.1%, 6 months, respectively) in this study were similar to those observed in the lomustine and carboplatin studies.[37] Together, these results indicate that different cytotoxic chemotherapies have similar minimal efficacy in the setting of recurrence after standard TMZ chemoradiotherapy.

Although other cytotoxic chemotherapy agents or alternative schedules or combinations of commonly used chemotherapy agents can be considered in GBM, it is the authors' opinion that all patients with recurrent GBM and a reasonable functional status should be considered for a clinical trial of an investigational agent given the

CHAPTER 10

Antiangiogenic Therapy for Glioblastoma

Arman Jahangiri, BS[1], Patrick Flanigan, BS[1], Manish K. Aghi, MD, PhD*

INTRODUCTION

This chapter reviews the history of angiogenesis and how it was recognized as an essential mechanism for tumor establishment and growth. From the initial recognition of tumor vascularity to the purification of vascular endothelial growth factor (VEGF), this chapter begins with a historical overview of the key scientific discoveries. Focusing on the development of the anti-VEGF monoclonal antibody, bevacizumab, it then discusses how it came to be used in glioblastoma and the ensuing clinical trials. It also covers the current state of the field, shortcomings of antiangiogenic therapy in glioblastoma as it relates to therapeutic resistance, and the future direction of antiangiogenic therapy in glioblastoma.

MOLECULAR BASIS FOR THE USE OF ANTIANGIOGENIC THERAPY IN GLIOBLASTOMA

History of Early Research in Angiogenesis

Angiogenesis, the process by which new blood vessels are formed from preexisting vessels, plays a major role in normal biology such as embryonic and adult development.[1] This process is also essential to pathologic states such as the development and proliferation of tumors.[2] The term angiogenesis is distinct from neovascularization, which is used to describe the formation of new vascular networks from vascular progenitor cells rather than from preexisting blood vessels as occurs with angiogenesis.

Scientists, including Rudolf Virchow, first made the link between tumor growth and their specific blood supply leading to increased vascularity more than a century ago.[3] In the late 1920s, Warren Lewis[4] was the first to describe that spontaneously growing tumors in rats had different types of vasculature depending on the type of tumor. This discovery was the first step toward the understanding that the tumor environment plays a crucial role in the morphologic characteristics as well the growth rate of each tumor's blood vessels.

Intravital analysis with transparent chambers, a process in which a transparent chamber is implanted into a rabbit's ear, allowing microscopic visualization of vessels, was an important tool that allowed the observation of angiogenesis, and was developed by J.C. Sandison[5] in 1928. Using this technique a decade later, Ide and colleagues[6] began to examine the relationship between growth rates of carcinoma in relation to its vascular supply in rabbits. They found that, as a tumor began to grow, a widespread and rapid establishment of blood vessels accompanied it, evolving as the tumor increased in size. The investigators made the important leap of establishing that not only did this blood vessel formation help the tumor grow because it provided a growing tumor with necessary nutrients and oxygen but that tumor growth depended on this vessel formation and without this new vessel formation a tumor would not grow. This observation was the foundation of attempts to inhibit angiogenesis decades later.

An important article from Algire and colleagues[7] at the National Cancer Institute further expanded on this hypothesis in 1945. Adapting the transparent chambers to a murine model, they counted the number of blood vessels daily, thereby advancing this technique to a quantitative modality for assessing blood vessel growth in relation to tumor proliferation. Similar to Ide and colleagues,[6] they too observed that it was the tumor and not the normal tissue that permitted increased blood vessel formation and growth. Furthermore, they observed that vascular growth took place before the tumor entering its rapid growth state.

Department of Neurological Surgery, University of California, 505 Parnassus Avenue, Room M779, San Francisco, CA 94143-0112, USA

[1]Contributed equally to the work.

* Corresponding author.

E-mail address: Manish.Aghi@ucsf.edu

They concluded that a tumor's ability for blood vessel formation is perhaps one of the most essential steps for tumor formation and growth,[7] a notion that eventually gave rise to the term angiogenic switch.

There were minimal advancements in this field until a renewed interest developed in the 1960s. Using a transplantable mammary gland carcinoma model, Tannock and colleagues[8] continued to explore the correlation between tumor-cell and endothelial-cell proliferation by applying newly arising autoradiographic techniques. They were able to show that, as tumor cells moved further away from endothelial cells, their mitotic index was decreased proportionally. This finding was the first direct evidence to show that tumors depend on the nutrients and oxygen diffused from endothelial cells, serving as the rate-liming step for the growth of tumor cells.

Defining Proangiogenic Tumor Secreted Factors

Although many investigators had speculated that a specific factor released by tumor cells led to neovascularization and tumor angiogenesis, direct experiments on this topic were not conducted until the late 1960s.[3] By adapting transparent chambers to a pouch inserted in hamster cheeks, Greenblatt and Shubi[9] at Chicago Medical School and Ehrmann and Knoth[10] from Harvard Medical School showed in parallel that choriocarcinoma or melanoma cells transplanted with a filter interposition between the host and the tumor still promoted the proliferation of blood vessels. Both groups concluded that the most conceivable explanation for the witnessed phenomenon was the diffusion of tumor-produced secreted factors driving tumor vessel formation.

In 1971, Judah Folkman[1] introduced the concept of anti-angiogenic compounds in order to combat human cancers. Folkman and colleagues[11] also published on their isolation attempts of a tumor angiogenesis factor (TAF) from animal and human tumors, which stimulated angiogenesis in the dorsal air-sac model of rats. In addition, they showed the in vitro production of TAF activity from cultured cells, by assessing its ability to stimulate new vessel development in the chick chorioallantoic membrane.[12] In the ensuing 15 years, several pro angiogenic molecules were discovered, including transforming growth factor-alpha, angiogenin, fibroblast growth factor 1 (FGF; also referred to as aFGF), and bFGF (basic fibroblast growth factor), although their specific roles in angiogenesis regulation remained a mystery.[13]

In 1983, Senger and colleagues[14] isolated a protein through partial purification from guinea pig cancer cell conditioned medium. The identified protein was named tumor vascular permeability factor, because of its ability to stimulate vascular leakage in the Miles assay. By 1989, Ferrara and colleagues[15] at Genentech successfully isolated and identified an endothelial-cell mitogen from medium conditioned by folliculostellate cells of bovine pituitary. Because of the high mitogenic levels present, they concluded that the isolated protein was most likely secreted, unlike bFGF, which is produced by the same cell line, but stored internally as previously reported.[16] The protein was named VEGF because of its vascular endothelial cell–specific growth stimulation.[3]

TRANSLATION OF ANTIANGIOGENIC THERAPY FROM OTHER ONCOLOGIC FIELDS TO GLIOBLASTOMA

It had become clear that the development of a VEGF inhibitor was crucial to establishing VEGF as an essential factor for tumor angiogenesis, with the underlying hypothesis that the antibody would inhibit tumor growth. By 1993, Ferrara and colleagues[17] developed a monoclonal antibody with the ability to target and neutralize VEGF-A, the VEGF family member specifically implicated in most angiogenic activity. This antibody decreased the growth rate of glioblastoma tumors implanted in athymic nude mice by 80%. The antibody was as efficient or more successful on other tumor types, including the aggressive rhabdomyosarcoma. As hypothesized, the anti-VEGF antibody did not have an impact on tumor cells in culture, confirming that inhibition of angiogenesis was the mechanism by which tumor cells were suppressed in vivo. These findings led Genentech to move forward with the development of the recombinant humanized VEGF-A–specific monoclonal antibody, bevacizumab (Avastin). By 1997, bevacizumab was being tested in patients with cancer and in 2004 the US Food and Drug Administration (FDA) granted approval for its use as the first line of treatment of metastatic colorectal cancer. Despite promising preclinical data,[17] investigators were hesitant to use bevacizumab for glioblastoma because of safety concerns over increased rates of stroke and intracerebral hemorrhage. During this time, the husband of a patient with glioblastoma in Texas advocated to his wife's oncologist that his wife be trialed on bevacizumab based on his independent research. His oncologist, Dr Stark-Vance, agreed and initiated treatment with bevacizumab in combination with irinotecan, a topoisomerase inhibitor.[18] Given her lack of complications and significant radiographic response, Dr Stark-Vance enrolled 21 patients with high-grade glioma (including 11 with glioblastoma and 10 with anaplastic astrocytoma) in a phase I trial, treating them with bevacizumab and irinotecan in combination. The results of this study were presented at the meeting of the European Association of Neuro-Oncology in 2005 as the first study to confirm the safety and efficacy of bevacizumab treatment in recurrent glioblastoma.[19] Furthermore, the results from this study proved to be encouraging, with a 43% response rate in the 21 patients included in the trial. A phase II trial examining the efficacy of the bevacizumab-irinotecan combination in recurrent glioblastoma soon followed, showing an improved 6-month progression-free survival (PFS) ranging from 30% to 60%,[20,21] compared with that of historical controls, which were between 9% and 21%.[22]

HISTORY OF CLINICAL TRIALS FOR BEVACIZUMAB FOR GLIOBLASTOMA
Bevacizumab as Monotherapy for Recurrent Glioblastoma
By 2009, several studies had been published that assessed bevacizumab as a monotherapy for recurrent glioblastoma. The results from these studies were promising, with the 6-month PFS in phase II trials ranging between 29% and 43%, whereas the overall response rate increased to 28%.[23–25] These results outperformed the findings of studies in which patients received the traditional treatment modality for recurrent glioblastoma, such as various chemotherapeutic regiments and radiation therapy with 6-month PFS ranging from 4% to 9% and 9% to 21%, respectively.[22,26–29] When treated with bevacizumab, patients with recurrent glioblastoma had a 35% radiological response rate under the Macdonald criteria, whereas this number increased to 71% when the assessment used the Levin criteria.[24] Taken together, these phase II clinical trial results proved the initial safety and efficacy of bevacizumab for recurrent glioblastoma and led to the FDA approving bevacizumab for recurrent glioblastoma in 2009.[23,24] This approval made bevacizumab only the second systemic drug to be approved for the treatment of glioblastoma in almost 4 decades. Unlike temozolomide and the locally applied carmustine wafers, bevacizumab's approval received an accelerated designation because of its FDA approval without a randomized phase III clinical trial.[30]

Bevacizumab in Combination with Other Treatments for Recurrent Glioblastoma
Although the numerous targets of VEGF receptor (VEGFR) inhibitors have allowed them to become effective as monotherapeutic agents, many clinicians consider bevacizumab and other VEGF-targeted therapeutics to perform with an increased efficacy when administered in combination with other agents.

When irinotecan, a topoisomerase I inhibitor, was administered as a monotherapy to patients with glioblastoma, its antitumoral effects were minimal, with response rates ranging from 0% to 17%.[31–34] These results were comparable with those of other chemotherapeutics targeting glioblastoma that were used at that time. Phase II clinical trials in which irinotecan and bevacizumab were administered concomitantly went on to show a significantly increased PFS ranging from 38% to 50.3% with the 6-month overall survival (OS) ranging between 72% and 77%.[20,21,23] Several explanations can account for the increased efficacy that ensued as a result of combining bevacizumab with irinotecan. In the presence of bevacizumab, irinotecan may benefit from an increased uptake into the central nervous system, and/or the ability of bevacizumab to target glioma stem cells, whereas irinotecan targets the differentiated tumor cells.[35] When comparing bevacizumab as monotherapy with bevacizumab and irinotecan combination therapy, the PFS was increased from 29% with monotherapy to 46% with combination therapy.[21,24] The radiological response rate using the Macdonald criteria also showed an increase from 35% for patients who received bevacizumab as a monotherapy to 57% for the combination trial, once again supporting the notion of an increased benefit when irinotecan is added to bevacizumab.[21,24] However, combining bevacizumab treatment with temozolomide in a study with 32 patients did not prove to be as promising as irinotecan, and the results were inferior compared with the bevacizumab monotherapy trial.[36] For this study, the 6-month PFS was only 18.8%, with a median PFS of 15.8 weeks. The 6-month OS was 62.5% with a 37-week median OS.[36]

The encouraging results from the irinotecan and bevacizumab combination study led to the search for other potential therapeutic partners for bevacizumab. Sorafenib, an inhibitor of Raf kinase and VEGFR, was of great interest because of the promising preclinical results it produced with antitumoral activity against gliomas.[37] Because sorafenib only proved to have a modest effect as a single agent, it was combined with bevacizumab to inhibit the VEGF/VEGFR axis.[38] However, sorafenib combined with bevacizumab did not improve the outcomes significantly, with 6-month PFS ranging from 17% to 26% compared with 18% with bevacizumab as a single agent or historical controls, which may have been attributed to sorafenib's inadequacy in crossing the blood-brain barrier.[39,40] At present, sorafenib is not recommended in combination with bevacizumab for glioblastoma. In addition to sorafenib, several other agents were combined with bevacizumab and studied for recurrent glioblastoma, including etoposide, erlotonib, fotemustine, carmustine, and carboplatin. Not only were the benefits minimal but these drugs were sources of potential side effects.[40–42]

A recently completed randomized trial in Europe made significant advances relative to the studies cited earlier in defining the role of bevacizumab in treating recurrent glioblastoma. This phase III trial, the European Organisation for Research and Treatment of Cancer (EORTC) 26101 trial, explored the combination of bevacizumab and lomustine in patients with a first recurrence of a glioblastoma. Results presented at the 2015 Society for Neuro-Oncology annual meeting revealed that OS was not superior in patients receiving lomustine plus bevacizumab (n = 149 patients) compared with those receiving lomustine alone (n = 288 patients; hazard ratio [HR], 0.95; confidence interval [CI], 0.74–1.21; P = .65), whereas locally assessed PFS was longer with the addition of bevacizumab to lomustine (HR, 0.49; CI, 0.39–0.61).[43]

Bevacizumab in Newly Diagnosed Glioblastoma

Most of the early studies of bevacizumab in glioblastoma were based on treatment of recurrent glioblastoma. In order to fully investigate the therapeutic potential of bevacizumab for patients with glioblastoma beyond its benefits for recurrent disease, the reasonable subsequent step was to determine the drug's efficacy earlier in the course of the disease. Phase II trials were conducted in which bevacizumab was given in addition to the Stupp protocol of temozolomide and radiation therapy. The results were not promising because there was little to no improvement on OS, the primary end point, which ranged from 19.6 to 23 months,[44,45] compared with an OS of 14.6 to 21.1 months[44,46] when the Stupp protocol was followed without the addition of bevacizumab. Although the OS was not affected with bevacizumab at diagnosis, the studies showed a significant improvement in PFS, a secondary end point, ranging from 13 to 13.6 months[44,45] compared with 6 to 9 months with the standard Stupp protocol without bevacizumab.[46] The 6-month PFS rate was also favorable when bevacizumab was added to the Stupp protocol, increasing to 85% to 88%,[44,45] a value far exceeding the 54% noted with the standard Stupp protocol.[47] These results

are consistent with those seen in the disease setting and suggest a short-term benefit of bevacizumab in delaying recurrence that fails to affect OS, perhaps because of the tumor that emerges on recurrence being more biologically aggressive than the originally treated tumor.[48]

The results were further confirmed in 2 randomized phase III trials, the Radiation Therapy Oncology Group (RTOG) 0825 trial and the Avastin in Glioblastoma (AVAglio) trial, which compared the OS (primary end point) and PFS (secondary end point) of patients with newly diagnosed glioblastoma receiving the Stupp protocol alone versus Stupp protocol plus bevacizumab. In the AVAglio phase III trial, median PFS was improved with the addition of bevacizumab to the Stupp protocol, reaching 10.6 months when bevacizumab was added to the Stupp protocol compared with 6.2 months with the Stupp protocol alone (P<.001).[49] The Stupp protocol plus bevacizumab group had a higher OS 1 year after initiation of treatment (72.4% vs 66.3%, respectively; P<.049), but by 2 years this difference had faded (33.9% vs 30.1%, respectively; P = .24). Median OS, the primary end point of the study, was 16.8 months in the Stupp protocol plus bevacizumab group compared with 16.7 months for patients treated with the Stupp protocol by itself (P = .1).[49]

The results from the RTOG 0825 phase III trial revealed a similar trend. The median PFS increased with the addition of bevacizumab to 10.7 months compared with 7.3 months in patients who were solely treated with the Stupp protocol (P = .007).[50] There was no significant difference in median OS observed with the Stupp protocol alone (16.1 months) compared with the Stupp protocol plus bevacizumab (15.7 months) (P = .21).[50] With the results from these phase III trials, investigators were able to confirm the trends and findings of phase II trials, which showed that bevacizumab given at the time of glioblastoma diagnosis carries a favorable PFS outcome, but that it fails to be of any benefit with regard to OS.

The combination of bevacizumab with the Stupp protocol at the time of diagnosis played a significant role in improving the baseline quality of life, as well as performance measures. The addition of bevacizumab to the Stupp protocol resulted in Karnofsky Performance Scale scores that remained greater than 70 for 9 months, whereas the group receiving the Stupp protocol alone were only able to maintain a score of more than 70 for 6 months.[49] Similarly, performance status was also preserved in the bevacizumab plus Stupp protocol group for a median of 9 months compared with 5.5 months in those treated with the Stupp protocol alone (P<.001). Furthermore, the time to clinical deterioration for patients receiving bevacizumab in addition to the Stupp protocol was 14.2 months, which was significantly longer than the 11.8 months it took for patients only treated with the Stupp protocol (*P* = .02). Note that there was a decreased requirement for glucocorticoid administration for patients who were treated with bevacizumab.[49] However, in the experimental group there was a greater number of complications and serious adverse events deemed attributable to bevacizumab as well as decreased quality of life outcomes and neurocognitive function. These results show that even though bevacizumab added to the standard Stupp protocol at the time of diagnosis has shown results that are promising for PFS in addition to certain clinical outcome measures, the OS for these patients was unchanged, and may be associated with a higher complication rate. These findings confirm the notion that bevacizumab carries limited additional benefits when administered earlier in the course of glioblastoma.

SUMMARY AND FUTURE DIRECTIONS
The results from the recently completed phase III trials suggest that bevacizumab combined with

standard therapy prolonged PFS without affecting OS when given at the time of diagnosis and at the time of recurrence. However, these findings temper the optimism for antiangiogenic therapy in glioblastoma that emerged from the preclinical laboratory studies and early clinical trials described earlier in this chapter. These findings also underscore the importance of identifying biomarkers for response and resistance so that appropriate candidates for treatment can continue to be identified, because the randomized trials and day-to-day clinical practice have revealed examples of patients who have experienced clinical benefit from bevacizumab and have also shown a poor prognosis once resistance becomes entrenched. For the time being, patients diagnosed with glioblastoma who are being treated with bevacizumab should be monitored diligently for radiological changes and treatment-related morbidity, with a recognition that progression during bevacizumab treatment may show unconventional imaging features such as lack of enhancement, a feature of this agent that has led to refinement of traditional radiographic definitions of glioblastoma recurrence (**Fig. 10.1**).[51] Clinicians using the agent must also have a low threshold for changing treatments early when imaging changes emerge

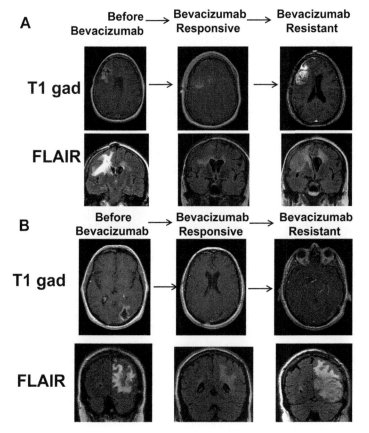

A Before Bevacizumab → Bevacizumab Responsive → Bevacizumab Resistant

T1 gad

FLAIR

B Before Bevacizumab → Bevacizumab Responsive → Bevacizumab Resistant

T1 gad

FLAIR

Fig. 10.1 Radiographic imaging of variations of bevacizumab resistance. Examples of enhancing (*A*) and nonenhancing (*B*) recurrence during bevacizumab treatment of recurrent glioblastomas. FLAIR, fluid-attenuated inversion recovery; T1 gad, T1 gadolinium enhanced.

because bevacizumab-resistant glioblastomas have a poor prognosis whether managed by chemotherapy or repeat surgery and timely identification of recurrence may prevent the phenotype from becoming entrenched.[48]

REFERENCES

1. Folkman J. Tumor angiogenesis: therapeutic implications. N Engl J Med 1971;285(21):1182–6.
2. Ferrara N, Adamis AP. Ten years of anti-vascular endothelial growth factor therapy. Nat Rev Drug Discov 2016;15(6):385–403.
3. Ferrara N. VEGF and the quest for tumour angiogenesis factors. Nat Rev Cancer 2002;2(10):795–803.
4. Lewis WH. The vascular pattern of tumors. Bulletin of the Johns Hopkins Hospital 1927;41:156–70.
5. Sandison JC. Observations on the growth of blood vessels as seen in the transparent chamber introduced into the rabbit's ear. Am J Anat 1928;41(3):475–96.
6. Ide AG, Baker NH, Warren SL. Vascularization of the Brown Pearce rabbit epithelioma transplant as seen in the transparent ear chamber. Am J Roentgenol 1939;42:891–9.
7. Algire GH, Chalkley HW, Legallais FY, et al. Vascular reactions of normal and malignant tissues in vivo. I. Vascular reactions of mice to wounds and to normal and neoplastic transplants. J Natl Cancer Inst 1945;6:73–85.
8. Tannock IF. The relation between cell proliferation and the vascular system in a transplanted mouse mammary tumour. Br J Cancer 1968;22(2):258–73.
9. Greenblatt M, Shubi P. Tumor angiogenesis: transfilter diffusion studies in the hamster by the transparent chamber technique. J Natl Cancer Inst 1968;41(1):111–24.
10. Ehrmann RL, Knoth M. Choriocarcinoma. Transfilter stimulation of vasoproliferation in the hamster cheek pouch. Studied by light and electron microscopy. J Natl Cancer Inst 1968;41(6):1329–41.
11. Folkman J, Merler E, Abernathy C, et al. Isolation of a tumor factor responsible for angiogenesis. J Exp Med 1971;133(2):275–88.
12. Klagsbrun M, Knighton D, Folkman J. Tumor angiogenesis activity in cells grown in tissue culture. Cancer Res 1976;36(1):110–4.
13. Klagsbrun M. Regulators of angiogenesis: stimulators, inhibitors, and extracellular matrix. J Cell Biochem 1991;47(3):199–200.
14. Senger DR, Galli SJ, Dvorak AM, et al. Tumor cells secrete a vascular permeability factor that promotes accumulation of ascites fluid. Science 1983;219(4587):983–5.
15. Ferrara N, Henzel WJ. Pituitary follicular cells secrete a novel heparin-binding growth factor specific for vascular endothelial cells. Biochem Biophys Res Commun 1989;161(2):851–8.
16. Ferrara N, Schweigerer L, Neufeld G, et al. Pituitary follicular cells produce basic fibroblast growth factor. Proc Natl Acad Sci U S A 1987;84(16):5773–7.
17. Kim KJ, Li B, Winer J, et al. Inhibition of vascular endothelial growth factor-induced angiogenesis suppresses tumour growth in vivo. Nature 1993;362(6423):841–4.
18. Kolata G, PA. Costly cancer drug offers hope, but also a dilemma. 2008. Available at: http://www.nytimes.com/2008/07/06/health/06avastin.html. Accessed October 2, 2014.
19. Stark-Vance V. Bevacizumab and CPT-11 in the treatment of relapsed malignant glioma. Presented at the World Federation of Neuro-Oncology. Neuro-Oncol 2005;7:369.
20. Vredenburgh JJ, Desjardins A, Herndon JE 2nd, et al. Phase II trial of bevacizumab and irinotecan in recurrent malignant glioma. Clin Cancer Res 2007;13(4):1253–9.
21. Vredenburgh JJ, Desjardins A, Herndon JE 2nd, et al. Bevacizumab plus irinotecan in recurrent glioblastoma multiforme. J Clin Oncol 2007;25(30):4722–9.
22. Ballman KV, Buckner JC, Brown PD, et al. The relationship between six-month progression-free survival and 12-month overall survival end points for phase II trials in patients with glioblastoma multiforme. Neuro Oncol 2007;9(1):29–38.
23. Friedman HS, Prados MD, Wen PY, et al. Bevacizumab alone and in combination with irinotecan in recurrent glioblastoma. J Clin Oncol 2009;27(28):4733–40.
24. Kreisl TN, Kim L, Moore K, et al. Phase II trial of single-agent bevacizumab followed by bevacizumab plus irinotecan at tumor progression in recurrent glioblastoma. J Clin Oncol 2009;27(5):740–5.
25. Nagane M, Nishikawa R, Narita Y, et al. Phase II study of single-agent bevacizumab in Japanese patients with recurrent malignant glioma. Jpn J Clin Oncol 2012;42(10):887–95.
26. Happold C, Roth P, Wick W, et al. ACNU-based chemotherapy for recurrent glioma in the temozolomide era. J Neurooncol 2009;92(1):45–8.
27. Lamborn KR, Yung WK, Chang SM, et al. Progression-free survival: an important end point in evaluating therapy for recurrent high-grade gliomas. Neuro Oncol 2008;10(2):162–70.
28. Wick W, Puduvalli VK, Chamberlain MC, et al. Phase III study of enzastaurin compared with lomustine in the treatment of recurrent intracranial glioblastoma. J Clin Oncol 2010;28(7):1168–74.
29. Yung WK, Albright RE, Olson J, et al. A phase II study of temozolomide vs. procarbazine in patients with glioblastoma multiforme at first relapse. Br J Cancer 2000;83(5):588–93.
30. Cohen MH, Shen YL, Keegan P, et al. FDA drug approval summary: bevacizumab (Avastin) as

treatment of recurrent glioblastoma multiforme. Oncologist 2009;14(11):1131–8.

31. Chamberlain MC. Salvage chemotherapy with CPT-11 for recurrent glioblastoma multiforme. J Neurooncol 2002;56(2):183–8.

32. Cloughesy TF, Filka E, Nelson G, et al. Irinotecan treatment for recurrent malignant glioma using an every-3-week regimen. Am J Clin Oncol 2002; 25(2):204–8.

33. Friedman HS, Petros WP, Friedman AH, et al. Irinotecan therapy in adults with recurrent or progressive malignant glioma. J Clin Oncol 1999;17(5):1516–25.

34. Prados MD, Lamborn K, Yung WK, et al. A phase 2 trial of irinotecan (CPT-11) in patients with recurrent malignant glioma: a North American Brain Tumor Consortium study. Neuro Oncol 2006;8(2):189–93.

35. Bao S, Wu Q, Sathornsumetee S, et al. Stem cell-like glioma cells promote tumor angiogenesis through vascular endothelial growth factor. Cancer Res 2006;66(16):7843–8.

36. Desjardins A, Reardon DA, Coan A, et al. Bevacizumab and daily temozolomide for recurrent glioblastoma. Cancer 2012;118(5):1302–12.

37. Siegelin MD, Raskett CM, Gilbert CA, et al. Sorafenib exerts anti-glioma activity in vitro and in vivo. Neurosci Lett 2010;478(3):165–70.

38. Nabors LB, Supko JG, Rosenfeld M, et al. Phase I trial of sorafenib in patients with recurrent or progressive malignant glioma. Neuro Oncol 2011; 13(12):1324–30.

39. Fischer I, Gagner JP, Law M, et al. Angiogenesis in gliomas: biology and molecular pathophysiology. Brain Pathol 2005;15(4):297–310.

40. Galanis E, Anderson SK, Lafky JM, et al. Phase II study of bevacizumab in combination with sorafenib in recurrent glioblastoma (N0776): a north central cancer treatment group trial. Clin Cancer Res 2013;19(17):4816–23.

41. Chamberlain MC. Bevacizumab for the treatment of recurrent glioblastoma. Clin Med Insights Oncol 2011;5:117–29.

42. Taal W, Oosterkamp HM, Walenkamp AM, et al. Single-agent bevacizumab or lomustine versus a combination of bevacizumab plus lomustine in patients with recurrent glioblastoma (BELOB trial): a randomised controlled phase 2 trial. Lancet Oncol 2014;15(9):943–53.

43. Wick W, Brandes AA, Gorlia T, et al. Phase III trial exploring the combination of bevacizumab and lomustine in patients with first recurrence of a glioblastoma: The EORTC 26101 Trial. Annual Scientific Meeting of the Society for Neuro-Oncology. San Antonio, Texas, 2015.

44. Lai A, Tran A, Nghiemphu PL, et al. Phase II study of bevacizumab plus temozolomide during and after radiation therapy for patients with newly diagnosed glioblastoma multiforme. J Clin Oncol 2011;29(2): 142–8.

45. Narayana A, Gruber D, Kunnakkat S, et al. A clinical trial of bevacizumab, temozolomide, and radiation for newly diagnosed glioblastoma. J Neurosurg 2012;116(2):341–5.

46. Stupp R, Hegi ME, Mason WP, et al. Effects of radiotherapy with concomitant and adjuvant temozolomide versus radiotherapy alone on survival in glioblastoma in a randomised phase III study: 5-year analysis of the EORTC-NCIC trial. Lancet Oncol 2009;10(5):459–66.

47. Stupp R, Mason WP, van den Bent MJ, et al. Radiotherapy plus concomitant and adjuvant temozolomide for glioblastoma. N Engl J Med 2005; 352(10):987–96.

48. Clark AJ, Lamborn KR, Butowski NA, et al. Neurosurgical management and prognosis of patients with glioblastoma that progress during bevacizumab treatment. Neurosurgery 2012;70(2):361–70.

49. Chinot OL, Wick W, Mason W, et al. Bevacizumab plus radiotherapy-temozolomide for newly diagnosed glioblastoma. N Engl J Med 2014;370(8): 709–22.

50. Gilbert MR, Dignam JJ, Armstrong TS, et al. A randomized trial of bevacizumab for newly diagnosed glioblastoma. N Engl J Med 2014;370(8): 699–708.

51. Wen PY, Macdonald DR, Reardon DA, et al. Updated response assessment criteria for high-grade gliomas: response assessment in neuro-oncology working group. J Clin Oncol 2010;28(11):1963–72.

CHAPTER 11

Recurrent Glioblastoma

Kalil G. Abdullah, MD[a], Jacob A. Miller, BS[b],
Corey Adamson, MD, PhD, MPH[c], Steven Brem, MD[a],*

Given the aggressive nature of glioblastoma, it is nearly a certainty that all patients will need to be evaluated for potential treatment of recurrent disease. There is currently no definitive standard of care for recurrent glioblastoma. Unlike in other solid tumors that have benefited from genomic or molecular profiling and targeted therapy, it is often the case that the recurrent tumor no longer reflects the index tumor. In the pre-bevacizumab era, the meidan overall survival was 30 weeks, and only 10 weeks for median progression-free survival.[1] This chapter discusses the definition of recurrence and gives a further breakdown of the treatment options and surgical and nonsurgical management, with a review of pertinent studies that have led to a better understanding of treatment options for recurrent disease. Other chapters provide expert opinion on the role of antiangiogenic agents (see Chapter 10) and tumor treating fields (See Chapter 17) as they pertain to recurrent glioblastoma and are only briefly discussed here.

DEFINING RECURRENCE

Before the decision to treat recurrent glioblastoma, it is essential to determine whether or not radiographic evidence of recurrent disease is secondary to glioblastoma progression or to radiographic pseudoprogression.[2] In order to standardize the assessment of response to initial glioblastoma treatment, the MacDonald Criteria organized response based on 4 categories: complete response (CR), partial response (PR), stable disease (SD), and progressive disease (PD)[3] (Table 11.1).

These criteria were initially formulated in 1990, and relied on the enhancing pattern of the tumor, which did not address the effects of chemoradiotherapy and antiangiogenic agents on radiographic imaging. Several factors compound the difficulty in determining pseudoprogression from true progression and include post–radiation treatment effects that increase contrast enhancement and T2 hyperintensity over the first month, which may increase vascular probability, and the use of bevacizumab, which may conversely decrease contrast enhancement. To address this, the Response Assessment in Neuro-Oncology Working Group (RANO) devised criteria for determination of the first progression, which depend on the timing from the initial chemoradiotherapy treatment. In general, these criteria added more restrictive parameters for diagnosing progressive disease within 90 days of chemoradiotherapy completion as well as consideration to corticosteroid use and T2/fluid-attenuated inversion recovery sequencing assessment.[4] At present, the RANO criteria are considered the most appropriate tools for evaluation of progression and response in glioblastoma.[5] Advances in MRI diagnostic capabilities have also been used to differentiate pseudoprogression from true progression, although these tools are suggested for guidance and not definitive diagnosis. Recently, Galldiks and colleagues[6] evaluated a group of 22 patients with glioblastoma with concern for new contrast-enhancing lesions or existing lesions showing increased enhancement on their routine MRI within first 4 months after completion of chemoradiotherapy and compared those findings with O-(2-(18)F-fluoroethyl)-L-tyrosine [(18)F-FET] PET scans done at the same time. In the 11 patients with available histopathologic confirmation, they found significantly lower compound uptake in those with necrosis or pseudoprogression than in those with confirmed tumor recurrence. Although this is

[a] Department of Neurosurgery, Hospital of the University of Pennsylvania, 3400 Spruce Street, Philadelphia, PA 19104, USA; [b] Cleveland Clinic Lerner College of Medicine, Cleveland Clinic, 9980 Carnegie Avenue, Cleveland, OH 44195, USA; [c] Department of Neurosurgery, Emory University Hospital, 1365-B Clifton Road, Atlanta, GA 30322, USA
* Corresponding author. Department of Neurosurgery, Hospital of the University of Pennsylvania, Silverstein 3, 3400 Spruce Street, Philadelphia, PA 19104.
E-mail address: Steven.Brem@uphs.upenn.edu

TABLE 11.1
MacDonald versus Response Assessment in Neuro-Oncology (RANO) Criteria for response in malignant gliomas

MacDonald	RANO
CR	
Complete disappearance of all enhancing measurable and nonmeasurable disease sustained for at least 4 wk	Disappearance of all enhancing measurable and nonmeasurable disease sustained for a minimum of 4 wk
	Stable or improved FLAIR/T2-weighted lesions
No new lesions	No new lesions
Stable or improved clinically	Stable or improved clinically
No corticosteroids	Patients cannot be receiving corticosteroids (physiologic replacement doses are acceptable)
PR	
≥50% decrease compared with baseline in the sum of products of perpendicular diameters of all measurable enhancing lesions sustained for at least 4 wk	≥50% decrease (compared with baseline) in the sum of products of perpendicular diameters of all measurable enhancing lesions sustained for a minimum of 4 wk
	No progression of nonmeasurable disease
No new lesions	No new lesions
Stable or reduced corticosteroid dose	Stable or improved FLAIR/T2-weighted lesions
Stable or improved clinically	Stable or improved clinically
	Corticosteroid dosage at the time of the scan should be no greater than the dosage at the time of the baseline scan
SD	
Does not qualify for CR, PR, or PD	Patient does not qualify for CR, PR, or progression
	Stable FLAIR/T2-weighted lesions on a corticosteroid dose no greater than at baseline
Stable clinically	Stable clinically
PD	
≥25% increase in sum of the products of perpendicular diameters of enhancing lesions relative to best previous scan	≥25% increase in sum of the products of perpendicular diameters of all measurable enhancing lesions compared with the smallest tumor measurement obtained either at baseline or best response following the initiation of therapy, while on a stable or increasing dose of corticosteroids. Significant increase in FLAIR T2-weighted lesions compared with baseline or best response following initiation of therapy, not caused by comorbid events (eg, radiation therapy, ischemic injury, seizures, postoperative changes, other treatment effects), while on a stable or increasing dose of corticosteroids
Any new lesion	New lesions
Clinical deterioration	Clinical deterioration not attributable to any causes apart from the tumor (eg, seizures, medication side effects, complications of therapy, cerebrovascular events, or infection) or decreases in corticosteroid dose. Failure to return for evaluation owing to death or deteriorating condition. Clear progression of nonmeasurable disease

Abbreviation: FLAIR, fluid-attenuated inversion recovery.
From Roy S, Lahiri D, Maji T, et al. Recurrent glioblastoma: where we stand. South Asian J Cancer 2015;4:164; with permission.

promising, this study and others have determined that labeled uptake remains a diagnostic option.[7]

SURGICAL INTERVENTION FOR RECURRENT DISEASE

The decision to proceed with surgical intervention on a patient with recurrent glioblastoma is not always clear. However, existing within the current literature are multiple prognostic factors that can guide the course of treatment of recurrent disease. There are many studies that have individually examined consecutive patients and their outcomes following repeat resection. This chapter describes what the authors think is the most relevant literature in assisting clinicians (and patients) in the decision to proceed with surgery.

One of the most important studies advocating gross total resection of recurrent glioblastoma was performed in 2012 by Bloch and colleagues.[8] A total of 107 patients were examined after repeat glioblastoma resection. Of that subset, 52 patients had an initial gross total resection, of whom 31 (60%) had gross resection at recurrence and a median survival of 20.4 months versus 18.4 months for patients with a subsequent subtotal resection. In patients who initially had a subtotal resection (55), 47% had gross total resection recurrence with a median survival of 19 months and 53% had a subtotal resection with a median survival of 15.9 months. These findings indicated that extensive initial resection was not necessarily correlated with survival for every presentation, but that gross total resection on recurrence was statistically associated with increased overall survival. In this study, as in several others, the Karnofsky Performance Scale (KPS) at the time of surgical intervention for recurrent disease was an independent predictor of survival. More recent studies have similarly found that low residual volume and increased extent of resection were consistent with longer overall survival and progression-free survival[9,10] (**Fig. 11.1**).

Studies that examine the overall survival for patients with current disease are sometimes intrinsically biased secondary to patient selection. For example, patients with a high KPS and noneloquent areas tend to be logical candidates for second, if not third or even fourth, resections of glioblastoma. For example, a study by Chaichana and colleagues[11] found that the median survival for patients who underwent 1, 2, 3, and 4 resections was 6.8, 15.5, 22.4, and 26.6 months. Although these patients were matched in a case-control evaluation, the specific tumor molecular heterogeneity was unable to be analyzed, and it may be more a reflection of underlying favorable molecular

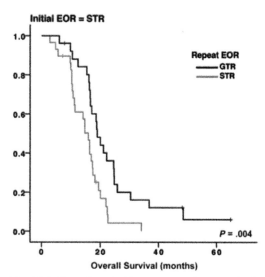

Fig. 11.1 Overall survival in patients with an initial subtotal resection, stratified by either gross total resection (GTR), or subtotal resection (STR) on recurrence. EOR, extent of resection. (*From* Bloch O, Han SJ, Cha S, et al. Impact of extent of resection for recurrent glioblastoma on overall survival: clinical article. J Neurosurg 2012;117:1036; with permission.)

profiling than simply surgical intervention that allowed these impressive extensions of life. These special patients are more likely to be included in studies and trials that result in publication. It is rare for a very old patient with a low KPS and highly aggressive course to benefit from second-stage or third-stage craniotomies. There is a growing body of literature that indicates that although the ideal patient may be of younger age, elderly patients when properly selected may also benefit from surgical resection.[12,13] Park and colleagues[14] devised a validated scale to predict survival after recurrent surgery and their findings were as expected: patients with Karnofsky performance statuses greater than 80, tumor volume less than 50 cm^3, and lack of involvement in cortical brain structures were all significantly associated with better postoperative survival. This scale was updated in 2010 and added the presence of ependymal involvement to further stratify patients by likelihood of prognosis following surgical resection.[15]

The use of carmustine wafers is discussed in detail elsewhere in this book (Chapter 16), but briefly these wafers were first approved by the US Food and Drug Administration (FDA) in the context of recurrent glioblastoma. This approval was based on a 1995 study of 222 patients with recurrent glioblastoma across 27 medical centers who underwent randomization to receive either carmustine wafers or placebo. The median survival of the 110 patients who received carmustine wafers was 31 weeks compared with 23 weeks for those who received placebo, and 6-month overall survival was 50% greater in those in the experimental group.[16] In 2008, a 10-year institutional analysis at Johns Hopkins reviewed 122 patients who underwent craniotomy and Gliadel wafer implantation for recurrent glioblastoma with a median survival of 11.3 months, and 13% were alive at 2 years, with an increasing trend to survival linked to the use of Gliadel.[17] The combination of Gliadel with other agents is challenging because of the exclusion of Gliadel wafers in many clinical trials evaluating novel agents, due in part to the confounding radiographic artifacts due to Gliadel. The complications noted by the Hopkins group were similar to a comparative cohort without wafers, and included cerebral edema, seizures, and wound infections. An advantage of the carmustine wafer is that it avoids the systemic toxicity (immunosuppression, bone marrow failure, gastrointestinal effects) of chemotherapy, as there is no detectable level of agent in the blood stream.

CHEMOTHERAPY AND RADIATION FOR THE TREATMENT OF RECURRENT GLIOBLASTOMA

Chemotherapy

Since 1996 there have been almost 100 studies to establish the ideal treatment of recurrent glioblastoma (Table 11.2). Most of these were phase I and II, single-arm studies with fewer than 50 patients in the experimental group. These studies examined chemotherapeutic, dietary, and mechanistic permutations that included, in chronologic order, tamoxifen, procarbazine, temozolomide, carboplatin, etoposide, RMP-7 (bradykinin anal-g, Cereport™), gefitinib, bis-chloroethylnitrosourea; carmustine (BCNU), irinotecan, temsirolimus, imatinib, hydroxyurea, tipifarnib, sirolimus, pioglitazone, rofecoxib, capecitabine, bevacizumab, cilengitide, erlotinib, vorinostat, everolimus, O-benzylguanine, sulfasalazine, cetuximab, cediranib, lapatinib, enzastaurin, lomustine, cintredekin, sorafenib, sagopilone, 6-Thioguanine (6-TG), capecitabine, celecoxib, bortezomib, lomustine, 1-2-chlorethyl-3-cyclohexyl-1-nitrosurea (CCNU), tumor treating fields, lonafarnib, sunitinib, ketogenic diet, temsirolimus, dasatinib, panobinostat, etirinotecan pegol, valparin, and afatinib.[18–80] Despite these investigations, there still exists no clear standard of care for recurrent disease.

Given its low side effect profile, ease of administration, and known improvement for patients with newly diagnosed glioblastoma, temozolomide has become for many centers the most commonly administered chemotherapeutic for recurrent disease. Several phase I and phase II studies on temozolomide for recurrent disease showed efficacy and safety that led to FDA approval.[81] Wei and colleagues[82] recently examined via meta-analysis the optimal regimen for temozolomide in the treatment of recurrent disease, although this is not a clinical consensus. In their review of 33 studies involving 1760 patients, the schedule of 7 days on and 7 days off was significantly superior to the standard regimen for progression-free survival at 6 months. Han and colleagues[69] examined the safety of this dose-dense 7-on/7-off schedule in 40 patients in order to examine the primary end point of progression-free survival at 6 months and the secondary outcome of correlation of o(6)-methylguanine-dna methyltransferase (MGMT) promoter status influence on survival. They found the progression-free survival at 6 months to be 10%, with a median overall survival of 21.6 weeks. There were trends, but no clear statistical significance of longer progression-free survival and overall survival with MGMT promoter methylation. Multiple attempts at evaluating temozolomide monotherapy via alternating metronomic schedules have been made. The DIRECTOR trial (Dose-intensified rechallenge with temozolomide), a randomized trial of patients with glioblastoma at first progression after standard temozolomide and radiation therapy randomized to either 1 week of 120 mg daily with 1 week off or 3 weeks of 80 mg of temozolomide, found that median time to failure in patients with MGMT methylated tumors was 3.2 months versus 1.8 months in unmethylated tumors, and the median progression-free survival rate at 6 months was 39.7 with methylation and 6.9% without.[80]

In general, before 1999, the nitrosoureas (lomustine, nimustine, carmustine) were used as first-line treatment of glioblastoma because of their ability to cross the left brain barrier as a result of their high lipophilicity. There have been several notable phase 3 trials of nitrosoureas used as salvage therapy for recurrent glioblastoma. In 2010, Wick and colleagues[51] completed an open-label phase 3 study comparing the efficacy and safety of enzastaurin versus lomustine, which was terminated at 266 patients because of futility, and found that although enzastaurin was well tolerated and had a beneficial hematologic toxicity profile, it did not have superior efficacy compared with lomustine. Temozolomide was compared with procarbazine, lomustine, and vincristine and found to have similar toxicity and no clear survival benefit between groups in a phase 3 study enrolling a total of 477 patients.[44] The use of immunotherapy with epidermal growth factor receptor targeting (See Chapter 19), small molecule targeting

TABLE 11.2
Studies of novel agents for the treatment of recurrent glioblastoma

Investigators, Year	Study Design	Patients Per Arm (N)	Interventions	Prior Adjuvant Therapy	Radiographic Response (%)	PFS (mo)	Median OS (mo)
Couldwell et al,[17] 1996	Phase II, single arm	20	Tamoxifen	RT + Chemo	CR or PR (20)	NA	7
Brandes et al,[18] 1999	Phase II, single arm	28	Procarbazine + tamoxifen	RT + Chemo	CR (4), PR (25), SD (32), PD (39)	Median 3	7
Yung et al,[19] 2000	Phase II, 2 randomized arms	112	TMZ	RT + Chemo	PR (5), SD (40)	6, 21%; median 4	4
		138	Procarbazine	RT + Chemo	PR (5), SD (27)	6, 8%; median 2	2
Watanabe et al,[20] 2002	Phase II, single arm	14	Carboplatin + etoposide	RT + Chemo	CR (0), PR (14), SD (43), PD (43)	Mean 4	9
Prados et al,[21] 2003	Phase II, 2 randomized arms	40	RMP-7 + carboplatin	RT + Chemo	CR (0), PR (8)	Median 2	6
		40	Placebo + carboplatin	RT + Chemo	CR (3), PR (10)	Median 2	5
Rich et al,[24] 2004	Phase II, single arm	53	Gefitinib	RT + Chemo	CR (0), PR (0), SD (42), PD (58)	6, 13%	9
Brandes et al,[22] 2004	Phase II, single arm	42	BCNU + irinotecan	RT + Chemo	CR (0), PR (21), SD (50), PD (29)	6, 17%; median 4	12
Prados et al,[23] 2004	Phase II, single arm	38	BCNU + TMZ	RT + Chemo	CR (0), PR (6), SD (6), PD (88)	6, 38%; median 3	9
Chang et al,[25] 2005	Phase II, single arm	43	Temsirolimus	RT at minimum	CR (0), PR (5), SD (47), PD (48)	6, 2%; median 2	NA
Dresemann,[26] 2005	Phase II, single arm	30	Imatinib + hydroxyurea	RT + Chemo	CR or PR (20)	6, 32%; 24, 16%	5
Galanis et al,[27] 2005	Phase II, single arm	65	Temsirolimus	RT + Chemo	CR or PR (0)	6, 8%; median 4	4
Reardon et al,[28] 2005	Phase II, single arm	33	Imatinib + hydroxyurea	Chemo at minimum	CR (3), PR (6), SD (42), PD (48)	6, 27%; median 4	12

(continued on next page)

TABLE 11.2 (continued)

Investigators, Year	Study Design	Patients Per Arm (N)	Interventions	Prior Adjuvant Therapy	Radiographic Response (%)	PFS (mo)	Median OS (mo)
Cloughesy et al,[29] 2006	Phase II, single arm	67	Tipifarnib	RT at minimum	CR (0), PR (7)	6, 9%	NA
Reardon et al,[30] 2006	Phase II, single arm	34	Gefitinib + sirolimus	RT + Chemo	CR (0), PR (5), SD (38), PD (47)	6, 23%	NA
Wen et al,[31] 2006	Phase II, single arm	34	Imatinib	Not specified	PR (6)	6, 3%	NA
Hau et al,[32] 2007	Phase II, single arm	14	Pioglitazone + rofecoxib + (capecitabine or TMZ)	RT + Chemo	CR (0), PR (20), SD (10), PD (70)	6, 20%	NA
Vredenburgh et al, 2007	Phase II, single arm	35	BEV + irinotecan	RT + Chemo	CR or PR (57)	6, 46%; median 6	10
Reardon et al,[34] 2008	Phase II, 2 randomized arms	40	Cilengitide high dose	RT + Chemo	CR (0), PR (13)	6, 15%; median 2	10
		41	Cilengitide low dose	RT + Chemo	CR (0), PR (5)	6, 10%; median 2	7
de Groot et al,[33] 2008	Phase II, single arm	44	Erlotinib + carboplatin	RT + Chemo	CR (0), PR (2), SD (47), PD (51)	6, 14%; median 2	7
Galanis et al,[36] 2009	Phase II, single arm	66	Vorinostat	Not specified	CR or PR (3)	6, 17%; median 2	6
Kreisl et al,[37] 2009	Phase II, single arm	22	Everolimus + gefitinib	Not specified	CR (0), PR (14), SD (36), PD (50)	6, 5%; median 3	6
Quinn et al,[39] 2009	Phase II, single arm	52	O-benzylguanine + gliadel wafers	RT + Chemo	NA	NA	13
Reardon et al,[40] 2009	Phase II, single arm	27	Etoposide + BEV	RT + Chemo	CR (4), PR (19), SD (70), PD (7)	6, 46%; median 5	12
Robe et al,[41] 2009	Phase II, single arm	10	Sulfasalazine	RT + Chemo	CR (0), PR (0), SD (10), PD (90)	Median 1	2
Friedman et al,[35] 2009	Phase II, 2 randomized arms	85	BEV	RT + Chemo	CR (1), PR (27)	6, 43%; median 4	9
		82	BEV + irinotecan	RT + Chemo	CR (2), PR (29)	6, 50%; median 6	9
van den Bent et al,[42] 2009	Phase II, 2 randomized arms	54	Erlotinib	RT + Chemo	CR (0), PR (4), SD (17)	6, 11%	8

		56	TMZ or carmustine (if failed TMZ)	RT + Chemo	CR (0), PR (10), SD (35)	6, 24%	7
Neyns et al,[38] 2009	Phase II, single arm	55	Cetuximab	RT + Chemo	CR (0), PR (5), SD (31)	6, 7%; median 2	5
Reardon et al,[48] 2009	Phase II, single arm	231	Imatinib + hydroxyurea	Not specified	CR or PR (8)	6, 11%; median 26	6
Batchelor et al,[43] 2010	Phase II, single arm	31	Cediranib	RT + Chemo	PR (57), SD (31)	6, 26%	8
Raizer et al,[47] 2010	Phase II, single arm	38	Erlotinib	RT + Chemo	CR (0), PR (0), SD (8), PD (92)	6, 3%; median 2	6
Reardon et al,[48] 2010	Phase II, single arm	32	Sirolimus + erlotinib	RT + Chemo	CR (0), PR (0), SD (47), PD (53)	6, 3%; median 2	9
Yung et al,[52] 2010	Phase II, single arm	48	Erlotinib	RT + Chemo	CR (2), PR (4), SD (16), PD (78)	6, 20%	9
Sathornsumetee et al,[49] 2010	Phase II, single arm	25	BEV + erlotinib	RT + Chemo	CR (4), PR (46), SD (42), PD (8)	6, 29%; median 4	11
Thiessen et al,[50] 2010	Phase II, single arm	17	Lapatinib	RT + Chemo	CR (0), PR (0), SD (25), PD (75)	NA	NA
Dresemann et al,[45] 2010	Phase III, 2 randomized arms	120	Hydroxyurea	Not specified	CR or PR (1)	6, 7%	5
		120	Imatinib + hydroxyurea	Not specified	CR or PR (2)	6, 5%	5
Wick et al,[51] 2010	Phase III, 2 randomized arms	174	Enzastaurin	Not specified	NA	6, 11%; median 2	7
		92	Lomustine	Not specified	NA	6, 19%; median 2	7
Kunwar et al, 2010	Phase III, 2 randomized arms	183	Cintredekin besudotox	RT + Chemo	NA	NA	9
		93	Gliadel wafers	RT + Chemo	NA	NA	9
Perry et al,[46] 2010	Phase II, single stratified arm. Stratified by prior TMZ failure timing	29	Dose-dense TMZ (progression before 6 cycles TMZ)	RT + Chemo	CR or PR (3), SD (24), PD (73)	6, 27%; median 4	27
		29	Dose-dense TMZ (progression after 6 cycles TMZ)	RT + Chemo	CR or PR (0), SD (8), PD (92)	6, 7%; median 2	15
		29	Dose-dense TMZ (progression after TMZ completion)	RT + Chemo	CR or PR (11), SD (26), PD (63)	6, 36%; median 4	29

(continued on next page)

TABLE 11.2 (continued)

Investigators, Year	Study Design	Patients Per Arm (N)	Interventions	Prior Adjuvant Therapy	Radiographic Response (%)	PFS (mo)	Median OS (mo)
Brada et al,[55] 2010	Phase II, 3 randomized arms	224	PCV	RT alone	NA	Median 4	7
		112	5-d TMZ	RT alone	NA	Median 5	9
		111	21-d TMZ	RT alone	NA	Median 4	7
Reardon et al,[54] 2011	Phase II, single arm	32	Sorafenib + TMZ	RT + Chemo	CR (0), PR (3), SD (47), PD (50)	6, 9%; median 6	10
Abacioglu et al,[53] 2011	Phase II, single arm	25	Dose-dense TMZ	RT + Chemo	CR (0), PR (10), SD (50), PD (40)	6, 17%; median 3	7
Stupp et al,[55] 2011	Phase II, single arm	38	Sagopilone	RT + Chemo	CR (0), PR (0), SD (25), PD (75)	6, 81%; median 2	8
Walbert et al,[56] 2011	Phase II, single stratified arm	43	6-TG + capecitabine + celecoxib + (TMZ or lomustine)	RT + Chemo	CR (2), PR (9), SD (33), PD (56)	6, 14%; median 2	8
Reardon et al,[54] 2011	Phase II, 2 randomized arms	10	Metronomic TMZ + BEV	RT + Chemo (BEV resistant)	CR (0), PR (0), SD (40), PD (60)	6, 0%; median 1	3
		13	Metronomic etoposide + BEV	RT + Chemo (BEV resistant)	CR (0), PR (0), SD (62), PD (31)	6, 10%; median 2	5
Friday et al,[58] 2012	Phase II, single arm	37	Vorinostat + bortezomib	Not specified	NA	6, 0%; median 2	3
Gilbert et al,[59] 2012	Phase II, single arm	30	Cilengitide + surgery	Not specified	NA	6, 12%; median 2	NA
Desjardins et al, 2012	Phase II, single arm	32	TMZ + BEV	RT + Chemo	CR (0), PR (28), SD (50), PD (22)	6, 19%; median 4	9
Franceschi et al,[57] 2012	Phase II, single arm	26	CCNU + dasatinib	RT + Chemo	CR (0), PR (4), SD (25), PD (71)	6, 6%; median 1	6
Lee et al,[60] 2012	Phase II, single arm	18	Sorafenib + temsirolimus	RT + Chemo	CR (0), PR (12)	6, 0%; median 2	NA
Pan et al,[61] 2012	Phase II, single arm	16	Sunitinib	RT + Chemo	CR (0), PR (0), SD (31), PD (69)	6, 17%; median 1	13

Study	Design	N	Treatment	Prior treatment	Response	PFS	OS
Stupp et al,[62] 2012	Phase III, 2 randomized arms	120	TTF	RT + Chemo	CR or PR 14	6, 21%; median 2	7
		117	Physician's choice Chemo	RT + Chemo	CR or PR 10	6, 15%; median 2	6
Batchelor et al,[63] 2013	Phase III, 3 randomized arms	131	Cediranib	RT + Chemo	CR (1), PR (14), SD (64), PD (9)	Median 3	8
		129	Cediranib + lomustine	RT + Chemo	CR (2), PR (16), SD (55), PD (16)	Median 4	9
		65	Lomustine + placebo	RT + Chemo	CR (0), PR (9), SD (41), PD (41)	Median 3	10
Yust-Katz et al,[67] 2013	Phase IB, single arm	34	Lonafarnib + TMZ	RT + Chemo	CR (6), PR (18), SD (47), PD (29)	6, 38%; median 4	14
Peereboom et al,[66] 2013	Phase II, single arm	56	Erlotinib + sorafenib	Not specified	CR (0), PR (5), SD (41), PD (45)	6, 14%; median 3	6
Zustovich et al,[68] 2013	Phase II, single arm	43	Sorafenib + TMZ	RT + Chemo	CR (0), PR (12), SD (48), PD (48)	6, 26%; median 3	7
Norden et al,[65] 2013	Phase II, single arm	58	Dose-dense TMZ	RT + Chemo	CR (0), PR (13), SD (35), PD (52)	6, 11%; median 2	12
Kreisl et al,[64] 2013	Phase II, single stratified arm. Stratified by prior BEV failure	31	Sunitinib (BEV resistant)	RT + Chemo (± BEV)	CR or PR (0)	6, 0%	4.4
		32	Sunitinib (BEV naive)	RT + Chemo (± BEV)	CR or PR (10)	6, 6%	9.4
Han et al,[69] 2014	Phase II, single arm	40	Dose-dense TMZ	RT + Chemo	CR or PR (3)	6, 10%; median 2	5
Rieger et al,[70] 2014	Phase II, single arm	20	Ketogenic diet	RT + Chemo	CR (0), PR (0), SD (8), PD (92)	Median 1	8
Wen et al,[72] 2014	Phase II, single arm	43	Erlotinib + temsirolimus	RT + Chemo	CR (0), PR (0), SD (29), PD (71)	6, 13%; median 2	NA
Taal et al,[71] 2014	Phase II, 3 randomized arms	50	BEV	RT + Chemo	CR or PR (38)	6, 16%; median 3	8
		46	Lomustine	RT + Chemo	CR or PR (5)	6, 13%; median 1	8
		52	BEV + lomustine	RT + Chemo	CR or PR (39)	6, 42%; median 4	12
Lassman et al,[73] 2015	Phase II, single arm	50	Dasatinib	RT + Chemo	CR (0), PR (0), SD (24), PD (76)	6, 6%; median 2	8

(continued on next page)

TABLE 11.2 (continued)

Investigators, Year	Study Design	Patients Per Arm (N)	Interventions	Prior Adjuvant Therapy	Radiographic Response (%)	PFS (mo)	Median OS (mo)
Lee et al,[74] 2015	Phase II, single arm	24	Panobinostat + BEV	RT + Chemo	CR (0), PR (29), SD (58), PD (12)	6, 30%; median 5	9
Nagpal et al,[75] 2015	Phase II, single arm	20	Etirinotecan pegol	RT + Chemo (BEV resistant)	CR (0), PR (17)	6, 11%; median 2	5
Odia et al,[76] 2015	Phase II, single arm	30	Bortezomib + tamoxifen	RT + Chemo	CR (0), PR (0), SD (0), PD (100)	6, 0%; median 1	4
Taylor et al,[79] 2015	Phase II, single arm	11	Bosutinib	RT + Chemo	CR (0), PR (0), SD (25), PD (75)	6, 0%; median 2	12
Weller et al,[80] 2015	Phase II, 2 randomized arms	52	Dose-intensified TMZ biweekly	RT + Chemo	CR (4), PR (4)	Median 2	10
		53	Dose-intensified TMZ monthly	RT + Chemo	CR (8), PR (8)	Median 2	10
Robins et al,[78] 2015	Phase II, 2 randomized arms. Stratified by BEV resistance	73	TMZ + veliparib 21-d, BEV naive	RT + Chemo	CR or PR (0)	Median 2	10
		73	TMZ + veliparib 5-d, BEV naive	RT + Chemo	CR or PR (4)	Median 2	11
		32	TMZ + veliparib 21-d, BEV resistant	RT + Chemo	CR or PR (5)	Median 2	5
		37	TMZ + veliparib 5-d, BEV resistant	RT + Chemo	CR or PR (0)	Median 2	5
Reardon et al,[77] 2015	Phase II, 3 randomized arms	41	Afatinib	RT + Chemo	CR (0), PR (2), SD (34), PD (56)	3%; median 1	10
		39	Afatinib + TMZ	RT + Chemo	CR (3), PR (5), SD (36), PD (44)	6, 10%; median 2	8
		39	TMZ	RT + Chemo	CR (0), PR (10), SD (54), PD (33)	6, 23%; median 2	11

Abbreviations: BEV, bevacizumab; Chemo, chemotherapy; NA, not available; OS, overall survival; PFS, progression-free survival; RT, radiation therapy; TMZ, temozolomide.

TABLE 11.3
Representative vaccine therapies: ongoing trials

	Phase	Study Intervention	Patient Population
Active Immunotherapy			
Peptide Vaccines			
DCVaX-L			
NCT00045968	III	DCVaX-L (autologous tumor lysate)	New GBM[a]
HSPPC-96 (Prophage)			
NCT01814813	II	HSPCC-96 w/BEV vs BEV	rGBM s/p GTR
NCT02122822	I	HSPCC-96	New GBM
Rindopepimut (CDX-110)			
NCT01480479 (ACT IV)	III	Rindopepimut/GM-CSF	New GBM, EGFRvIII+
NCT01498328 (ReACT)	II	Rindopepimut	rGBM, EGFRvIII+
Viral Vaccines			
DNX-2401[b]			
NCT01956734	I	DNX-2401 + TMZ	rGBM
NCT00805376	I	DNX-2401	rHGG
NCT02197169 (TARGET-1)	Ib	DNX-2401 + INF-γ	rGBM or gliosarcoma
PSVRIPO	—	—	—
NCT01491893	I	PSVRIPO	rGBM
Adoptive Immunotherapy			
CMV			
NCT00693095 (ERaDICATE)	I	CMV-ALT ± skin injections of DC pulsed w/pp65 RNA	New GBM w/therapeutic TMZ-induced lymphopenia
NCT00626483 (REGULATE)	I	CMV-ALT + basiliximab (Simulect) + GM-CSF	New GBM w/therapeutic TMZ-induced lymphopenia
NCT01109095 (HERT-GBM)	I	Genetically modified CMV-specific T cells w/HER2 antibody + CD28	rGBM
EGFRvIII			
NCT01454596	I/II	Anti-EGFRvIII CAR transduced CTL + aldesleukin	rGBM or progressive GBM
ICT-107			
NCT01280552	II	ICT-107	New or rGBM
Other DC vaccines			
NCT01759810	II–III	DC vaccine + CTL + hematopoietic stem cells	rGBM
NCT02010606	I	DC vaccine + RT/TMZ ± BEV if rGBM	New or rGBM
NCT02287428	I	Neoantigen vaccine	New GBM w/MGMT unmethylated

Abbreviations: ALT, autologous lymphocyte transfer; CAR, chimeric antigen receptor; CMV, cytomegalovirus; GBM, glioblastoma; GM-CSF, granulocyte-macrophage colony-stimulating factor; GTR, gross total resection; rGBM, recurrent glioblastoma; rHGG, recurrent high grade glioma; s/p, status post.
[a] Newly diagnosed GBM.
[b] Oncolytic adenovirus (Delta-24-RGD).

TABLE 11.4
Alternative delivery methods

Delivery Method	Example	Current Trials in GBM
Convection-enhanced delivery	Poliovirus vaccine	NCT01491893
Nanoparticles	Cilengitide	NCT00979862, NCT00085254, NCT01122888
	Liposomal irinotecan	NCT02022644
	Nanoliposomal CPT-11	NCT00734682
Stem cell delivery	—	—
Intranasal delivery	—	—
LRP-1	GRN1005, ANG1005	NCT01967810
Retroviral replicating vector	Toca 511	NCT01156584, NCT01470794, NCT01985256

Abbreviation: CPT-11, irinotecan (Camptosar®); LRP-1, lipoprotein receptor–related protein-1.

(See Chapter 5), tumor treating fields (See Chapter 17), and bevacizumab (See Chapter 10) are discussed in separate chapters.

In addition to chemotherapy and radiation, many molecular targeting trials via vaccines and alternative delivery methods have also been undertaken, mostly for recurrent glioblastoma. Other chapters specifically address this, but **Tables 11.3** and **11.4** provide a summary of these efforts.

Radiotherapy

In some cases, reirradiation of recurrent disease may be an option. With the onset of more precise radiotherapy techniques, including stereotactic radiosurgery, radiation oncologists have greater opportunity to specifically target and map areas of the brain without committing as many collateral adjacent structures to irradiation. Hasan and colleagues[83] reviewed 19 patients with recurrent glioblastoma following resection chemoradiation who received 18 to 35 Gy in 3 to 5 factions via CyberKnife (Accuray Inc, Sunnyvale, CA) focused stereotactic radiotherapy and found the overall median survival from date of recurrence to be 8 months, and 5.3 months from the end of radiosurgery. The overall survival at 6 months and 12 months was 47% and 32%, respectively. The study was confounded by 16 patients receiving some individual or combination adjuvant systemic therapy with bevacizumab, temozolomide, or anti–epidermal growth factor receptor treatment. In addition, many of these patients had smaller frontal lobe tumors.[83] Niranjan and colleagues[84] reviewed 297 patients with glioblastomas that were either unresectable or had recurred after initial resection. Although this population was heterogeneous, the overall survival was 2 years, which is far more than would be expected in this

cohort, and suggestive of a larger necessary role in adjuvant or salvage radiosurgery. Yazici and colleagues[85] presented 37 patients with recurrent glioblastoma who underwent CyberKnife therapy who underwent doses between 14 and 32 Gy (median, 30 Gy) and reported a median survival of 16.8 months in patients who underwent stereotactic radiotherapy and chemotherapy, and 9.7 months in patients who were not prescribed any chemotherapy. Lower gross tumor volume ($\leq$24 cm^3) was associated with significantly longer survival following radiotherapy compared with those lesions with a large volume.

REFERENCES

1. Wong ET, Hess KR, Gleason MJ, et al. Outcomes and prognostic factors in recurrent glioma patients enrolled onto phase II clinical trials. J Clin Oncol 1999;17:2572–8.
2. Kamiya-Matsuoka C, Gilbert MR. Treating recurrent glioblastoma: an update. CNS Oncol 2015;4: 91–104.
3. Macdonald DR, Cascino TL, Schold SC Jr, et al. Response criteria for phase II studies of supratentorial malignant glioma. J Clin Oncol 1990;8: 1277–80.
4. Seystahl K, Wick W, Weller M. Therapeutic options in recurrent glioblastoma–An update. Crit Rev Oncol Hematol 2016;99:389–408.
5. Ellingson BM, Bendszus M, Boxerman J, et al. Consensus recommendations for a standardized brain tumor imaging protocol in clinical trials. Neuro Oncol 2015;17:1188–98.
6. Galldiks N, Dunkl V, Stoffels G, et al. Diagnosis of pseudoprogression in patients with glioblastoma using O-(2-[18F]fluoroethyl)-L-tyrosine PET. Eur J Nucl Med Mol Imaging 2015;42: 685–95.

7. Dankbaar JW, Snijders TJ, Robe PA, et al. The use of (18)F-FDG PET to differentiate progressive disease from treatment induced necrosis in high grade glioma. J Neurooncol 2015;125:167–75.

8. Bloch O, Han SJ, Cha S, et al. Impact of extent of resection for recurrent glioblastoma on overall survival: clinical article. J Neurosurg 2012;117:1032–8.

9. Chaichana KL, Cabrera-Aldana EE, Jusue-Torres I, et al. When gross total resection of a glioblastoma is possible, how much resection should be achieved? World Neurosurg 2014;82:e257–65.

10. Grabowski MM, Recinos PF, Nowacki AS, et al. Residual tumor volume versus extent of resection: predictors of survival after surgery for glioblastoma. J Neurosurg 2014;121:1115–23.

11. Chaichana KL, Zadnik P, Weingart JD, et al. Multiple resections for patients with glioblastoma: prolonging survival. J Neurosurg 2013;118:812–20.

12. D'Amico RS, Cloney MB, Sonabend AM, et al. The safety of surgery in elderly patients with primary and recurrent glioblastoma. World Neurosurg 2015;84:913–9.

13. Abdullah KG, Ramayya A, Thawani JP, et al. Factors associated with increased survival after surgical resection of glioblastoma in octogenarians. PLoS One 2015;10:e0127202.

14. Park JK, Hodges T, Arko L, et al. Scale to predict survival after surgery for recurrent glioblastoma multiforme. J Clin Oncol 2010;28:3838–43.

15. Park CK, Kim JH, Nam DH, et al. A practical scoring system to determine whether to proceed with surgical resection in recurrent glioblastoma. Neuro Oncol 2013;15:1096–101.

16. Brem H, Piantadosi S, Burger PC, et al. Placebo-controlled trial of safety and efficacy of intraoperative controlled delivery by biodegradable polymers of chemotherapy for recurrent gliomas. The Polymer-brain Tumor Treatment Group. Lancet 1995;345:1008–12.

17. Attenello FJ, Mukherjee D, Datoo G, et al. Use of Gliadel (BCNU) wafer in the surgical treatment of malignant glioma: a 10-year institutional experience. Ann Surg Oncol 2008;15:2887–93.

18. Couldwell WT, Hinton DR, Surnock AA, et al. Treatment of recurrent malignant gliomas with chronic oral high-dose tamoxifen. Clin Cancer Res 1996;2:619–22.

19. Brandes AA, Ermani M, Turazzi S, et al. Procarbazine and high-dose tamoxifen as a second-line regimen in recurrent high-grade gliomas: a phase II study. J Clin Oncol 1999;17:645–50.

20. Yung WK, Albright RE, Olson J, et al. A phase II study of temozolomide vs. procarbazine in patients with glioblastoma multiforme at first relapse. Br J Cancer 2000;83:588–93.

21. Watanabe K, Kanaya H, Fujiyama Y, et al. Combination chemotherapy using carboplatin (JM-8) and etoposide (JET therapy) for recurrent malignant gliomas: a phase II study. Acta Neurochir 2002;144:1265–70 [discussion: 70].

22. Prados MD, Schold SC Jr, Fine HA, et al. A randomized, double-blind, placebo-controlled, phase 2 study of RMP-7 in combination with carboplatin administered intravenously for the treatment of recurrent malignant glioma. Neuro Oncol 2003;5:96–103.

23. Brandes AA, Tosoni A, Basso U, et al. Second-line chemotherapy with irinotecan plus carmustine in glioblastoma recurrent or progressive after first-line temozolomide chemotherapy: a phase II study of the Gruppo Italiano Cooperativo di Neuro-Oncologia (GICNO). J Clin Oncol 2004;22:4779–86.

24. Prados MD, Yung WKA, Fine HA, et al. Phase 2 study of BCNU and temozolomide for recurrent glioblastoma multiforme: North American Brain Tumor Consortium study. Neuro Oncol 2004;6:33–7.

25. Rich JN, Reardon DA, Peery T, et al. Phase II trial of gefitinib in recurrent glioblastoma. J Clin Oncol 2004;22:133–42.

26. Dresemann G. Imatinib and hydroxyurea in pretreated progressive glioblastoma multiforme: a patient series. Ann Oncol 2005;16:1702–8.

27. Galanis E, Buckner JC, Maurer MJ, et al. Phase II trial of temsirolimus (CCI-779) in recurrent glioblastoma multiforme: a North Central Cancer Treatment Group Study. J Clin Oncol 2005;23:5294–304.

28. Reardon DA, Egorin MJ, Quinn JA, et al. Phase II study of imatinib mesylate plus hydroxyurea in adults with recurrent glioblastoma multiforme. J Clin Oncol 2005;23:9359–68.

29. Cloughesy TF, Wen PY, Robins HI, et al. Phase II trial of tipifarnib in patients with recurrent malignant glioma either receiving or not receiving enzyme-inducing antiepileptic drugs: a North American Brain Tumor Consortium Study. J Clin Oncol 2006;24:3651–6.

30. Reardon DA, Quinn JA, Vredenburgh JJ, et al. Phase 1 trial of gefitinib plus sirolimus in adults with recurrent malignant glioma. Clin Cancer Res 2006;12:860–8.

31. Wen PY, Yung WKA, Lamborn KR, et al. Phase I/II study of imatinib mesylate for recurrent malignant gliomas: North American Brain Tumor Consortium Study 99-08. Clin Cancer Res 2006;12:4899–907.

32. Hau P, Kunz-Schughart L, Bogdahn U, et al. Low-dose chemotherapy in combination with COX-2 inhibitors and PPAR-gamma agonists in recurrent high-grade gliomas - a phase II study. Oncology 2007;73:21–5.

33. de Groot JF, Gilbert MR, Aldape K, et al. Phase II study of carboplatin and erlotinib (Tarceva, OSI-774) in patients with recurrent glioblastoma. J Neurooncol 2008;90:89–97.

34. Reardon DA, Fink KL, Mikkelsen T, et al. Random-ized phase II study of cilengitide, an integrin-targeting arginine-glycine-aspartic acid peptide, in recurrent glioblastoma multiforme. J Clin Oncol 2008;26:5610–7.

35. Friedman HS, Prados MD, Wen PY, et al. Bevacizu-mab alone and in combination with irinotecan in recurrent glioblastoma. J Clin Oncol 2009;27:4733–40.

36. Galanis E, Jaeckle KA, Maurer MJ, et al. Phase II trial of vorinostat in recurrent glioblastoma multiforme: a North Central Cancer Treatment Group study. J Clin Oncol 2009;27:2052–8.

37. Kreisl TN, Lassman AB, Mischel PS, et al. A pilot study of everolimus and gefitinib in the treatment of recurrent glioblastoma (GBM). J Neurooncol 2009;92:99–105.

38. Neyns B, Sadones J, Joosens E, et al. Stratified phase II trial of cetuximab in patients with recurrent high-grade glioma. Ann Oncol 2009;20:1596–603.

39. Quinn JA, Jiang SX, Carter J, et al. Phase II trial of Gliadel plus O6-benzylguanine in adults with recur-rent glioblastoma multiforme. Clin Cancer Res 2009;15:1064–8.

40. Reardon DA, Dresemann G, Taillibert S, et al. Multi-centre phase II studies evaluating imatinib plus hy-droxyurea in patients with progressive glioblastoma. Br J Cancer 2009;101:1995–2004.

41. Robe PA, Martin DH, Nguyen-Khac MT, et al. Early termination of ISRCTN45828668, a phase 1/2 pro-spective, randomized study of sulfasalazine for the treatment of progressing malignant gliomas in adults. BMC Cancer 2009;9:372.

42. van den Bent MJ, Brandes AA, Rampling R, et al. Randomized phase II trial of erlotinib versus temo-zolomide or carmustine in recurrent glioblastoma: EORTC brain tumor group study 26034. J Clin Oncol 2009;27:1268–74.

43. Batchelor TT, Duda DG, di Tomaso E, et al. Phase II study of cediranib, an oral pan-vascular endothelial growth factor receptor tyrosine kinase inhibitor, in patients with recurrent glioblastoma. J Clin Oncol 2010;28:2817–23.

44. Brada M, Stenning S, Gabe R, et al. Temozolomide versus procarbazine, lomustine, and vincristine in recurrent high-grade glioma. J Clin Oncol 2010;28:4601–8.

45. Dresemann G, Weller M, Rosenthal MA, et al. Ima-tinib in combination with hydroxyurea versus hy-droxyurea alone as oral therapy in patients with progressive pretreated glioblastoma resistant to standard dose temozolomide. J Neurooncol 2010;96:393–402.

46. Perry JR, Bélanger K, Mason WP, et al. Phase II trial of continuous dose-intense temozolomide in recur-rent malignant glioma: RESCUE study. J Clin Oncol 2010;28:2051–7.

47. Raizer JJ, Abrey LE, Lassman AB, et al. A phase II trial of erlotinib in patients with recurrent malignant gli-omas and nonprogressive glioblastoma multiforme postradiation therapy. Neuro Oncol 2010;12:95–103.

48. Reardon DA, Desjardins A, Vredenburgh JJ, et al. Phase 2 trial of erlotinib plus sirolimus in adults with recurrent glioblastoma. J Neurooncol 2010;96:219–30.

49. Sathornsumetee S, Desjardins A, Vredenburgh JJ, et al. Phase II trial of bevacizumab and erlotinib in patients with recurrent malignant glioma. Neuro Oncol 2010;12:1300–10.

50. Thiessen B, Stewart C, Tsao M, et al. A phase I/II trial of GW572016 (lapatinib) in recurrent glioblastoma multiforme: clinical outcomes, pharmacokinetics and molecular correlation. Cancer Chemother Phar-macol 2010;65:353–61.

51. Wick W, Puduvalli VK, Chamberlain MC, et al. Phase III study of enzastaurin compared with lomustine in the treatment of recurrent intracranial glioblastoma. J Clin Oncol 2010;28:1168–74.

52. Yung WKA, Vredenburgh JJ, Cloughesy TF, et al. Safety and efficacy of erlotinib in first-relapse glio-blastoma: a phase II open-label study. Neuro Oncol 2010;12:1061–70.

53. Abacioglu U, Caglar HB, Yumuk PF, et al. Efficacy of protracted dose-dense temozolomide in patients with recurrent high-grade glioma. J Neurooncol 2011;103:585–93.

54. Reardon DA, Vredenburgh JJ, Desjardins A, et al. Effect of CYP3A-inducing anti-epileptics on sorafe-nib exposure: results of a phase II study of sorafenib plus daily temozolomide in adults with recurrent glioblastoma. J Neurooncol 2011;101:57–66.

55. Stupp R, Tosoni A, Bromberg JEC, et al. Sagopilone (ZK-EPO, ZK 219477) for recurrent glioblastoma. A phase II multicenter trial by the European Organisa-tion for Research and Treatment of Cancer (EORTC) Brain Tumor Group. Ann Oncol 2011;22:2144–9.

56. Walbert T, Gilbert MR, Groves MD, et al. Combina-tion of 6-thioguanine, capecitabine, and celecoxib with temozolomide or lomustine for recurrent high-grade glioma. J Neurooncol 2011;102:273–80.

57. Franceschi E, Stupp R, van den Bent MJ, et al. EORTC 26083 phase I/II trial of dasatinib in combi-nation with CCNU in patients with recurrent glio-blastoma. Neuro Oncol 2012;14:1503–10.

58. Friday BB, Anderson SK, Buckner J, et al. Phase II trial of vorinostat in combination with bortezomib in recurrent glioblastoma: a North Central Cancer Treatment Group study. Neuro Oncol 2012;14:215–21.

59. Gilbert MR, Kuhn J, Lamborn KR, et al. Cilengitide in patients with recurrent glioblastoma: the results of NABTC 03-02, a phase II trial with measures of treatment delivery. J Neurooncol 2012;106:147–53.

60. Lee EQ, Kuhn J, Lamborn KR, et al. Phase I/II study of sorafenib in combination with temsirolimus for recurrent glioblastoma or gliosarcoma: North American Brain Tumor Consortium study 05-02. Neuro Oncol 2012;14:1511–8.

61. Pan E, Yu D, Yue B, et al. A prospective phase II single-institution trial of sunitinib for recurrent malignant glioma. J Neurooncol 2012;110:111–8.

62. Stupp R, Wong ET, Kanner AA, et al. NovoTTF-100A versus physician's choice chemotherapy in recurrent glioblastoma: a randomised phase III trial of a novel treatment modality. Eur J Cancer 2012;48:2192–202.

63. Batchelor TT, Mulholland P, Neyns B, et al. Phase III randomized trial comparing the efficacy of cediranib as monotherapy, and in combination with lomustine, versus lomustine alone in patients with recurrent glioblastoma. J Clin Oncol 2013;31:3212–8.

64. Kreisl TN, Smith P, Sul J, et al. Continuous daily sunitinib for recurrent glioblastoma. J Neurooncol 2013;111:41–8.

65. Norden AD, Lesser GJ, Drappatz J, et al. Phase 2 study of dose-intense temozolomide in recurrent glioblastoma. Neuro Oncol 2013;15:930–5.

66. Peereboom DM, Ahluwalia MS, Ye X, et al. NABTT 0502: a phase II and pharmacokinetic study of erlotinib and sorafenib for patients with progressive or recurrent glioblastoma multiforme. Neuro Oncol 2013;15:490–6.

67. Yust-Katz S, Liu D, Yuan Y, et al. Phase 1/1b study of lonafarnib and temozolomide in patients with recurrent or temozolomide refractory glioblastoma. Cancer 2013;119:2747–53.

68. Zustovich F, Landi L, Lombardi G, et al. Sorafenib plus daily low-dose temozolomide for relapsed glioblastoma: a phase II study. Anticancer Res 2013;33:3487–94.

69. Han SJ, Rolston JD, Molinaro AM, et al. Phase II trial of 7 days on/7 days off temozolmide for recurrent high-grade glioma. Neuro Oncol 2014;16:1255–62.

70. Rieger J, Bähr O, Maurer GD, et al. ERGO: a pilot study of ketogenic diet in recurrent glioblastoma. Int J Oncol 2014;44:1843–52.

71. Taal W, Oosterkamp HM, Walenkamp AME, et al. Single-agent bevacizumab or lomustine versus a combination of bevacizumab plus lomustine in patients with recurrent glioblastoma (BELOB trial): a randomised controlled phase 2 trial. Lancet Oncol 2014;15:943–53.

72. Wen PY, Chang SM, Lamborn KR, et al. Phase I/II study of erlotinib and temsirolimus for patients with recurrent malignant gliomas: North American Brain Tumor Consortium trial 04-02. Neuro Oncol 2014;16:567–78.

73. Lassman AB, Pugh SL, Gilbert MR, et al. Phase 2 trial of dasatinib in target-selected patients with recurrent glioblastoma (RTOG 0627). Neuro Oncol 2015;17:992–8.

74. Lee EQ, Reardon DA, Schiff D, et al. Phase II study of panobinostat in combination with bevacizumab for recurrent glioblastoma and anaplastic glioma. Neuro Oncol 2015;17:862–7.

75. Nagpal S, Recht CK, Bertrand S, et al. Phase II pilot study of single-agent etirinotecan pegol (NKTR-102) in bevacizumab-resistant high grade glioma. J Neurooncol 2015;123:277–82.

76. Odia Y, Kreisl TN, Aregawi D, et al. A phase II trial of tamoxifen and bortezomib in patients with recurrent malignant gliomas. J Neurooncol 2015;125:191–5.

77. Reardon DA, Nabors LB, Mason WP, et al. Phase I/randomized phase II study of afatinib, an irreversible ErbB family blocker, with or without protracted temozolomide in adults with recurrent glioblastoma. Neuro Oncol 2015;17:430–9.

78. Robins HI, Zhang P, Gilbert MR, et al. A randomized phase I/II study of ABT-888 in combination with temozolomide in recurrent temozolomide resistant glioblastoma: an NRG oncology RTOG group study. J Neurooncol 2015;126(2):309–16.

79. Taylor JW, Dietrich J, Gerstner ER, et al. Phase 2 study of bosutinib, a Src inhibitor, in adults with recurrent glioblastoma. J Neurooncol 2015;121:557–63.

80. Weller M, Tabatabai G, Kästner B, et al. MGMT promoter methylation is a strong prognostic biomarker for benefit from dose-intensified temozolomide rechallenge in progressive glioblastoma: the DIRECTOR trial. Clin Cancer Res 2015;21:2057–64.

81. Wick W, Steinbach JP, Kuker WM, et al. One week on/one week off: a novel active regimen of temozolomide for recurrent glioblastoma. Neurology 2004;62:2113–5.

82. Wei W, Chen X, Ma X, et al. The efficacy and safety of various dose-dense regimens of temozolomide for recurrent high-grade glioma: a systematic review with meta-analysis. J Neurooncol 2015;125:339–49.

83. Hasan S, Chen E, Lanciano R, et al. Salvage fractionated stereotactic radiotherapy with or without chemotherapy and immunotherapy for recurrent glioblastoma multiforme: a single institution experience. Front Oncol 2015;5:106.

84. Niranjan A, Kano H, Iyer A, et al. Role of adjuvant or salvage radiosurgery in the management of unresected residual or progressive glioblastoma multiforme in the pre-bevacizumab era. J Neurosurg 2015;122:757–65.

85. Yazici G, Cengiz M, Ozyigit G, et al. Hypofractionated stereotactic reirradiation for recurrent glioblastoma. J Neurooncol 2014;120:117–23.

CHAPTER 12

Principles of Surgical Treatment

Shawn L. Hervey-Jumper, MD[a],*, Mitchel S. Berger, MD[b]

PREOPERATIVE SURGICAL EVALUATION

The initial evaluation of a patient with suspected glioblastoma includes history and physical examination, anatomic imaging, and symptom management with seizure medications and corticosteroids. Clinical presentation of glioblastoma is highly variable, depending on tumor size, location, and the amount of peritumoral edema. Glioblastomas are rarely discovered incidentally (3.8% of patients).[1] Seizures and neurocognitive changes are the most common presenting symptom, occurring in more than 70% of patients.[2–4] Blunted affect, changes in personality, and neurocognitive dysfunction may be more prevalent in patients with frontal tumors. Speech and language deficits occur in 58% of patients from tumors affecting cortical or subcortical language pathways in the dominant hemisphere.[5] Additional symptoms include headaches, memory loss, sensory dysfunction, and visual field deficits.[3]

Initial imaging of patients with suspected glioblastoma begins with brain MRI with and without enhancement. T1-weighted images with and without gadolinium enhancement are critical, because they allow the estimation of anatomic localization, tumor necrosis, vascularity, and amount of mass effect. T2-weighted, fluid-attenuated inversion recovery (FLAIR) images and diffusion-weighted MRI sequences show the extent of surrounding vasogenic edema. Glioblastomas are typically avidly enhancing on FLAIR signals outside of tumor boundaries, showing the degree of surrounding peritumoral edema. Structural and functional imaging, such as functional MRI (fMRI), diffusion tensor imaging (DTI), and magnetoencephalography (MEG), may be useful when evaluating tumors within presumed functional areas.

Corticosteroids are commonly used to control tumor-associated vasogenic edema. Dexamethasone is commonly used, with doses ranging between 2 and 24 mg daily. Corticosteroids may improve focal neurologic deficits and level of consciousness, and relieve headaches. Major side effects of corticosteroids include depression, osteoporosis, and immunosuppression; therefore, they should be administered only if necessary and at the lowest dose possible.[6] Recent data suggest that higher doses of corticosteroids may lead to resistance to alkylating chemotherapy such as temozolomide.[7] Patients presenting with seizures should be started on an anticonvulsant while balancing side-effect profiles and drug-to-drug interactions.[8,9] Phenytoin was historically the first-line antiepileptic agent; however, levetiracetam is now commonly used because of its low toxicity, lack of need to monitor serum levels, and minor side-effect profile.

PREOPERATIVE PLANNING

Management of intrinsic brain tumors begins with surgery intended to establish the diagnosis and maximal safe resection. In order to minimize perioperative risk, careful planning should occur before the patient is taken to the operating room. High-quality contrast MRI scans with and without enhancement are vital for developing the optimal operative plan. Preoperative imaging provides knowledge about glioblastoma location as well as its relationship to vascular structures and potential functional areas. Structural MRI and fMRI can be reconstructed to create three-dimensional models to establish a safe surgical corridor during surgery. fMRI, DTI tractography, and MEG MRI provide valuable information

Disclosures: The authors have no conflicts of interest to declare.
a Department of Neurosurgery, University of Michigan, 1500 East Medical Center Drive, Taubman Health Center SPC 5338, Ann Arbor, MI 48109, USA; b Department of Neurological Surgery, University of California San Francisco, 505 Parnassus Avenue, Room 779M, San Francisco, CA 94143, USA
* Corresponding author.
E-mail address: herveyju@med.umich.edu

regarding the interface of tumor tissue with adjacent functional cortical and subcortical pathways (**Fig. 12.1**). fMRI produces the blood oxygenation level–dependent (BOLD) signal, which marks cortical regions associated with task performance (motor, expressive language, receptive language).[10,11] DTI tractography establishes white matter tracts surrounding the glioblastoma and can be helpful in determining whether functional pathways are infiltrated or displaced by tumor mass effect.[12–14] DTI of white matter pathways is particularly important for language pathways, including corticospinal tract, superior longitudinal fasciculus, arcuate fasciculus, uncinate fasciculus, inferior orbitofrontal fasciculus, and optic pathways. Preoperative clinical evaluation should include baseline language and sensorimotor assessment performed 24 to 48 hours before surgery.[15] Many glioblastomas are within or adjacent to potential functional areas, making it difficult to balance achieving an excellent extent of resection with minimizing postoperative deficits. Preoperative planning must therefore take into consideration the range of available approaches, including awake language and motor brain mapping craniotomy, asleep motor mapping craniotomy, image-guided resection, and use of the intraoperative MRI (iMRI).

INTRAOPERATIVE STANDARDS OF RESECTION

Over the past 2 decades, numerous studies have enhanced the understanding of the impact of extent of resection on overall and progression-free survival in patients with glioblastoma.[16] The decision to offer maximal safe resection depends on factors such as performance status, patient age, and tumor location and size. There are several intraoperative tools and strategies that have been developed to both enhance safety and improve the extent of tumor resection. These options include neuronavigation, intraoperative brain mapping, use of iMRI, and fluorescence-guided surgical resection.

Neuronavigation

Functional and anatomic image guidance (neuronavigation) is an important part of both preoperative planning and intraoperative tumor resection. It is used to plan size and location of the craniotomy, and to estimate extent of resection during glioblastoma resection. Image guidance allows a generalized assessment of vascular and functional pathway displacement in relation to the tumor. Functional neuronavigation refers to the integration of DTI tractography, transcranial magnet stimulation, MEG, or fMRI for the identification of cortical and subcortical areas of functional significance (**Fig. 12.2**).[17] Intraoperative functional neuronavigation can therefore display plots of functional areas and their relationships to the tumor using preoperative gadolinium-enhanced MRI. However, these studies are tend to be inaccurate because of distortion caused by mass effect, individual anatomic variability, or functional reorganization caused by cortical and subcortical plasticity.[18,19] fMRI has a sensitivity and specificity of 91% and 64% for identification of Broca area, 93% and 18% for identification of Wernicke area, and close to 100% for identification of the primary motor cortex.[20] Uncoupling of the BOLD signal in highly vascular tumors such as glioblastoma makes

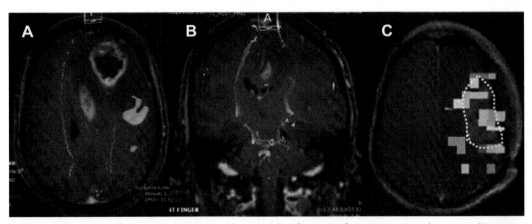

Fig. 12.1 Structural and functional imaging provides valuable information for preoperative planning and intraoperative use. (*A*) fMRI for motor language tasks reveals language activation sites lateral to the tumor (*yellow*). (*B*) DTI tractography identifies corticospinal fibers (*purple*) running lateral to the posterior margin of the tumor. (*C*) MEG similarly identifies areas of high functional connectivity (*red*) and low connectivity (*yellow*) around the tumor (*dotted outline*).

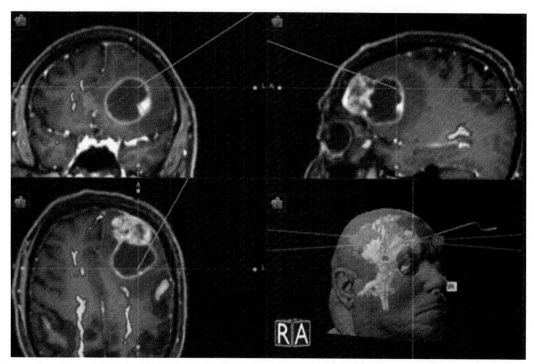

Fig. 12.2 Intraoperative functional neuronavigation can display functional areas and their relationships to the tumor bases on preoperative gadolinium-enhanced MRI. This study shows cortical motor language activation by fMRI, which is pushed posterior by the tumor (*green*), and cortical motor activation in purple.

interpretation of fMRI results difficult. Resting state coherence measured with MEG is a noninvasive measure of functional connectivity of the brain. Glioblastomas with decreased resting state connectivity have a low risk of postoperative neurologic deficits, whereas those with increased resting state connectivity are associated with higher risk of postoperative neurologic deficits.[21] It is advantageous to preoperatively and intraoperatively visualize functional pathways and their spatial relationships to a glioblastoma.

Awake Craniotomy and Intraoperative Brain Mapping

Direct cortical and subcortical stimulation mapping allows the identification of language, sensorimotor, and cognitive functions during surgery.[15] Proper patient selection is critical and patients are considered for an awake craniotomy if they have a supratentorial intrinsic brain tumor located within or adjacent to regions presumed to have language or sensorimotor function on preoperative imaging. Proper patient selection is critical to maximizing perioperative safety.[15] Given the limitations of structural and functional imaging, glioblastomas presumed to be within functional sites on preoperative anatomic imaging are never an absolute contraindication to attempting intraoperative mapping.

Several factors are associated with increased perioperative risk during awake brain tumor surgery.[15,22] Absolute contraindications to an awake craniotomy include an uncontrolled persistent cough, severe dysphasia (ie, >25% naming errors despite a trial of preoperative dexamethasone and mannitol), large glioblastomas with mass effect resulting in more than 2 cm of midline shift, or hemiplegia with less than antigravity motor function. In the remainder of circumstances there are solutions and strategies to these obstacles. Patients with severely impaired preoperative language or motor function (>25% naming errors and <2 of 5 motor function) may be treated with high-dose corticosteroids (dexamethasone, 4–8 mg intravenously every 6 hours) and/or osmotic diuretics (mannitol 20%, 30 g every 6 hours for 48–72 hours) followed by reassessment of preoperative function. Obese patients, including individuals with body mass index greater than 35, may be treated with a laryngeal mask airway to prevent hypercapnia. Patients with generalized anxiety or severe untreated psychiatric history should be treated with antidepressant and mood-stabilizing medications before surgery. All seizures should be well controlled before an awake craniotomy, given the risk of intraoperative stimulation-induced seizures during intraoperative mapping. Intraoperative seizures may be treated with topical iced Ringer solution applied to the cortex. In addition, intravenous (IV) propofol, diazepam, or lorazepam should be ready for rapid administration as needed. Nausea should be treated with antiemetic medications such as ondansetron hydrochloride or scopolamine.

Preoperative evaluation before an awake craniotomy for glioblastoma includes functional and anatomic imaging, baseline language and sensorimotor testing, neuroanesthesia evaluation, and patient counseling and education. Baseline language assessments are performed by surgical neurophysiology or speech pathology 24 to 48 hours before surgery for tasks including picture naming, responsive naming, or reading, depending on tumor location.[15,23]

Specialized neuroanesthesia is critical for completion of a safe awake craniotomy, because it ensures clear communication between neurosurgeon, anesthesiologist, speech pathologist, and other members of the mapping team.[24] Surgery commences with the appropriate patient monitoring and premedicating with midazolam, fentanyl, or dexmedetomidine before positioning.[15] Sedation is achieved with propofol (up to 100 µg/kg/min) or dexmedetomidine (up to 1 µg/kg/min) and remifentanil (0.07–2.0 µg/kg/h).[25–27] Sedation begins during Foley catheter insertion and Mayfield head holder pin placement. A scalp block using a mixture of 1% lidocaine with 1:100,000 epinephrine and 0.5% bupivacaine is applied by the surgical team. Optimal head positioning usually involves a small amount of neck extension (for airway patency), which allows ease of operation, patient comfort, and optimal airway patency. A dedicated IV line is filled with a 1-mg/kg bolus of propofol if needed for suppression of an intraoperative grand mal seizure. Topical ice-cold Ringer lactate solution is available on the surgical field at all times for seizure suppression. After skin incision and removal of the bone flap, all sedatives are held or reduced before dural opening.

Intraoperative mapping originally involved large craniotomies with the goal of finding positive language and motor sites. The overall goal was to perform a focused exposure encompassing the lesion plus a 2-cm margin. Craniotomies are now focused to open only the dura overlying the lesion with a reliance on negative mapping, which avoids cortical injury to the surrounding brain. A dural block can be placed using a 30-gauge needle with 1% lidocaine to infiltrate the region around the middle meningeal artery. Following removal of the bone flap, sedating medications are discontinued or greatly reduced to ensure that the patient is cooperative before dural opening. If the brain is tense, the patient is asked to take additional controlled breaths, mannitol is given, and the head of the bed raised.

Cortical stimulation depolarizes a focal area of brain, which excites local neurons via diffusion of current using both orthodromic and antidromic propagation. Bipolar stimulation using a 2-mm tip with 5 mm of separation allows for local diffusion and more precise mapping.[28] Mapping begins with a stimulation current of 1.5 to 2 mA using a constant-current generator that delivers 1.25-millisecond biphasic square waves in trains of 2 to 4 seconds at 50 or 60 Hz. Numerical markers are placed on the surgical field spaced 1 cm apart (**Fig. 12.3**). Electrocorticography is used to monitor for subclinical seizure activity and detect after-discharge potentials, which improves mapping accuracy. All language tasks are repeated at least 3 times per cortical site, and a positive site is defined as the inability to count, name objects, or read words during stimulation at least 66% of times. Language mapping seeks to identify sites responsible for speech arrest, anomia, and alexia with stimulation testing. Speech arrest is defined as discontinuation in number counting without simultaneous motor response. Dysarthria can be distinguished from speech arrest by an absence of involuntary muscle contractions affecting speech.[5]

Intraoperative MRI

MRI-guided surgery has been shown to enhance the extent of glioblastoma resection and therefore patient survival. Neuronavigation becomes less reliable during surgery. Therefore the rationale for the use of iMRI combined with conventional neuronavigation-guided resection is the avoidance of brain shift caused by cerebrospinal fluid loss and tissue edema.[29] Numerous studies have attempted to quantify the effect of iMRI on extent of glioblastoma resection.[30,31] Both iMRI and awake craniotomy are tools to maximize extent of resection while limiting neurologic deficits; however, there have been no head-to-head comparison studies. Both approaches have been proved safe and effective, but patient selection is critical. Awake brain mapping surgery allows real-time language and sensorimotor mapping and monitoring. However, patients with relative or absolute contraindications might be at increased risk. The primary advantage of iMRI is the ability to acquire updated anatomic and structural imaging throughout the procedure. Patients with cardiac comorbidities might be at increased risk during iMRI surgery given interference between telemetry and the operating room MRI equipment. It is becoming increasingly customary

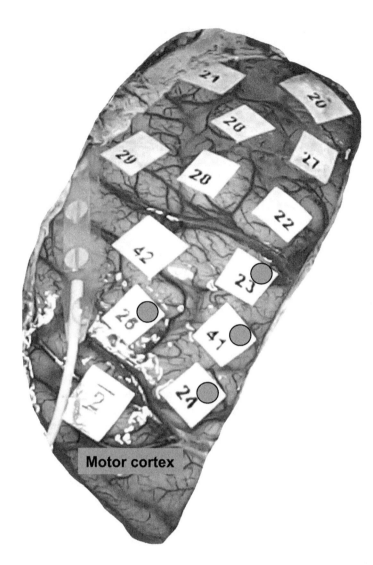

Fig. 12.3 Direct cortical stimulation mapping is the gold standard for identification of functional areas. Mapping is performed in 1-cm intervals. In this intraoperative case the primary motor cortex was posterior to the tumor, and positive language sites (a change in language function during stimulation) are identified with gray circles. These sites are retained during the resection.

to use awake brain mapping within an MRI operating suite. Extent of tumor resection must be measured against perioperative risks, quality of life, and long-term neurologic disability.

Fluorescence-guided Surgery Using 5-Aminolevulinic Acid

It has been well established that most glioblastoma recurrences occur within a centimeter of the tumor resection cavity. In addition, most neurosurgeons overestimate the degree of resection they are able to achieve and do not have access to iMRI. 5-Aminolevulinic acid (5-ALA) is an inexpensive nonfluorescent amino acid precursor that produces an accumulation of fluorescent protoporphyrin IX in glioblastoma cells.[32] Intracellular protoporphyrin IX level peaks 6 hours after administration and remains increased for 12 hours.[33]

Protoporphyrin IX has an absorption band strongest in the 380 ± 420 nm spectrum, emitting red fluorescence at 635 nm and 704 nm in the brain. A long-pass filter mounted to the surgical microscope allows tumor visualization as the operator switches between white and violet light. The use of 5-ALA as an adjuvant to glioblastoma surgery improves extent of resection. A phase III clinical trial of patients with suspected glioblastoma receiving surgery using either conventional white light microsurgery or fluorescence-guided surgery assisted with 5-ALA found that 65% of patients treated with 5-ALA received a gross total resection compared with 36% of patients treated with conventional white light microsurgery. Study patients therefore experienced a 50% improvement in 6-month progression-free survival (41.0% vs 21.1%).[32] Complete removal of all fluorescent tissue (also known as a 5-ALA complete resection) results in improved overall survival without an increase in postoperative neurologic deficits.[32]

EXTENT OF RESECTION AND ITS INFLUENCE ON OUTCOME

Glioblastoma represents the most common and most difficult-to-treat primary brain tumor because of its ability to invade brain parenchyma and recur after initial treatment. Patients with glioblastoma have a median survival ranging from 12.2 to 18.2 months.[34,35] Microsurgery plays a central role in management, and there is increasing evidence regarding the value of extent of tumor resection to improve both survival and quality of life. Gross total resection of contrast-enhanced tumor can be difficult to achieve in many cases because of proximity to eloquent structures. However, cumulative evidence suggests that a more extensive surgical resection is associated with longer survival and improved quality of life. To this end, extent of tumor resection, in addition to patient age, tumor histology, performance status, and tumor genetics, is predictive of patient outcome. Over the past 3 decades there has been an enhanced understanding of the value of extent of resection on survival.

The impact of extent of resection to enhance survival of patients with primary and recurrent high-grade gliomas has been studied in 33 published reports.[35–67] Although most studies are retrospective single-institution series, the preponderance of evidence supports extent of resection as a predictor of overall and progression-free survival in glioblastoma. After gross total or near-total resection, overall survival improves from 64.9 to 75.2 months for World Health Organization (WHO) grade III gliomas, and from 11.3 to 14.5 months for WHO grade IV gliomas.

SURGICAL TENETS OF RECURRENT GLIOBLASTOMA RESECTION

The value of extent of resection at the point of glioblastoma recurrence is less well defined. There is no agreement in the literature regarding the role of reoperation. A total of 31 studies have addressed this question in a systematic manner, of which 29 showed either a survival benefit or improved functional status following reoperation. Common indications for reoperation include the presence of new neurologic deficits, tumor mass effect, signs of increased intracranial pressure, headaches, increased seizure frequency, and radiographic asymptomatic tumor progression.

Although fraught with selection bias, the following criteria are suggestive of a survival benefit after reoperation: (1) time interval of 6 to 12 months between operations, (2) patient age, and (3) Karnofsky Performance Status score greater than 70. Extent of resection at reoperation improves survival, even in patients with subtotal resection at initial operation. A retrospective analysis of 107 patients with recurrent glioblastoma revealed that patients who received an initial subtotal resection experienced a survival benefit when gross total resection was achieved at recurrence (19 months overall survival for gross total resection vs 15.9 months overall survival for subtotal resection).[37] It has recently been recognized that an extent of resection threshold of at least 80% at the time of reoperation offers a survival benefit.[55] Although available data are limited to retrospective analysis and selection bias, carefully selected patients seem to benefit from reoperation at the time of glioblastoma recurrence.

SUMMARY

Glioblastomas are a major cause of morbidity in the United States. Although glioblastomas are aggressive, patients experience enhanced survival after maximal extent of resection. Several techniques have been developed to enhance extent while minimizing morbidity. The pursuit of maximal extent of resection must be balanced with preservation of language, motor, and cognitive functional networks, which have a profound impact on quality of life.

REFERENCES

1. Pallud J, Fontaine D, Duffau H, et al. Natural history of incidental World Health Organization grade II gliomas. Ann Neurol 2010;68(5):727–33.
2. Chang EF, Potts MB, Keles GE, et al. Seizure characteristics and control following resection in 332 patients with low-grade gliomas. J Neurosurg 2008; 108(2):227–35.
3. Smith JS, Chang EF, Lamborn KR, et al. Role of extent of resection in the long-term outcome of low-grade hemispheric gliomas. J Clin Oncol 2008;26(8):1338–45.
4. Taphoorn MJ, Klein M. Cognitive deficits in adult patients with brain tumours. Lancet Neurol 2004; 3(3):159–68.
5. Sanai N, Mirzadeh Z, Berger MS. Functional outcome after language mapping for glioma resection. N Engl J Med 2008;358(1):18–27.
6. Roth P, Wick W, Weller M. Steroids in neurooncology: actions, indications, side-effects. Curr Opin Neurol 2010;23(6):597–602.

7. Weiler M, Blaes J, Pusch S, et al. mTOR target NDRG1 confers MGMT-dependent resistance to alkylating chemotherapy. Proc Natl Acad Sci U S A 2014;111(1):409–14.

8. Weller M, Gorlia T, Cairncross JG, et al. Prolonged survival with valproic acid use in the EORTC/NCIC temozolomide trial for glioblastoma. Neurology 2011;77(12):1156–64.

9. Weller M, Stupp R, Wick W. Epilepsy meets cancer: when, why, and what to do about it? Lancet Oncol 2012;13(9):70266–8.

10. Bogomolny DL, Petrovich NM, Hou BL, et al. Functional MRI in the brain tumor patient. Top Magn Reson Imaging 2004;15(5):325–35.

11. Nimsky C, Ganslandt O, Von Keller B, et al. Intraoperative high-field-strength MR imaging: implementation and experience in 200 patients. Radiology 2004;233(1):67–78.

12. Alexander AL, Lee JE, Lazar M, et al. Diffusion tensor imaging of the brain. Neurotherapeutics 2007;4(3):316–29.

13. Bello L, Gambini A, Castellano A, et al. Motor and language DTI fiber tracking combined with intraoperative subcortical mapping for surgical removal of gliomas. Neuroimage 2008;39(1):369–82.

14. Berman JI, Berger MS, Chung SW, et al. Accuracy of diffusion tensor magnetic resonance imaging tractography assessed using intraoperative subcortical stimulation mapping and magnetic source imaging. J Neurosurg 2007;107(3):488–94.

15. Hervey-Jumper SL, Li J, Lau D, et al. Awake craniotomy to maximize glioma resection: methods and technical nuances over a 27-year period. J Neurosurg 2015;24:1–15.

16. Hervey-Jumper SL, Berger MS. Role of surgical resection in low- and high-grade gliomas. Curr Treat Options Neurol 2014;16(4):014–0284.

17. Trinh VT, Fahim DK, Maldaun MV, et al. Impact of preoperative functional magnetic resonance imaging during awake craniotomy procedures for intraoperative guidance and complication avoidance. Stereotact Funct Neurosurg 2014;92(5):315–22.

18. Duffau H. New concepts in surgery of WHO grade II gliomas: functional brain mapping, connectionism and plasticity–a review. J Neurooncol 2006;79(1):77–115.

19. Thiel A, Herholz K, Koyuncu A, et al. Plasticity of language networks in patients with brain tumors: a positron emission tomography activation study. Ann Neurol 2001;50(5):620–9.

20. Bizzi A, Blasi V, Falini A, et al. Presurgical functional MR imaging of language and motor functions: validation with intraoperative electrocortical mapping. Radiology 2008;248(2):579–89.

21. Guggisberg AG, Honma SM, Findlay AM, et al. Mapping functional connectivity in patients with brain lesions. Ann Neurol 2008;63(2):193–203.

22. Berger MS. Lesions in functional ("eloquent") cortex and subcortical white matter. Clin Neurosurg 1994;41:444–63.

23. Fernandez Coello A, Moritz-Gasser S, Martino J, et al. Selection of intraoperative tasks for awake mapping based on relationships between tumor location and functional networks. J Neurosurg 2013;119(6):1380–94.

24. Taylor MD, Bernstein M. Awake craniotomy with brain mapping as the routine surgical approach to treating patients with supratentorial intraaxial tumors: a prospective trial of 200 cases. J Neurosurg 1999;90(1):35–41.

25. Bekker AY, Kaufman B, Samir H, et al. The use of dexmedetomidine infusion for awake craniotomy. Anesth Analg 2001;92(5):1251–3.

26. Herrick IA, Craen RA, Gelb AW, et al. Propofol sedation during awake craniotomy for seizures: patient-controlled administration versus neurolept analgesia. Anesth Analg 1997;84(6):1285–91.

27. Olsen KS. The asleep-awake technique using propofol-remifentanil anaesthesia for awake craniotomy for cerebral tumours. Eur J Anaesthesiol 2008;25(8):662–9.

28. Nathan SS, Sinha SR, Gordon B, et al. Determination of current density distributions generated by electrical stimulation of the human cerebral cortex. Electroencephalogr Clin Neurophysiol 1993;86(3):183–92.

29. Nimsky C, Ganslandt O, Tomandl B, et al. Low-field magnetic resonance imaging for intraoperative use in neurosurgery: a 5-year experience. Eur Radiol 2002;12(11):2690–703.

30. Knauth M, Wirtz CR, Tronnier VM, et al. Intraoperative MR imaging increases the extent of tumor resection in patients with high-grade gliomas. AJNR Am J Neuroradiol 1999;20(9):1642–6.

31. Wirtz CR, Knauth M, Staubert A, et al. Clinical evaluation and follow-up results for intraoperative magnetic resonance imaging in neurosurgery. Neurosurgery 2000;46(5):1112–20.

32. Stummer W, Pichlmeier U, Meinel T, et al. Fluorescence-guided surgery with 5-aminolevulinic acid for resection of malignant glioma: a randomised controlled multicentre phase III trial. Lancet Oncol 2006;7(5):392–401.

33. Stummer W, Reulen HJ, Novotny A, et al. Fluorescence-guided resections of malignant gliomas–an overview. Acta Neurochir Suppl 2003;88:9–12.

34. Hegi ME, Diserens AC, Gorlia T, et al. MGMT gene silencing and benefit from temozolomide in glioblastoma. N Engl J Med 2005;352(10):997–1003.

35. Keles GE, Chang EF, Lamborn KR, et al. Volumetric extent of resection and residual contrast enhancement on initial surgery as predictors of outcome in adult patients with hemispheric anaplastic astrocytoma. J Neurosurg 2006;105(1):34–40.

36. Barker FG 2nd, Prados MD, Chang SM, et al. Radiation response and survival time in patients with glioblastoma multiforme. J Neurosurg 1996;84(3):442–8.

37. Bloch O, Han SJ, Cha S, et al. Impact of extent of resection for recurrent glioblastoma on overall survival: clinical article. J Neurosurg 2012;117(6):1032–8.

38. Brown PD, Ballman KV, Rummans TA, et al. Prospective study of quality of life in adults with newly diagnosed high-grade gliomas. J Neurooncol 2006;76(3):283–91.

39. Buckner JC, Schomberg PJ, McGinnis WL, et al. A phase III study of radiation therapy plus carmustine with or without recombinant interferon-alpha in the treatment of patients with newly diagnosed high-grade glioma. Cancer 2001;92(2):420–33.

40. Curran WJ Jr, Scott CB, Horton J, et al. Does extent of surgery influence outcome for astrocytoma with atypical or anaplastic foci (AAF)? A report from three Radiation Therapy Oncology Group (RTOG) trials. J Neurooncol 1992;12(3):219–27.

41. Dinapoli RP, Brown LD, Arusell RM, et al. Phase III comparative evaluation of PCNU and carmustine combined with radiation therapy for high-grade glioma. J Clin Oncol 1993;11(7):1316–21.

42. Duncan GG, Goodman GB, Ludgate CM, et al. The treatment of adult supratentorial high grade astrocytomas. J Neurooncol 1992;13(1):63–72.

43. Hervey-Jumper SL, Berger MS. Reoperation for recurrent high-grade glioma: a current perspective of the literature. Neurosurgery 2014;75(5):491–9.

44. Hollerhage HG, Zumkeller M, Becker M, et al. Influence of type and extent of surgery on early results and survival time in glioblastoma multiforme. Acta Neurochir 1991;113(1–2):31–7.

45. Huber A, Beran H, Becherer A, et al. Supratentorial glioma: analysis of clinical and temporal parameters in 163 cases. Neurochirurgia 1993;36(6):189–93 [in German].

46. Jeremic B, Grujicic D, Antunovic V, et al. Influence of extent of surgery and tumor location on treatment outcome of patients with glioblastoma multiforme treated with combined modality approach. J Neurooncol 1994;21(2):177–85.

47. Keles GE, Anderson B, Berger MS. The effect of extent of resection on time to tumor progression and survival in patients with glioblastoma multiforme of the cerebral hemisphere. Surg Neurol 1999;52(4):371–9.

48. Kowalczuk A, Macdonald RL, Amidei C, et al. Quantitative imaging study of extent of surgical resection and prognosis of malignant astrocytomas. Neurosurgery 1997;41(5):1028–36.

49. Lacroix M, Abi-Said D, Fourney DR, et al. A multivariate analysis of 416 patients with glioblastoma multiforme: prognosis, extent of resection, and survival. J Neurosurg 2001;95(2):190–8.

50. Lamborn KR, Chang SM, Prados MD. Prognostic factors for survival of patients with glioblastoma: recursive partitioning analysis. Neuro Oncol 2004;6(3):227–35.

51. Levin VA, Yung WK, Bruner J, et al. Phase II study of accelerated fractionation radiation therapy with carboplatin followed by PCV chemotherapy for the treatment of anaplastic gliomas. Int J Radiat Oncol Biol Phys 2002;53(1):58–66.

52. McGirt MJ, Chaichana KL, Gathinji M, et al. Independent association of extent of resection with survival in patients with malignant brain astrocytoma. J Neurosurg 2009;110(1):156–62.

53. Nitta T, Sato K. Prognostic implications of the extent of surgical resection in patients with intracranial malignant gliomas. Cancer 1995;75(11):2727–31.

54. Nomiya T, Nemoto K, Kumabe T, et al. Prognostic significance of surgery and radiation therapy in cases of anaplastic astrocytoma: retrospective analysis of 170 cases. J Neurosurg 2007;106(4):575–81.

55. Oppenlander ME, Wolf AB, Snyder LA, et al. An extent of resection threshold for recurrent glioblastoma and its risk for neurological morbidity. J Neurosurg 2014;120(4):846–53.

56. Oszvald A, Guresir E, Setzer M, et al. Glioblastoma therapy in the elderly and the importance of the extent of resection regardless of age. J Neurosurg 2012;116(2):357–64.

57. Phillips TL, Levin VA, Ahn DK, et al. Evaluation of bromodeoxyuridine in glioblastoma multiforme: a Northern California Cancer Center Phase II study. Int J Radiat Oncol Biol Phys 1991;21(3):709–14.

58. Pope WB, Sayre J, Perlina A, et al. MR imaging correlates of survival in patients with high-grade gliomas. AJNR Am J Neuroradiol 2005;26(10):2466–74.

59. Prados MD, Gutin PH, Phillips TL, et al. Highly anaplastic astrocytoma: a review of 357 patients treated between 1977 and 1989. Int J Radiat Oncol Biol Phys 1992;23(1):3–8.

60. Puduvalli VK, Hashmi M, McAllister LD, et al. Anaplastic oligodendrogliomas: prognostic factors for tumor recurrence and survival. Oncology 2003;65(3):259–66.

61. Sanai N, Polley MY, McDermott MW, et al. An extent of resection threshold for newly diagnosed glioblastomas. J Neurosurg 2011;115(1):3–8.

62. Sandberg-Wollheim M, Malmstrom P, Stromblad LG, et al. A randomized study of chemotherapy with procarbazine, vincristine, and lomustine with and without

radiation therapy for astrocytoma grades 3 and/or 4. Cancer 1991;68(1):22–9.

63. Shibamoto Y, Yamashita J, Takahashi M, et al. Supratentorial malignant glioma: an analysis of radiation therapy in 178 cases. Radiother Oncol 1990; 18(1):9–17.

64. Simpson JR, Horton J, Scott C, et al. Influence of location and extent of surgical resection on survival of patients with glioblastoma multiforme: results of three consecutive Radiation Therapy Oncology Group (RTOG) clinical trials. Int J Radiat Oncol Biol Phys 1993;26(2):239–44.

65. Stark AM, Nabavi A, Mehdorn HM, et al. Glioblastoma multiforme–report of 267 cases treated at a single institution. Surg Neurol 2005;63(2):162–9.

66. Ushio Y, Kochi M, Hamada J, et al. Effect of surgical removal on survival and quality of life in patients with supratentorial glioblastoma. Neurol Med Chir 2005;45(9):454–60.

67. Vecht CJ, Avezaat CJ, van Putten WL, et al. The influence of the extent of surgery on the neurological function and survival in malignant glioma. A retrospective analysis in 243 patients. J Neurol Neurosurg Psychiatry 1990;53(6):466–71.

CHAPTER 13

Awake Craniotomy for Glioblastoma

Roberto Jose Diaz, MD, PhD, FRCS(C), Stephanie Chen, MD, Anelia Kassi, BSc, Ricardo J. Komotar, MD*, Michael E. Ivan, MD, MBS

INTRODUCTION

The goal of modern surgery for glioblastoma is maximal safe resection. Neurosurgeons are keenly aware of the dramatic negative effects that postoperative neurologic deficits have on survival[1] and quality of life.[2] In contrast, achieving a complete or near-complete resection of enhancing tumor has been associated with improved survival in patients with glioblastoma.[3–5] Tumor resection using the technique of awake craniotomy may allow oncologic surgeons to enhance the extent of resection while minimizing the risks of neurologic deficit. Nevertheless, like any other surgical techniques, a thorough understanding of its indication, application, limitations, and outcomes is necessary for the surgeon undertaking its use. This chapter reviews the surgical decision making and technical points, and discusses outcomes related to awake craniotomy in patients with glioblastoma.

INDICATIONS FOR AWAKE CRANIOTOMY IN GLIOBLASTOMA

Glioblastoma is an invasive and rapidly growing primary brain tumor that can arise de novo or by transformation from a low-grade astrocytoma. In many cases, secondary glioblastoma arising from a preexisting low-grade astrocytoma occurs in eloquent regions.[6] Those patients with long-standing preexisting tumors may show shift of critical eloquent brain function to different anatomic locations, thereby potentially rendering a greater extent of resection possible than that predicted based on preoperative imaging and knowledge of expected functional anatomy.[7] De-novo tumors may be confined to a non-eloquent gyrus and displace adjacent eloquent

cortex by respecting the sulcal margin. Resection of the affected gyrus with preservation of adjacent eloquent cortex can be achieved with cortical mapping. Glioblastomas migrate via the white matter tracts and therefore subcortical stimulation to identify the location of corticospinal tract fibers can further assist in resection of tumors extending to the corona radiate and centrum semiovale and near corticospinal and speech/language fibers. In common practice, awake craniotomy has been used for tumors in or adjacent to the paracentral lobule, insula, posterior dominant frontal lobe, dominant temporal lobe, dominant perisylvian region, and dominant angular gyrus.[8–11] Other surgeons have also reported the use of awake craniotomy for dominant parietal tumors,[12–14] tumors near the optic radiations,[15–17] and tumors near the visual cortex.[18]

PATIENT SELECTION AND PREOPERATIVE EVALUATION

Patients with preserved or partially preserved eloquent cortex function are ideal candidates for awake craniotomy because the goal is to maintain or improve on preoperative function with tumor resection. When considering age appropriateness, it is important to factor whether the patient has the age-appropriate cognitive capacity to understand the elements of the procedure and follow directions. Elderly patients with early dementia, prior stroke, or with multiple comorbidities that have affected their cognitive performance are often excluded from participation. Furthermore, patients with prior psychiatric comorbidities, such as severe anxiety or claustrophobia, may find it difficult to tolerate the procedure. Preoperative

University of Miami Miller School of Medicine, Department of Neurological Surgery, University of Miami Hospital, 1321 NW 14th Street, West Building Suite 306, Miami, FL 33125, USA
* Corresponding author.
E-mail address: RKomotar@med.miami.edu

evaluation includes a detailed neuropsychiatric history to rule out claustrophobia, posttraumatic stress disorder, delusional thoughts, hallucinations, dissociative states, and severe anxiety. Furthermore, it is important to assess medical risk factors for altered response to anesthetic agents, such as alcoholism, drug abuse, polypharmacy, benzodiazepine or narcotic dependence, respiratory illness, obesity, obstructive sleep apnea, uncontrolled seizures, and prior lack of effect of local anesthetics.

The ideal patient is motivated, mature, and able to tolerate a strange and stressful environment for an extended period of time.[19] General rules for patient preparation include providing honest information about the steps of the procedure without overuse of medical jargon as well as straightforward discussion of risks, complications, and outcomes.[20] Some clinicians suggest proper counseling augmented with other forms of information, such as short films.[21] Other centers perform a test run of patient positioning and language testing the day before surgery.[22] In our center, an additional brief overview of the procedure and what the patient will experience is provided in the preoperative area on the day of surgery because the patient may have forgotten the information from the preoperative clinic visit. The patient is reminded to report any discomfort, even minor discomfort or pain, at any point during the procedure and is reassured that the team will be responsive. Regardless of the patient education strategy used, the most important factor in patient satisfaction seems to be the time spent preoperatively with members of the clinical team establishing a trusting alliance.[20] The importance of this factor is understandable in that patients experience a sense of powerlessness and loss of control before the procedure and this can be reduced by open communication.[22,23]

ANESTHETIC CONSIDERATIONS

Although the awake craniotomy is generally a well-tolerated procedure, its success depends heavily on specialized anesthetic management. It requires extensive knowledge in local anesthesia for scalp block, advanced airway management, sedation sequences, management of hemodynamics, and patient coaching.

Premedication

Premedication is intended to relieve anxiety without oversedation, as well as preventing nausea, seizures, reflux, pain, or other adverse events. Midazolam or alprazolam are short-acting benzodiazepines, which can be used to provide anxiolysis and prevent nausea before positioning.[24] Pretreatment with metoclopramide and ondansetron also helps to prevent nausea.[19,25,26] Dexamethasone is routinely given to reduce brain edema and prevent nausea.[26,27] Although mannitol can be given after urinary catheter placement to reduce intracranial pressure, the authors have found that patients often complain of excessive thirst, which may interfere with language evaluation. Therefore, we only administer mannitol in cases in which other methods to reduce intracranial pressure have not worked. To prevent seizures, patients are usually pretreated with anticonvulsants as well. The 2 anticonvulsants of choice are levetiracetam (Keppra) and phenytoin (Dilantin).[28]

Local Anesthesia

Initially, awake neurosurgery was done with only local anesthesia to the scalp and dura.[29] However, with the discovery of neuroleptics such as propofol, local anesthesia and general anesthesia are now used in combination for greater patient comfort and amnesia during awake craniotomies. Local anesthetic is injected to reversibly reduce pain sensation in either a regional field block or complete scalp block. The scalp block targets 6 nerves: the auriculotemporal nerve, zygomaticotemporal nerve, supraorbital nerve, supratrochlear nerve, greater occipital nerve, and lesser occipital nerve.[30] Additional injection of the pin sites and surgical skin incision line is associated with improved pain scores[31–33] and has minimal risks for systemic toxicity. Furthermore, there is evidence that local anesthesia also serves to blunt the hemodynamic response to cranial fixation and incision, such as increased heart rate and blood pressure,[34,35] which in turn may prevent increased intracranial pressure. Bupivacaine, levobupivacaine, and ropivacaine are chosen for their long duration of action.[36] They may be administered in combination with epinephrine in concentrations of 1:200,000 or 1:400,000.[37]

Asleep-Awake-Asleep Technique

The asleep-awake-asleep monitored anesthesia technique entails general anesthesia with or without the use of an airway for deep sedation during the opening and closing portions of the surgery, with the awakening of the patients during the critical portion of tumor resection.[38] The following drug regimens are used for intraoperative sedation and analgesia: propofol-fentanyl, propofol-remifentanil, dexmedetomidine-remifentanil.[39] In intubated patients, some anesthesiologists add a volatile anesthetic such as nitrous oxide for craniotomy opening.[28]

Propofol is widely used for awake craniotomy because of its rapid onset of action and rapid redistribution and metabolism, which allow easy sedation titration.[40] Furthermore, propofol decreases cerebral oxygen consumption, reduces intracranial pressure, and has antiseizure properties and antiemetic effects.[41–43] Typically, a propofol infusion is used during the asleep segment of the procedure and then turned off 15 minutes before the awake portion.[28]

In recent years, many anesthesiologists have been combining propofol with an opioid analgesic such as fentanyl or remifentanil. Both fentanyl and remifentanil have favorable pharmacokinetics with very short half-lives, which facilitates the transition to wakefulness.[44] Remifentanil seems to be associated with fewer intraoperative seizures than other opioid analgesics[19,45]; however, remifentanil may cause bradycardia, which is a concern in patients taking β-blockers.[28]

Dexmedetomidine is a newer alternative to propofol. Dexmedetomidine is a highly selective alpha-2 adrenoreceptor agonist with dose-dependent sedative, anxiolytic, and analgesic effects without respiratory suppression. Multiple studies have shown that the sedative effect of dexmedetomidine causes somnolence that can be easily reversed without subsequent agitation or confusion, as well as analgesia that reduces the necessary amounts of other drugs. In general, a dexmedetomidine load of 0.5 to 1 µg/kg/h over 20 minutes is followed by infusion at rates of 0.1 to 0.7 µg/kg/h to 20 minutes before testing.[39]

In the case series presented by Hervey-Jumper and Berger[46] there was no correlation between the various drug regimens for sedation and tumor grade, tumor site, stimulation-induced seizures, laryngeal mask airway (LMA) use, patient body mass index, or aborted procedure. One study found fewer stimulated seizures with propofol versus dexmedetomidine[47]; however, no drug regimen has been shown to be superior.

In most patients undergoing awake craniotomy a secured airway is not necessary. A low threshold for placement of a nasal trumpet occurs if the patient shows signs of airway obstruction or snoring with sedation, and noninvasive supplemental oxygen can be delivered via a nasal cannula. Nevertheless, oversedation during the sleep portion of surgery can lead to apnea, oxygen desaturation, and carbon dioxide retention. An LMA is an airway device that can be used in this event because of its ease of insertion and removal without manipulating the head. It is generally well tolerated by awake patients while in place,[48] and can be removed easily during the awake portion so that the patient can verbalize

clearly. In one case series, LMA was only required in 1% of patients as a result of tumors with significant mass effect and the need for hyperventilation caused by tumor vascularity and venous engorgement secondary to hypercapnia.[46] Endotracheal intubation is preferred to LMA in the rare patients with risk of pulmonary aspiration, because the LMA does not protect against aspiration from gastric contents. A fiberoptic bronchoscope should be used to emergently intubate patients in this situation in order to minimize head movement.

Monitored Anesthesia Care

Monitored anesthesia care (MAC) is a sedation protocol in which the patient is sedated but breathing spontaneously, and responsive to name-calling throughout the procedure. MAC uses similar medications in lower doses in order to achieve conscious sedation with spontaneous ventilation. Theoretically, the light sedation during the opening and closing portions of the surgery allow a shorter time to full alertness and smoother transitions, but require a more cooperative patient. Propofol doses are often between 30 and 180 µg/kg/min and remifentanil doses range from 0.03 to 0.09 µg/kg/min.[25,42,49] Once the dura is open, a low-dose infusion of remifentanil 0 µg/kg/min to 0.01 µg/kg/min or dexmedetomidine 0 µg/kg/h to 0.5 µg/kg/h can be used to achieve relaxation.[19,42,50–53]

Complications

Anesthetic complications vary depending on anesthetic technique. There is a risk for airway complications and desaturations during awake-asleep-awake craniotomy given the use of sedation with an unprotected airway.[19,22,54,55] However proper patient selection, preoperative airway evaluation, patient positioning, close monitoring of end-tidal carbon dioxide, and a readily available nasal trumpet, LMA, and endotracheal tube can prevent adverse sequelae. In some cases, hypoventilation results in increased brain volume during an awake craniotomy.[22,55] Mannitol can be used before dural opening to minimize cerebral edema and herniation during dural opening. However, emergent intubation and conversion to general anesthesia may be required for significant brain swelling.[22,46]

Intraoperative seizure is a dangerous complication when a patient is fixed in pins without a secured airway, occurring in 3% to 20% of patients.[46,47,56–58] In one of the largest reviews of awake craniotomies, Hervey-Jumper and colleagues[59] noted that in 859 cases the overall perioperative complication rate was 10%, in which there were only 2 intraoperative seizures reported and in 0.5% of the cases the awake mapping was aborted. Seizures stimulated by cortical mapping can usually be aborted by stopping the stimulation or delivering ice-cold saline directly onto the cortical surface.[57] Resistant seizures may require immediate dosing of benzodiazepine or propofol, which may interfere with subsequent neurocognitive testing.[28] Having propofol loaded into a syringe and attached to within 15 cm (6 inches) of intravenous tubing to the patient can ensure a quick response to uncontrolled seizure activity.

Hemodynamic instability, including hypertension, hypotension, and tachycardia, can be encountered. An arterial line for close monitoring and prompt treatment with the appropriate medications may prevent associated adverse outcomes. Patient agitation and movement can be resolved by altering sedative medication and adjusting the patient's environment, such as temperature, light source, and padding.[28] However, some patients experience severe emergence delirium, which can result in serious injury to themselves and members of the operating room team. A practice wake-up before making the incision can be used to preemptively assess the patient's transition from asleep to awake in order to optimize patient safety. If the patient cannot tolerate the procedure or agitation cannot be controlled, the procedure can then be converted to general anesthesia.

SURGICAL TECHNIQUE
Positioning and Pinning
Positioning of awake patients is a crucial step in a successful awake craniotomy surgery. In addition to the usual considerations of optimizing tumor access and minimizing brain retraction, bleeding, intracranial pressure, and venous obstruction, there must be adequate space for the neurologic examination and an emergency airway.

With the patient lying supine on the operative table and sedated, local anesthetic is infiltrated into the scalp in a complete ring block. Following administration of the local anesthetic the patient is moved into position and pinned into the head frame. The patient should be positioned supine on the operative table with or without the use of a soft shoulder roll and pillows under the knees. The ankles, wrists, and elbows are padded with soft egg-crate foam. The neck is placed in a position of comfort, avoiding excessive flexion or rotation (no more than 20° of flexion or 30° of rotation). For lateral lesions the authors find that using a large shoulder roll and bolstering the

ipsilateral hip with pillows is sufficient and avoids placing the patient in a lateral position. The ipsilateral arm is placed in a crossed-arm position over the body and supported with tape so that the ipsilateral shoulder does not slump. The contralateral arm is free for patient assessment and supported on an arm board. Complete visualization of the contralateral arm and leg should be maintained to allow for observation of any motor stimulation during surgery. The patient is secured to the table with multiple Velcro belts and tape to allow for table rotation to bring the craniotomy site to the apex of the surgeon's view. At least 15° of reverse Trendelenburg position is used. The authors place a foot rest for patients who require greater than 30° of reverse Trendelenburg or who are obese, to eliminate traction on the neck. Body temperature is maintained at 36°C to 37°C to prevent shivering and allow rapid metabolism of anesthetic agents.

Surgical Incision and Draping
After registering the neuronavigation system the borders of the tumor are mapped on the scalp surface. A linear incision is devised, preserving the scalp vascularization and allowing an appropriately sized craniotomy. The craniotomy is designed based on the margins of the tumor and not for exposure of eloquent areas. The goal is to minimize exposure of eloquent brain not involved with tumor. Safe resection with negative mapping has previously been shown so that exposure of eloquent noninvolved brain for positive mapping is not required.[9,11,60] A hair-sparing incision technique is used in virgin cases[61,62] and minimal strip shave with clippers[63] is used for reoperative cases or patients with short (<2.5 cm [1 inch]) hair. A Layla bar is used to prop up the sterile towels and overdrape to allow face exposure. Access to the patient's airway under the drapes is further provided by a flexible loop attached to the bed frame. The surgical drapes should be arranged in a wide-open geometry to minimize claustrophobia and allow eye contact with patient as well as a view of the patient's face, arms, and legs for neurologic examination. A portable microphone is attached to the patient's neck to allow the surgeon to hear the patient from under the drapes.[64] In order to confirm that the patient will tolerate the head frame and desired surgical position during tumor resection a wake-up test is performed before sterile preparation of the incision. Adjustments are made if the patient reports any discomfort. If the patient arouses in an agitated state with inability to follow commands the procedure is performed under continuous sedation with only

biopsy of tumors in eloquent perisylvian cortex or with direct cortical/subcortical stimulation and motor evoke potential monitoring for tumors in or near the rolandic cortex or extending toward the corticospinal tract.

Language Mapping

Expressive speech is tested by having the patient count serial numbers from 1 to 50, name objects, and read a word out loud while the cortex is stimulated for 4 seconds at the start of the task. Receptive speech is tested by having the patient repeat a complex sentence stated by the examiner. A bipolar stimulating electrode with 5-mm spacing is used with square-wave pulse at 60 Hz and pulse duration of 2 milliseconds. The current is initially set at 1.5 to 2 mA and increased by 1-mA steps up to a maximum of 6 mA.[11,65] Afterdischarges recorded on a 4-contact or 6-contact strip electrode or a Montreal frame in adjacent cortex indicate the need to reduce the stimulating current by 0.5 to 1 mA.[66] Stimulation sites are distributed 1 cm apart, tested 3 times, and identified with sterile labels.[11] The patient's speech is assessed for speech arrest, slowing, dysnomia, or paraphasias elicited by the cortical stimulation. Speech arrest is characterized by the loss of speech production in the absence of involuntary muscle contraction affecting speech. Between stimulation episodes the patient is tested to determine recovery before continuation of testing. Localization of speech areas may be affected by the stimulation procedure used, extent of language testing, and differences in functional distribution between individual patients and languages. These factors may account for the higher rate of negative speech mapping compared with motor mapping.[67] Preoperative fMRI may allow identification of language areas for craniotomy and surgical approach planning; however, brain shift during tumor removal requires the use of awake mapping to ensure safety during resection (**Fig. 13.1**).

Cortical Motor Mapping

Preservation of motor function can be achieved in more than 90% of patients when the primary motor cortex is identified during awake craniotomy.[65,68,69] Determination of the primary motor cortex is achieved by use of somatosensory evoked potential phase reversal[70] or identifying the postcentral gyrus by obtaining sensory responses from the tongue area, which is located in a characteristic triangular region posterior to the central sulcus and superior to the sylvian fissure.[71] Preoperative diffusion tensor imaging can also assist in the guidance toward the motor

cortex but should be confirmed with direct stimulation. Direct cortical stimulation over the primary motor cortex is achieved with either monopolar anodal high-frequency stimulation or bipolar low-frequency stimulation. For bipolar stimulation, spherical poles (2.5-mm diameter) with 5-mm distance are used with a stimulus duration of 1 millisecond in trains of 2 to 4 seconds at 50 to 60 Hz with a starting current at 2 mA and progressing up at 1-mA steps. Up to 10 mA may be required to produce cortical motor stimulation with this type of bipolar stimulator, which is explained by the finding that D-wave responses are difficult to elicit with interpolar distances of less than 10 mm.[72] Bipolar stimulation is equally effective as monopolar anodal stimulation at eliciting a response in the primary motor cortex.[73] Monopolar anodal stimulation elicits direct waves in corticospinal tract axons by depolarization of the pyramidal cell body and the initial part of the axon; this results in a required stimulus duration that is much shorter (1.2 milliseconds) than that for bipolar stimulation (2–4 milliseconds).[73] Thus, monopolar anodal stimulation may be more efficient for repeated stimulation of the primary motor cortex and corticospinal tract during tumor resection.[73–75] Short-duration high-frequency stimulation has a lower risk of seizure induction than 50-Hz to 60-Hz stimulation, which makes use of monopolar stimulation preferable in patients with frequent seizures and rolandic or perirolandic glioblastoma.[76] A prospective study of high-frequency monopolar motor stimulation during awake craniotomy for malignant gliomas has not been conducted.

Subcortical Motor Mapping

Stimulation of white matter motor tracts can be performed with either bipolar or monopolar stimulation parameters. Subcortical bipolar stimulation is performed at 5 mA to allow a safe margin of error to stop resection before injury of descending corticospinal tract fibers or optic radiations. A recent study in patients under general anesthesia has shown that monopolar cathodal stimulation is more effective than bipolar stimulation at eliciting responses from the corticospinal tract during glioblastoma resection.[75] A comparative study during awake subcortical mapping has not been conducted. It is important to remember that the ultrasonic aspiration and bipolar cautery can mask functional sites so these tools should not be simultaneously used during stimulation.[77] However, standard suction can be used in tandem with subcortical stimulation to permit efficient tumor resection.

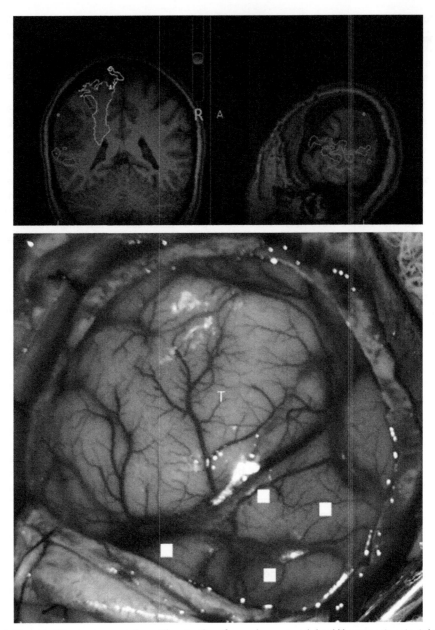

Fig. 13.1 A 55-year-old woman presenting with episodes of speech arrest and shocklike sensations in right arm. Preoperative fMRI and diffusion tensor imaging showing relationship of tumor to reading areas (*teal, right upper panel*) and corticospinal tract (*green, left upper panel*). Regions showing fMRI signal during foot movement (*yellow*) and hand movement (*purple*) are also shown. Tailored craniotomy showing the tumor (T) and relationship to positive direct cortical stimulation mapping of speech disturbance at 3 mA (*white boxes*). Subcortical stimulation to detect corticospinal tract proximity and arcuate fasciculus was performed at 5 mA with bipolar stimulation during the course of tumor resection. Red dot is used as a reference marker of the exposed brain in relation to the navigation images.

PATIENT OUTCOMES

Although awake craniotomy is a well-tolerated option for tumor resection, the literature provides scarce information about patients' experiences with this type of surgery compared with the standard craniotomy under general anesthesia. In a study comparing the two methods, Gupta and colleagues[78] found that patients who underwent surgery under general anesthesia had better outcomes, but the results were not statistically significant.[78] In contrast, Shinoura and colleagues[69] reported fewer deficits in the awake craniotomy group because of better localization of eloquent brain areas. Nine out of 14 patients with general anesthesia had poorer motor function postoperatively compared with 4 of 21 in the awake craniotomy group.[69] Continuous monitoring of neurologic function during awake craniotomy allows surgeons to stop tumor resection if new deficits occur and preserves as much function as possible.[69,78,79] When the tumor is in proximity to or invades eloquent regions, this inevitably results in limited resection of the tumor.[69]

Complete tumor resections correlate better with Karnofsky performance status (KPS) than partial resections.[4,80] Although several studies report KPS for preselection criteria, postoperative KPS was not recorded.[68,81,82] However, Gupta and colleagues[78] found no significant change in KPS after complete tumor resection in both standard and awake craniotomy. The challenge for surgeons in eloquent areas is to not only preserve function but also to remove the greatest amount of tumor tissue. Although transient deficits can range from 14% to 50%, 30 days after surgery 78% to 100% of these patient return to their preoperative baseline function. In addition, at 3 months, 25% of patients experience an improvement in their language function compared with before surgery.[11,83] Resections closer to eloquent areas increased the possibility of developing permanent motor and speech deficits and decreased quality of life.[69,79,84] Gil-Robles and Duffau[85] observed recovery of neurologic function at 6 to 12 months after partial deficit following resection up to the tumor-eloquent cortex boundary in low-grade gliomas, but the portability of this result to glioblastoma patients is uncertain. Transient postoperative language deficits have been reported in 24% to 36% of English-speaking patients undergoing awake craniotomy for glioma.[9,11] The risk of new postoperative deficits after awake craniotomy may be higher in Sino-Tibetan language family speakers because of differences in language networks compared with English speakers.[66,86,87]

Overall, patients who undergo awake craniotomies have a very high satisfaction rate and would even agree to do it again if needed.[81] The number of patients who recall the surgery varies.[79,81,88–91] In general, most patients have partial to total recollection.[79,81,88,90,91] Patients who remember the whole procedure range from 19% to 80%.[79,91] The reasons for a negative experience are anxiety, seizures, pain, and discomfort. In separate studies, significant anxiety was observed only in a minority of patients (13%–15%).[81,90,91] This finding could be related to intraoperative seizures or inability to perform a task when requested during the surgery.[88] A major cause of complaint was pain and discomfort. It was mostly associated with head clamps as well as incision and suturing of the scalp and could be relieved with local anesthesia.[79,88,91] Between 22% and 73% of patients experienced no pain during awake surgery.[49,81] The different techniques available in awake surgeries (asleep-awake-asleep, conscious sedation, and awake-awake-awake) as well as administration of anesthetics during surgery could account for the wide range in pain scores among patients. Another important parameter for variability is the small sample size in most of the studies on patients' experience of awake craniotomy.[49,79,81,91] Beez and colleagues[92] used the 10-cm visual analog score to rate pain and anxiety at the beginning, in the middle, and at the end of awake surgery. Mean pain and anxiety scores progressively increased from the beginning to the end of surgery, ranging from 1.3 to 2.1 (characterized as mild pain) and 2.2 to 2.6, respectively.[92] Increases in these values were not significant. Furthermore, women and patients less than 60 years of age experienced more pain and anxiety; these results require further attention. No cases of posttraumatic stress disorder following awake surgery have been reported.[23,79] Nevertheless, 87.5% of patients had 1 or more psychological symptoms related to the surgery, including vivid recollections or dreams, increased arousal, and need for stability.[23]

SUMMARY

Designed to avoid damage in eloquent areas, awake craniotomy is a highly rated surgical technique for glioblastoma surgery. Several studies report fewer sensorimotor and speech deficits with awake craniotomies. Furthermore, among the patients who remember the surgery, only a small number report pain or discomfort. Intraoperative complications can be minimized by adherence to key surgical principles and expertise with direct cortical stimulation techniques.

REFERENCES

1. McGirt MJ, Mukherjee D, Chaichana KL, et al. Association of surgically acquired motor and language deficits on overall survival after resection of glioblastoma multiforme. Neurosurgery 2009;65:463–9 [discussion: 469–70].

2. Osoba D, Aaronson NK, Muller M, et al. Effect of neurological dysfunction on health-related quality of life in patients with high-grade glioma. J Neurooncol 1997;34:263–78.

3. Chaichana KL, Jusue-Torres I, Navarro-Ramirez R, et al. Establishing percent resection and residual volume thresholds affecting survival and recurrence

for patients with newly diagnosed intracranial glioblastoma. Neuro Oncol 2014;16:113–22.

4. Li YM, Suki D, Hess K, et al. The influence of maximum safe resection of glioblastoma on survival in 1229 patients: can we do better than gross-total resection? J Neurosurg 2016;124(4):977–88.

5. Oppenlander ME, Wolf AB, Snyder LA, et al. An extent of resection threshold for recurrent glioblastoma and its risk for neurological morbidity. J Neurosurg 2014;120:846–53.

6. Duffau H, Capelle L. Preferential brain locations of low-grade gliomas. Cancer 2004;100:2622–6.

7. Signorelli F, Guyotat J, Isnard J, et al. The value of cortical stimulation applied to the surgery of malignant gliomas in language areas. Neurol Sci 2001; 22:3–10.

8. Duffau H, Denvil D, Lopes M, et al. Intraoperative mapping of the cortical areas involved in multiplication and subtraction: an electrostimulation study in a patient with a left parietal glioma. J Neurol Neurosurg Psychiatry 2002;73:733–8.

9. Kim SS, McCutcheon IE, Suki D, et al. Awake craniotomy for brain tumors near eloquent cortex: correlation of intraoperative cortical mapping with neurological outcomes in 309 consecutive patients. Neurosurgery 2009;64:836–45 [discussion: 345–6].

10. Rey-Dios R, Cohen-Gadol AA. Technical nuances for surgery of insular gliomas: lessons learned. Neurosurg Focus 2013;34:E6.

11. Sanai N, Mirzadeh Z, Berger MS. Functional outcome after language mapping for glioma resection. N Engl J Med 2008;358:18–27.

12. Della Puppa A, De Pellegrin S, d'Avella E, et al. Right parietal cortex and calculation processing: intraoperative functional mapping of multiplication and addition in patients affected by a brain tumor. J Neurosurg 2013;119:1107–11.

13. Magrassi L, Bongetta D, Bianchini S, et al. Central and peripheral components of writing critically depend on a defined area of the dominant superior parietal gyrus. Brain Res 2010;1346:145–54.

14. Maldonado IL, Moritz-Gasser S, de Champfleur NM, et al. Surgery for gliomas involving the left inferior parietal lobule: new insights into the functional anatomy provided by stimulation mapping in awake patients. J Neurosurg 2011;115:770–9.

15. Duffau H, Velut S, Mitchell MC, et al. Intra-operative mapping of the subcortical visual pathways using direct electrical stimulations. Acta Neurochir 2004; 146:265–9 [discussion: 269–70].

16. Gras-Combe G, Moritz-Gasser S, Herbet G, et al. Intraoperative subcortical electrical mapping of optic radiations in awake surgery for glioma involving visual pathways. J Neurosurg 2012;117:466–73.

17. Steno A, Karlik M, Mendel P, et al. Navigated three-dimensional intraoperative ultrasound-guided awake resection of low-grade glioma partially infiltrating optic radiation. Acta Neurochir 2012; 154:1255–62.

18. Nguyen HS, Sundaram SV, Mosier KM, et al. A method to map the visual cortex during an awake craniotomy. J Neurosurg 2011;114:922–6.

19. Sarang A, Dinsmore J. Anaesthesia for awake craniotomy–evolution of a technique that facilitates awake neurological testing. Br J Anaesth 2003;90: 161–5.

20. Milian M, Tatagiba M, Feigl GC. Patient response to awake craniotomy - a summary overview. Acta Neurochir 2014;156:1063–70.

21. Jaaskelainen J, Randell T. Awake craniotomy in glioma surgery. Acta Neurochir Suppl 2003;88:31–5.

22. Picht T, Kombos T, Gramm HJ, et al. Multimodal protocol for awake craniotomy in language cortex tumour surgery. Acta Neurochir 2006;148:127–37 [discussion: 137–8].

23. Milian M, Luerding R, Ploppa A, et al. "Imagine your neighbor mows the lawn": a pilot study of psychological sequelae due to awake craniotomy: clinical article. J Neurosurg 2013;118:1288–95.

24. Bauer KP, Dom PM, Ramirez AM, et al. Preoperative intravenous midazolam: benefits beyond anxiolysis. J Clin Anesth 2004;16:177–83.

25. Keifer JC, Dentchev D, Little K, et al. A retrospective analysis of a remifentanil/propofol general anesthetic for craniotomy before awake functional brain mapping. Anesth Analg 2005;101:502–8.

26. Tobias JD, Jimenez DF. Anaesthetic management during awake craniotomy in a 12-year-old boy. Paediatr Anaesth 1997;7:341–4.

27. Chen MS, Hong CL, Chung HS, et al. Dexamethasone effectively reduces postoperative nausea and vomiting in a general surgical adult patient population. Chang Gung Med J 2006;29:175–81.

28. Erickson KM, Cole DJ. Anesthetic considerations for awake craniotomy for epilepsy and functional neurosurgery. Anesthesiol Clin 2012;30:241–68.

29. Bulsara KR, Johnson J, Villavicencio AT. Improvements in brain tumor surgery: the modern history of awake craniotomies. Neurosurg Focus 2005;18:e5.

30. Girvin JP. Neurosurgical considerations and general methods for craniotomy under local anesthesia. Int Anesthesiol Clin 1986;24:89–114.

31. Bloomfield EL, Schubert A, Secic M, et al. The influence of scalp infiltration with bupivacaine on hemodynamics and postoperative pain in adult patients undergoing craniotomy. Anesth Analg 1998;87: 579–82.

32. Honnma T, Imaizumi T, Chiba M, et al. Preemptive analgesia for postoperative pain after frontotemporal craniotomy. No Shinkei Geka 2002;30:171–4 [in Japanese].

33. Sinha PK, Koshy T, Gayatri P, et al. Anesthesia for awake craniotomy: a retrospective study. Neurol India 2007;55:376–81.

34. Geze S, Yilmaz AA, Tuzuner F. The effect of scalp block and local infiltration on the haemodynamic and stress response to skull-pin placement for craniotomy. Eur J Anaesthesiol 2009;26:298–303.

35. Lee EJ, Lee MY, Shyr MH, et al. Adjuvant bupivacaine scalp block facilitates stabilization of hemodynamics in patients undergoing craniotomy with general anesthesia: a preliminary report. J Clin Anesth 2006;18:490–4.

36. Kerscher C, Zimmermann M, Graf BM, et al. Scalp blocks. A useful technique for neurosurgery, dermatology, plastic surgery and pain therapy. Anaesthesist 2009;58:949–58 [quiz: 959–60]. [in German].

37. Papangelou A, Radzik BR, Smith T, et al. A review of scalp blockade for cranial surgery. J Clin Anesth 2013;25:150–9.

38. Huncke K, Van de Wiele B, Fried I, et al. The asleep-awake-asleep anesthetic technique for intraoperative language mapping. Neurosurgery 1998;42:1312–6 [discussion: 1316–7].

39. Piccioni F, Fanzio M. Management of anesthesia in awake craniotomy. Minerva Anestesiol 2008;74:393–408.

40. Hans P, Bonhomme V. Why we still use intravenous drugs as the basic regimen for neurosurgical anaesthesia. Curr Opin Anaesthesiol 2006;19:498–503.

41. Hans P, Bonhomme V, Born JD, et al. Target-controlled infusion of propofol and remifentanil combined with bispectral index monitoring for awake craniotomy. Anaesthesia 2000;55:255–9.

42. Johnson KB, Egan TD. Remifentanil and propofol combination for awake craniotomy: case report with pharmacokinetic simulations. J Neurosurg Anesthesiol 1998;10:25–9.

43. Marik PE. Propofol: therapeutic indications and side-effects. Curr Pharm Des 2004;10:3639–49.

44. Herrick IA, Craen RA, Blume WT, et al. Sedative doses of remifentanil have minimal effect on ECoG spike activity during awake epilepsy surgery. J Neurosurg Anesthesiol 2002;14:55–8.

45. Luders JC, Steinmetz MP, Mayberg MR. Awake craniotomy for microsurgical obliteration of mycotic aneurysms: technical report of three cases. Neurosurgery 2005;56:E201 [discussion: E201].

46. Hervey-Jumper SL, Berger MS. Technical nuances of awake brain tumor surgery and the role of maximum safe resection. J Neurosurg Sci 2015;59:351–60.

47. Sokhal N, Rath GP, Chaturvedi A, et al. Anaesthesia for awake craniotomy: a retrospective study of 54 cases. Indian J Anaesth 2015;59:300–5.

48. Brimacombe J, Tucker P, Simons S. The laryngeal mask airway for awake diagnostic bronchoscopy. A retrospective study of 200 consecutive patients. Eur J Anaesthesiol 1995;12:357–61.

49. Manninen PH, Balki M, Lukitto K, et al. Patient satisfaction with awake craniotomy for tumor surgery: a comparison of remifentanil and fentanyl in conjunction with propofol. Anesth Analg 2006;102:237–42.

50. Almeida AN, Tavares C, Tibano A, et al. Dexmedetomidine for awake craniotomy without laryngeal mask. Arq Neuropsiquiatr 2005;63:748–50.

51. Ard JL Jr, Bekker AY, Doyle WK. Dexmedetomidine in awake craniotomy: a technical note. Surg Neurol 2005;63:114–6 [discussion: 116–7].

52. Mack PF, Perrine K, Kobylarz E, et al. Dexmedetomidine and neurocognitive testing in awake craniotomy. J Neurosurg Anesthesiol 2004;16:20–5.

53. Moore TA 2nd, Markert JM, Knowlton RC. Dexmedetomidine as rescue drug during awake craniotomy for cortical motor mapping and tumor resection. Anesth Analg 2006;102:1556–8.

54. Rajan S, Cata JP, Nada E, et al. Asleep-awake-asleep craniotomy: a comparison with general anesthesia for resection of supratentorial tumors. J Clin Neurosci 2013;20:1068–73.

55. Skucas AP, Artru AA. Anesthetic complications of awake craniotomies for epilepsy surgery. Anesth Analg 2006;102:882–7.

56. Boetto J, Bertram L, Moulinie G, et al. Low rate of intraoperative seizures during awake craniotomy in a prospective cohort with 374 supratentorial brain lesions: electrocorticography is not mandatory. World Neurosurg 2015;84:1838–44.

57. Sartorius CJ, Berger MS. Rapid termination of intraoperative stimulation-evoked seizures with application of cold Ringer's lactate to the cortex. Technical note. J Neurosurg 1998;88:349–51.

58. Taylor MD, Bernstein M. Awake craniotomy with brain mapping as the routine surgical approach to treating patients with supratentorial intraaxial tumors: a prospective trial of 200 cases. J Neurosurg 1999;90:35–41.

59. Hervey-Jumper SL, Li J, Lau D, et al. Awake craniotomy to maximize glioma resection: methods and technical nuances over a 27-year period. J Neurosurg 2015;123:325–39.

60. Sanai N, Berger MS. Intraoperative stimulation techniques for functional pathway preservation and glioma resection. Neurosurg Focus 2010;28:E1.

61. Bekar A, Korfali E, Dogan S, et al. The effect of hair on infection after cranial surgery. Acta Neurochir 2001;143:533–6 [discussion: 537].

62. Sheinberg MA, Ross DA. Cranial procedures without hair removal. Neurosurgery 1999;44:1263–5 [discussion: 1265–6].

63. Tanner J, Norrie P, Melen K. Preoperative hair removal to reduce surgical site infection. Cochrane Database Syst Rev 2011;(11):CD004122.

64. Bernstein M. Outpatient craniotomy for brain tumor: a pilot feasibility study in 46 patients. Can J Neurol Sci 2001;28:120–4.

65. Chacko AG, Thomas SG, Babu KS, et al. Awake craniotomy and electrophysiological mapping for

eloquent area tumours. Clin Neurol Neurosurg 2013;115:329–34.

66. Lu J, Wu J, Yao C, et al. Awake language mapping and 3-Tesla intraoperative MRI-guided volumetric resection for gliomas in language areas. J Clin Neurosci 2013;20:1280–7.

67. Paldor I, Drummond KJ, Awad M, et al. Is a wake-up call in order? Review of the evidence for awake craniotomy. J Clin Neurosci 2016;23:1–7.

68. Pereira LC, Oliveira KM, L'Abbate GL, et al. Outcome of fully awake craniotomy for lesions near the eloquent cortex: analysis of a prospective surgical series of 79 supratentorial primary brain tumors with long follow-up. Acta Neurochir 2009;151: 1215–30.

69. Shinoura N, Yamada R, Tabei Y, et al. Advantages and disadvantages of awake surgery for brain tumours in the primary motor cortex: institutional experience and review of literature. Br J Neurosurg 2011;25:218–24.

70. Cedzich C, Taniguchi M, Schafer S, et al. Somatosensory evoked potential phase reversal and direct motor cortex stimulation during surgery in and around the central region. Neurosurgery 1996;38:962–70.

71. Picard C, Olivier A. Sensory cortical tongue representation in man. J Neurosurg 1983;59:781–9.

72. Katayama Y, Tsubokawa T, Maejima S, et al. Corticospinal direct response in humans: identification of the motor cortex during intracranial surgery under general anaesthesia. J Neurol Neurosurg Psychiatry 1988;51:50–9.

73. Kombos T, Suess O, Kern BC, et al. Comparison between monopolar and bipolar electrical stimulation of the motor cortex. Acta Neurochir 1999;141: 1295–301.

74. Seidel K, Beck J, Stieglitz L, et al. Low-threshold monopolar motor mapping for resection of primary motor cortex tumors. Neurosurgery 2012;71:104–14 [discussion: 114–5].

75. Szelenyi A, Senft C, Jardan M, et al. Intra-operative subcortical electrical stimulation: a comparison of two methods. Clin Neurophysiol 2011;122:1470–5.

76. Szelenyi A, Joksimovic B, Seifert V. Intraoperative risk of seizures associated with transient direct cortical stimulation in patients with symptomatic epilepsy. J Clin Neurophysiol 2007;24:39–43.

77. Szelenyi A, Bello L, Duffau H, et al. Intraoperative electrical stimulation in awake craniotomy: methodological aspects of current practice. Neurosurg Focus 2010;28:E7.

78. Gupta DK, Chandra PS, Ojha BK, et al. Awake craniotomy versus surgery under general anesthesia for resection of intrinsic lesions of eloquent cortex–a prospective randomised study. Clin Neurol Neurosurg 2007;109:335–43.

79. Danks RA, Rogers M, Aglio LS, et al. Patient tolerance of craniotomy performed with the patient under

local anesthesia and monitored conscious sedation. Neurosurgery 1998;42:28–34 [discussion: 34–6].

80. Schneider JP, Trantakis C, Rubach M, et al. Intraoperative MRI to guide the resection of primary supratentorial glioblastoma multiforme–a quantitative radiological analysis. Neuroradiology 2005;47: 489–500.

81. Manchella S, Khurana VG, Duke D, et al. The experience of patients undergoing awake craniotomy for intracranial masses: expectations, recall, satisfaction and functional outcome. Br J Neurosurg 2011; 25(3):391–400.

82. Peruzzi P, Bergese SD, Viloria A, et al. A retrospective cohort-matched comparison of conscious sedation versus general anesthesia for supratentorial glioma resection. Clinical article. J Neurosurg 2011;114:633–9.

83. Duffau H, Moritz-Gasser S, Gatignol P. Functional outcome after language mapping for insular World Health Organization Grade II gliomas in the dominant hemisphere: experience with 24 patients. Neurosurg Focus 2009;27:E7.

84. Haglund MM, Berger MS, Shamseldin M, et al. Cortical localization of temporal lobe language sites in patients with gliomas. Neurosurgery 1994; 34:567–76 [discussion: 576].

85. Gil-Robles S, Duffau H. Surgical management of World Health Organization grade II gliomas in eloquent areas: the necessity of preserving a margin around functional structures. Neurosurg Focus 2010;28:E8.

86. Tan LH, Laird AR, Li K, et al. Neuroanatomical correlates of phonological processing of Chinese characters and alphabetic words: a meta-analysis. Hum Brain Mapp 2005;25:83–91.

87. Tan LH, Spinks JA, Gao JH, et al. Brain activation in the processing of Chinese characters and words: a functional MRI study. Hum Brain Mapp 2000;10:16–27.

88. Goebel S, Nabavi A, Schubert S, et al. Patient perception of combined awake brain tumor surgery and intraoperative 1.5-T magnetic resonance imaging: the Kiel experience. Neurosurgery 2010;67: 594–600 [discussion: 600].

89. Khu KJ, Doglietto F, Radovanovic I, et al. Patients' perceptions of awake and outpatient craniotomy for brain tumor: a qualitative study. J Neurosurg 2010;112:1056–60.

90. Wahab SS, Grundy PL, Weidmann C. Patient experience and satisfaction with awake craniotomy for brain tumours. Br J Neurosurg 2011;25:606–13.

91. Whittle IR, Midgley S, Georges H, et al. Patient perceptions of "awake" brain tumour surgery. Acta Neurochir 2005;147:275–7 [discussion: 277].

92. Beez T, Boge K, Wager M, et al. Tolerance of awake surgery for glioma: a prospective European Low Grade Glioma Network multicenter study. Acta Neurochir 2013;155:1301–8.

CHAPTER 14

Intraoperative Imaging of Glioblastoma

Christopher A. Sarkiss, MD, Jonathan J. Rasouli, MD,
Constantinos G. Hadjipanayis, MD, PhD*

INTRODUCTION

Glioblastoma (GBM) is one of the deadliest forms of cancer, with a median survival of approximately 15 months.[1,2] Standard of care treatment of GBM includes maximal safe surgical resection, fractionated radiotherapy, temozolomide chemotherapy, and, most recently, tumor treatment fields. Despite this combination treatment regimen, tumor progression or recurrence occurs after a median of 7 months.[3,4] Overall survival of patients with GBM is determined by multiple factors, including the patient's performance status (Karnofsky performance status [KPS]), age, tumor DNA repair status, and extent of surgical resection.

Despite advances in surgical techniques and radiographic imaging, maximal resection has been shown to be achieved in only 35% of cases.[5,6] Intraoperative brain shift, poorly demarcated tumor margins, and proximity to eloquent brain all affect the surgeon's ability to achieve the maximal extent of resection (EOR).[6] Therefore, there is renewed focus on improving the intraoperative imaging and visualization of GBM to overcome these inherent limitations during surgery. This chapter investigates the various surgical adjuncts available to aid in the surgical resection of GBM, namely neuronavigation with MRI, diffusion tensor imaging (DTI), functional MRI (fMRI), intraoperative MRI (iMRI), and intraoperative tumor visualization for fluorescence-guided surgery (FGS).

MRI NEURONAVIGATION

Frameless stereotactic navigation devices have been an indispensable tool for tumor removal by neurosurgeons since they were described by Barnett and colleagues[7] in 1993. At present, 2 commonly used devices are the StealthStation S7 (Medtronic, Minneapolis, MN) and the Brainlab Curve (Brainlab AG, Germany) (**Fig. 14.1**). Patients undergo high-resolution MRI before surgery. Typical sequences used are postcontrast three-dimensional, T1-weighted gradient-echo (magnetization-prepared rapid gradient-echo) and T1-weighted spin echo.[8] These preoperative MRI scans are subsequently uploaded to the device and registration is performed after the patient's head is immobilized by 3-pin fixation. Registration is accomplished through the use of skin fiducials (paired-point method) or laser surface registration.[9] The surgeon uses a metal pointer on the scalp to assist with planning for the craniotomy and incision. Intraoperative guidance is performed by using a sterile metal pointer in the surgical field to identify anatomic structures and tumor boundaries (**Fig. 14.2**). When applied in the surgical field, the average radial accuracy has been reported to be 2.4 ± 1.7 mm. Lesions in the frontal lobe have the highest navigation accuracy, whereas infratentorial lesions have the highest rate of error.[9] Periventricular tumors and those with a volume greater than 30 mL also have a higher rate of registration error.[10]

Because frameless stereotactic neuronavigation devices have been present for more than 2 decades at the time of this writing, the main advantages are their time-tested nature and ease of use. Despite these advantages, there are several significant limitations with neuronavigation during GBM resection. First, patient registration can be imprecise, causing delays in operating room workflow.[6,9] Second, the entry of atmospheric air into the cranial vault, tumor debulking, and the use of hyperosmolar solutions can potentiate brain shift, which exacerbate errors in registration.[6] Navigation errors of a centimeter or more have been reported.[11] These discrepancies can limit the neurosurgeon's ability to precisely

Department of Neurosurgery, Mount Sinai Health System, New York, NY, USA
* Corresponding author. Department of Neurosurgery, Phillips Ambulatory Care Center, 5th Floor, Suite 5E, 10 Union Square East, New York, NY 10003.
E-mail address: constantinos.hadjipanayis@mountsinai.org

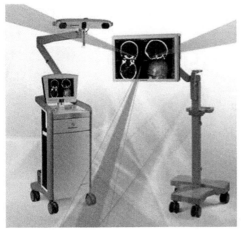 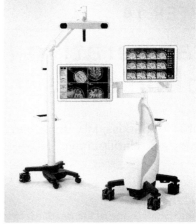

Fig. 14.1 Medtronic StealthStation S7 (*left*) and Brainlab Curve (*right*). (*Courtesy of* Medtronic Inc, Minneapolis, MN, with permission; and Brainlab AG Corp, Feldkirchen, Germany, with permission.)

excise the tumor, and increase the frequency of subtotal resections. In addition, the risk of inadvertent violation of eloquent brain is increased with imprecise navigation. Third, there are currently no reliable methods to account for the inaccuracies in navigation caused by brain shift.[6,12]

With these limitations in mind, tumor neurosurgeons have been progressively examining the use of advanced intraoperative imaging techniques such as DTI,[13] and fMRI (blood oxygen level–dependent fMRI).[14] These advanced magnetic resonance (MR) techniques, which are discussed further in this chapter, have shown promise in improving the EOR and functional outcomes after GBM surgery.

DIFFUSION TENSOR IMAGING
A defining characteristic of GBM is its ability to aggressively infiltrate surrounding white-matter tracts in the brain.[15] Although conventional MR

techniques can readily detect the enhancing portions of GBM, they are poor at detecting areas of microscopic invasion at the tumor periphery.[6,16] These areas of brain invasion at the tumor margin can involve both eloquent and noneloquent white-matter tracts and are not readily visible on conventional T1-weighted/T2-weighted imaging.[13,16] Because the degree of safe cytoreduction after surgery directly correlates with overall prognosis, the use of DTI has been proposed to address these shortcomings.[13,17] DTI is a type of diffusion-weighted MR technique that characterizes the molecular diffusion of water to estimate the topographic organization of white matter throughout the brain (**Fig. 14.3**).[16] This technique provides valuable patient-specific information about subcortical connectivity in relation to the GBM tumor.

The prior characterization of brain tumors with DTI has been well described. Coenen and colleagues[18] first described the intraoperative use of DTI in 2001 in patients with low-grade gliomas

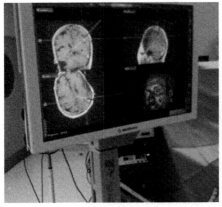 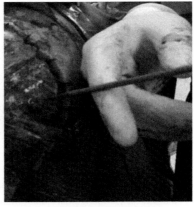

Fig. 14.2 A representative example of the intraoperative use of the StealthStation S7. After satisfactory patient registration is confirmed (*left*), the sterile pointer is placed over an area of interest (*right*), which corresponds with the patient's preoperative MRI scans. (Medtronic Inc, Minneapolis, MN.)

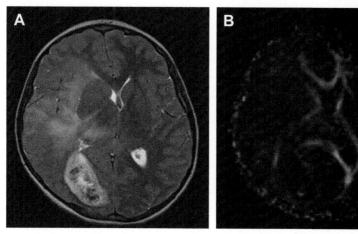

Fig. 14.3 DTI in a patient with GBM affecting the right hemisphere. (*A*) T2-weighted MRI showing an occipital GBM tumor with surrounding peritumoral edema. (*B*) DTI (fractional anisotropy map) showing shifting and disruption of surrounding white-matter tracts. (*Adapted from* Peet AC, Arvanitis TN, Leach MO, et al. Functional imaging in adult and paediatric brain tumours. Nat Rev Clin Oncol. 2012;9(12):702; with permission.)

and meningiomas. This description was followed by a 2004 study by Berman and colleagues,[19] showing a high correlation between white-matter tracts depicted by DTI and direct cortical stimulation during glioma surgery. In 2007, Wu and colleagues[13] published a randomized controlled trial comparing DTI-guided versus standard frameless stereotactic neuronavigation in patients with gliomas involving corticospinal motor pathways. For high-grade gliomas, the investigators showed improved EOR, decreased incidence of postoperative neurologic deficits (15.3% vs 32.8%), improved 6-month Karnofsky performance score (77 ± 27 vs 53 ± 32), and improved median survival (21.2 months vs 14 months). This study showed class I evidence for the benefit of using DTI versus standard MRI sequences to guide glioma resection involving eloquent cortex. DTI has also shown diagnostic value in differentiating between GBM and metastasis.[16]

The main advantage of DTI is its ability to accurately depict the true extent of tumor margins and surrounding central nervous system connectivity.[17] With this information, neurosurgeons are better equipped to plan a more patient-tailored approach to tumor resection. One of the major disadvantages of DTI is its reliance on region-of-interest (ROI) selection to reconstruct fiber pathways. ROI analysis can be time consuming and difficult in the setting of brain shift and edema caused by tumor.[17] As these processes become increasingly automated, this cumbersome postacquisition analysis will likely improve. Similar to conventional neuronavigation, another disadvantage of DTI is its inability to account for dynamic changes in the operating room, such as brain shift caused by

pneumocephalus.[13] Therefore, there is increased focus in using multimodal techniques such as fluorescence-guided surgery (FGS) in conjunction with advanced imaging techniques to improve outcomes in GBM surgery.

FUNCTIONAL AND INTRAOPERATIVE MRI

The use of iMRI has been more widely implemented for GBM resection over the past decade, since its introduction in the late 1990s.[20] The main objectives of iMRI are to update source imaging for neuronavigation use (minimize brain shift) and to identify any remaining contrast-enhancing tissue.[21] Several retrospective studies have been reported in the literature over the past decade that offer the potential advantages of iMRI use. Hirschberg and colleagues[12] provided a retrospective analysis of 32 patients with GBM and showed that the iMRI group had a median survival of 14.5 months compared with 12.1 months for the control group. Lenaburg and colleagues[22] reported on 35 GBM cases in 29 patients in whom the use of iMRI led to further resection in 72% of cases and thereby resulted in a tumor resection of greater than 95% in 27 out of 35 cases. Senft and colleagues[23] published a retrospective report on 41 patients with GBM in which they compared the use of iMRI in 10 patients with conventional neuronavigation in 31 patients. Gross total resection (GTR) was observed in all 10 iMRI cases versus 19 of 31 conventional cases, which translated to a median survival of 74 weeks for the GTR group compared with 46 weeks for the subtotal resection group (*P*<.001). This finding in turn led to a median survival of 88 weeks for the iMRI group versus 68 weeks for the conventional group ($P = .07$). Napolitano and colleagues[24] reported on 94 GBM resections over a 5-year period. They compared the use of iMRI versus conventional imaging and found that the rate of resection increased by 17.8% up to 73.2% of GTR/near-total resection (NTR). This greater EOR, in turn, led to greater overall survival, with a median survival of 15.26 months for the GTR/NTR group versus 10.26 months for the partial resection group ($P = .049$). Another study investigating tumor EOR and iMRI use for 135 patients with GBM showed that iMRI found residual tumor volume in 88 patients, leading to further surgical resection in 19 of those patients and GTR for 9 of those patients. This finding led to a survival benefit in those patients with an EOR greater than or equal to 98% and a median survival of 14 months compared with 9 months for patients with an EOR less than 98% ($P<.0001$).[25] Regardless, Kuhnt and colleagues[25] showed the influence of iMRI on EOR, as shown in **Table 14.1**.

A randomized, prospective trial by Senft and colleagues[26] of 58 patients with newly diagnosed GBM underwent resection with either the use of iMRI or conventional computer-assisted neuronavigation. The control group had a 68% GTR rate compared with 96% GTR for the iMRI group on blinded neuroradiological assessment ($P = .023$). This study provided level 1 evidence supporting a higher GTR of GBM tumors with the use of iMRI. However, this difference in EOR did not lead to a significant difference in progression-free survival (PFS) at 6 months. It is worth noting a recent study by Zhang and colleagues,[27] in which they combined the use of iMRI and functional neuronavigation with preoperative fMRI and DTI.

They studied 198 patients with glioma; 112 underwent surgery combined with iMRI and functional neuronavigation, and 86 patients were in the control group. The study group had a greater EOR (95.5% vs 89.9%; $P<.001$) and GTR rate (69.6% vs 47.7%; $P = .002$) in addition to greater language preservation as graded by the aphasia quotient. Moreover, they also showed greater overall survival for their study group (19.6 months vs 13.0 months; $P<.001$) with PFS double that of the control group (12.5 months vs 6.6 months; $P = .003$). Therefore, they showed a potential role for this combined preoperative functional neuronavigation assessment with the use of iMRI. Future studies are needed to assess whether factors such as the dose and timing of the contrast agent, the MRI field strength, and the location of the tumor play a role in achieving greater efficacy for iMRI use.[21]

Most recently, the use of whole-brain proton spectroscopic MRI (sMRI) was used to define the tumor margin in patients with GBM in combination with 5-aminolevulinic acid (5-ALA) tumor fluorescence and histopathology.[28] Whole-brain sMRI metabolite maps were coregistered with MRI neuronavigation to guide neurosurgical tumor sampling. sMRI metabolite abnormalities were located centimeters away from the contrast-enhancing border of GBM tumors, confirming the infiltrative border of GBM tumors and providing a basis for understanding recurrence patterns of GBM tumors.

INTRAOPERATIVE VISUALIZATION AND FLUORESCENCE-GUIDED SURGERY

Intraoperative tumor visualization and FGS has emerged as another important surgical adjunct for GBM resection. It is most commonly achieved by the use of 5-ALA, which is a natural metabolite found in the human body in the hemoglobin metabolic pathway. Once orally ingested, it penetrates the blood-brain barrier (BBB) and is taken up by glioma cells and metabolized into its fluorescent metabolite, protoporphyrin IX (PpIX). Accumulation of PpIX in glioma cells occurs because of lower levels of ferrochelatase PpIX present and decreased outflow from cells. PpIX emits violet-red fluorescence after excitation with 405-nm wavelength blue light (**Fig. 14.4**).[6,29,30] Numerous studies have consistently shown a greater than 90% sensitivity, specificity, and positive predictive value of 5-ALA tissue fluorescence and the presence of malignant tumor.[31–38] Moreover, another study confirmed that 5-ALA has a high positive predictive value

TABLE 14.1
Influence of iMRI on EOR

Resected Tumor Volume (%)	First iMRI (# of Patients)	Final iMRI (# of Patients)
100	0	9
99.9–98.0	0	1
97.9–95.0	3	0
94.9–90.0	1	1
<90.0	15	8

Adapted from Kuhnt D, Becker A, Ganslandt O, et al. Correlation of the extent of tumor volume resection and patient survival in surgery of glioblastoma multiforme with high-field intraoperative MRI guidance. Neuro Oncol 2011;13(12):1339–48.

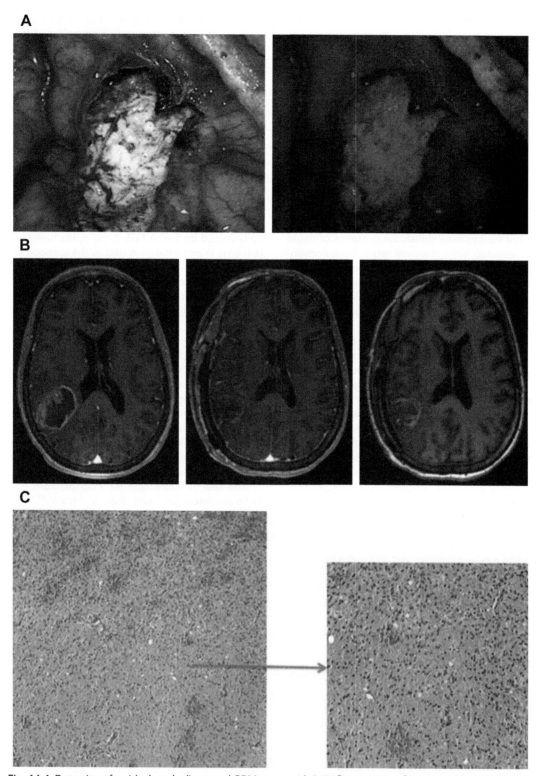

Fig. 14.4 Detection of residual newly diagnosed GBM tumor with PpIX fluorescence after maximal white-light conventional resection. (*A, left*) Microsurgical white-light visualization of GBM resection cavity after maximal conventional resection. (*A, right*) Visualization of PpIX fluorescence at tumor margin after conventional microsurgical resection. (*B, left*) Preoperative MRI scan with gadolinium enhancement in right parietal lobe consistent with malignant glioma. (*B, center and right*) Postoperative MRI scans with and without gadolinium enhancement confirming complete

in detecting neoplastic cells in both grossly pathologic and grossly normal-appearing tissues under white light, which is another indicator of the high sensitivity of the technique for tumor detection and visualization.[39]

The benefit of 5-ALA fluorescence-guided microsurgical resection of newly diagnosed GBM has been documented in a large, randomized controlled, multicenter phase III trial, which showed a complete resection rate of 65% with 5-ALA use compared with 36% in the non–5-ALA group, showing a statistically significant difference of 29% (P<.0001). A significant 20% advantage in 6-month PFS was seen for the 5-ALA group (41% vs 21.1%; P = .0003).[40] More recent studies have shown the presence of tissue fluorescence after maximal white-light conventional microsurgical resections and the subsequent presence of tumor within the fluorescent tissue.[6] Stummer and colleagues[35] reported on 33 patients with newly diagnosed malignant gliomas, 76% of whom had positive fluorescence and presence of tumor but were not detectable by conventional white-light microscopy. In a study by Nabavi and colleagues,[39] fluorescent but normal-appearing tissue under white light had a positive predictive value of 92% for the presence of malignant glioma in 22 of 24 patients. Panciani and colleagues[31] reported that 78% (18 of 23) of patients had tissue fluorescence outside the neuronavigation area that was positive for the presence of tumor, which further shows the added benefit of 5-ALA use. Another study by Coburger and colleagues[38] combined the use of 5-ALA and iMRI and showed higher sensitivity and specificity with 5-ALA compared with iMRI in detection of tumor. Another combined study of 5-ALA and iMRI by Yamada and colleagues[37] showed a 92% positive predictive value for 5-ALA and the presence of malignant glioma as confirmed by histology.

It is important to note the association between greater extent of tumor resection and 5-ALA FGS. Although newer series have reported an approximate 35% complete resection rate for the contrast-enhancing portion of tumors without the use of 5-ALA or MRI, this rate can be significantly augmented by 5-ALA use.[5] The initial randomized multicenter trial with the use of 5-ALA FGS reported a 65%

complete resection rate, with most importantly no difference in postoperative neurologic function compared with conventional white-light surgery.[40] More recent studies have shown as high as 89% complete resection and 73% rate of complete resection with tumors in eloquent cortex.[41–43] Eljamel[36] performed a meta-analysis of 565 patients and showed a gross total tumor resection rate of 75%.

The reported studies have all shown high sensitivity, specificity, and positive predictive value for fluorescence and presence of tumor tissue, as well as the identification of residual tumor tissue after presumed maximal resection with conventional white-light microscopy. Perhaps the greatest utility provided by 5-ALA FGS is the opportunity for real-time information provided to the surgeon independent of neuronavigation and brain shift, which allows better identification and differentiation of tumor from normal brain tissue, thereby allowing higher rates of more complete tumor resection.

In cases of reoperation for recurrent GBM, false-positive tumor fluorescence has been described after 5-ALA administration.[44] In contrast, false-negative fluorescence can also occur and is attributed to 4 major factors: the infiltrative nature of malignant gliomas in which low-density tumor cell infiltration and fluorescence can occur, the necrotic portions of malignant gliomas, structural barriers such as blood or overlying brain tissue, and timing of 5-ALA administration.[6,45]

The use of fluorescein for FGS of GBM has been reported for more than a decade.[46] The method consists of intravenous injection of fluorescein sodium (20 mg/kg) after dural opening, resulting in staining the tumor yellow. Fluorescein tumor fluorescence is limited to several hours. A major difference between fluorescein and 5-ALA is that fluorescein is not metabolized by glioma cells and remains extracellular. Fluorescein accumulates at sites of brain tumors because of the breakdown of the BBB and is cleared several hours later. The yellow staining of tumors can be visualized with a special filter attachment on the microscope in the presence of normal ambient light.[47] Several recent studies have investigated the use of fluorescein FGS for high-grade gliomas. A recent report of a phase II trial of 20 patients

resection of the enhancing tumor. (C) Histopathologic examination of fluorescent tissue at tumor margin confirming the presence of infiltrating tumor extending away from tumor bulk (hematoxylin-eosin, original magnification ×10 [*left*] and ×20 [*right*]). (*Adapted from* Hadjipanayis CG, Widhalm G, Stummer W. What is the surgical benefit of using 5-aminolevulinic acid for fluorescence-guided surgery of malignant gliomas? Neurosurg 2015;77(5):670; with permission.)

with high-grade gliomas showed a gross total resection of 80% with a 6-month PFS of 71.4%.[48] Studies have also shown that there is both high sensitivity (79%–82.2%) and high specificity (90.9%–100%) in fluorescein fluorescence.[49,50] In addition, Koc and colleagues[51] compared 47 patients with fluorescein FGS with 33 patients who did not undergo fluorescein injection and found that although there was no statistically significant difference in median survival between the two groups, the fluorescein group had greater rates of GTR (83% vs 55%), which in turn led to greater survival; patients with GTR had survival of 46.5 weeks compared with 34.3 weeks after partial resection.

SUMMARY

Although the use of MRI neuronavigation has become a gold standard in the process of GBM neurosurgical resection, newer modalities such as DTI, fMRI, iMRI, and FGS have emerged over the past decade as surgical adjuncts. Studies have shown the benefit of each as a tool in assisting neurosurgeons with GBM resection. Another tool that will become important for neurosurgeons is the use of imaging biomarkers (eg, sMRI metabolic abnormalities) to guide resections. Understanding the location of metabolically active tumor regions not currently visualized by conventional MRI sequences will allow neurosurgeons to further maximize tumor resection when safely possible.

REFERENCES

1. Grossman SA, Ye X, Piantadosi S, et al. Survival of patients with newly diagnosed glioblastoma treated with radiation and temozolomide in research studies in the United States. Clin Cancer Res 2010;16(8):2443–9.
2. Darefsky AS, King JT Jr, Dubrow R. Adult glioblastoma multiforme survival in the temozolomide era: a population-based analysis of Surveillance, Epidemiology, and End Results registries. Cancer 2012; 118(8):2163–72.
3. Stupp R, Mason WP, van den Bent MJ, et al. Radiotherapy plus concomitant and adjuvant temozolomide for glioblastoma. N Engl J Med 2005; 352(10):987–96.
4. Olson JJ, Fadul CE, Brat DJ, et al. Management of newly diagnosed glioblastoma: guidelines development, value and application. J Neurooncol 2009;93(1):1–23.
5. McGirt MJ, Chaichana KL, Gathinji M, et al. Independent association of extent of resection with survival in patients with malignant brain astrocytoma. J Neurosurg 2009;110(1):156–62.
6. Hadjipanayis CG, Widhalm G, Stummer W. What is the surgical benefit of utilizing 5-aminolevulinic acid for fluorescence-guided surgery of malignant gliomas? Neurosurgery 2015;77(5):663–73.
7. Barnett GH, Kormos DW, Steiner CP, et al. Use of a frameless, armless stereotactic wand for brain tumor localization with two-dimensional and three-dimensional neuroimaging. Neurosurgery 1993; 33(4):674–8.
8. Brant-Zawadzki M, Gillan GD, Nitz WR. MP RAGE: a three-dimensional, T1-weighted, gradient-echo sequence–initial experience in the brain. Radiology 1992;182(3):769–75.
9. Raabe A, Krishnan R, Wolff R, et al. Laser surface scanning for patient registration in intracranial image-guided surgery. Neurosurgery 2002;50(4): 797–801 [discussion: 802–3].
10. Benveniste R, Germano IM. Evaluation of factors predicting accurate resection of high-grade gliomas by using frameless image-guided stereotactic guidance. Neurosurg Focus 2003;14(2):e5.
11. Nimsky C, Ganslandt O, Cerny S, et al. Quantification of, visualization of, and compensation for brain shift using intraoperative magnetic resonance imaging. Neurosurgery 2000;47(5):1070–9 [discussion: 1079–80].
12. Hirschberg H, Samset E, Hol PK, et al. Impact of intraoperative MRI on the surgical results for high-grade gliomas. Minim Invasive Neurosurg 2005; 48(2):77–84.
13. Wu JS, Zhou LF, Tang WJ, et al. Clinical evaluation and follow-up outcome of diffusion tensor imaging-based functional neuronavigation: a prospective, controlled study in patients with gliomas involving pyramidal tracts. Neurosurgery 2007;61(5):935–48 [discussion: 948–9].
14. Holodny AI, Schulder M, Liu WC, et al. Decreased BOLD functional MR activation of the motor and sensory cortices adjacent to a glioblastoma multiforme: implications for image-guided neurosurgery. AJNR Am J Neuroradiol 1999;20(4):609–12.
15. Nakada M, Okada Y, Yamashita J. The role of matrix metalloproteinases in glioma invasion. Front Biosci 2003;8:e261–9.
16. Wang W, Steward CE, Desmond PM. Diffusion tensor imaging in glioblastoma multiforme and brain metastases: the role of p, q, L, and fractional anisotropy. AJNR Am J Neuroradiol 2009;30(1): 203–8.
17. Abdullah KG, Lubelski D, Nucifora PG, et al. Use of diffusion tensor imaging in glioma resection. Neurosurg Focus 2013;34(4):E1.
18. Coenen VA, Krings T, Mayfrank L, et al. Three-dimensional visualization of the pyramidal tract in a neuronavigation system during brain tumor surgery: first experiences and technical note. Neurosurgery 2001;49(1):86–92 [discussion: 92–3].

19. Berman JI, Berger MS, Mukherjee P, et al. Diffusion-tensor imaging-guided tracking of fibers of the pyramidal tract combined with intraoperative cortical stimulation mapping in patients with gliomas. J Neurosurg 2004;101(1):66–72.

20. Black PM, Moriarty T, Alexander E 3rd, et al. Development and implementation of intraoperative magnetic resonance imaging and its neurosurgical applications. Neurosurgery 1997;41(4):831–42 [discussion: 842–5].

21. Kubben PL, ter Meulen KJ, Schijns OE, et al. Intraoperative MRI-guided resection of glioblastoma multiforme: a systematic review. Lancet Oncol 2011; 12(11):1062–70.

22. Lenaburg HJ, Inkabi KE, Vitaz TW. The use of intraoperative MRI for the treatment of glioblastoma multiforme. Technol Cancer Res Treat 2009;8(2): 159–62.

23. Senft C, Franz K, Blasel S, et al. Influence of iMRI-guidance on the extent of resection and survival of patients with glioblastoma multiforme. Technol Cancer Res Treat 2010;9(4):339–46.

24. Napolitano M, Vaz G, Lawson TM, et al. Glioblastoma surgery with and without intraoperative MRI at 3.0T. Neurochirurgie 2014;60(4):143–50.

25. Kuhnt D, Becker A, Ganslandt O, et al. Correlation of the extent of tumor volume resection and patient survival in surgery of glioblastoma multiforme with high-field intraoperative MRI guidance. Neuro Oncol 2011;13(12):1339–48.

26. Senft C, Bink A, Franz K, et al. Intraoperative MRI guidance and extent of resection in glioma surgery: a randomised, controlled trial. The Lancet. Oncology 2011;12(11):997–1003.

27. Zhang J, Chen X, Zhao Y, et al. Impact of intraoperative magnetic resonance imaging and functional neuronavigation on surgical outcome in patients with gliomas involving language areas. Neurosurg Rev 2015;38(2):319–30 [discussion: 330].

28. Cordova JS, Shu HG, Liang Z, et al. Whole-brain spectroscopic MRI biomarkers identify infiltrating margins in glioblastoma patients. Neuro Oncol 2016;18(8):1180–9.

29. Stummer W, Stocker S, Novotny A, et al. In vitro and in vivo porphyrin accumulation by C6 glioma cells after exposure to 5-aminolevulinic acid. J Photochem Photobiol B 1998;45(2–3):160–9.

30. Collaud S, Juzeniene A, Moan J, et al. On the selectivity of 5-aminolevulinic acid-induced protoporphyrin IX formation. Curr Med Chem Anticancer Agents 2004;4(3):301–16.

31. Panciani PP, Fontanella M, Schatlo B, et al. Fluorescence and image guided resection in high grade glioma. Clin Neurol Neurosurg 2012; 114(1):37–41.

32. Diez Valle R, Tejada Solis S, Idoate Gastearena MA, et al. Surgery guided by 5-aminolevulinic fluorescence in glioblastoma: volumetric analysis of extent of resection in single-center experience. J Neurooncol 2011;102(1):105–13.

33. Roberts DW, Valdes PA, Harris BT, et al. Coregistered fluorescence-enhanced tumor resection of malignant glioma: relationships between delta-aminolevulinic acid-induced protoporphyrin IX fluorescence, magnetic resonance imaging enhancement, and neuropathological parameters. Clinical article. J Neurosurg 2011;114(3):595–603.

34. Hefti M, von Campe G, Moschopulos M, et al. 5-aminolevulinic acid induced protoporphyrin IX fluorescence in high-grade glioma surgery: a one-year experience at a single institution. Swiss Med Wkly 2008;138(11–12):180–5.

35. Stummer W, Tonn JC, Goetz C, et al. 5-Aminolevulinic acid-derived tumor fluorescence: the diagnostic accuracy of visible fluorescence qualities as corroborated by spectrometry and histology and postoperative imaging. Neurosurgery 2014;74(3): 310–9 [discussion: 319–20].

36. Eljamel S. 5-ALA fluorescence image guided resection of glioblastoma multiforme: a meta-analysis of the literature. Int J Mol Sci 2015;16(5):10443–56.

37. Yamada S, Muragaki Y, Maruyama T, et al. Role of neurochemical navigation with 5-aminolevulinic acid during intraoperative MRI-guided resection of intracranial malignant gliomas. Clin Neurol Neurosurg 2015;130:134–9.

38. Coburger J, Engelke J, Scheuerle A, et al. Tumor detection with 5-aminolevulinic acid fluorescence and Gd-DTPA-enhanced intraoperative MRI at the border of contrast-enhancing lesions: a prospective study based on histopathological assessment. Neurosurg Focus 2014;36(2):E3.

39. Nabavi A, Thurm H, Zountsas B, et al. Five-aminolevulinic acid for fluorescence-guided resection of recurrent malignant gliomas: a phase II study. Neurosurgery 2009;65(6):1070–6 [discussion: 1076–7].

40. Stummer W, Pichlmeier U, Meinel T, et al. Fluorescence-guided surgery with 5-aminolevulinic acid for resection of malignant glioma: a randomised controlled multicentre phase III trial. Lancet Oncol 2006;7(5):392–401.

41. Schucht P, Seidel K, Beck J, et al. Intraoperative monopolar mapping during 5-ALA-guided resections of glioblastomas adjacent to motor eloquent areas: evaluation of resection rates and neurological outcome. Neurosurg Focus 2014;37(6):E16.

42. Schucht P, Beck J, Abu-Isa J, et al. Gross total resection rates in contemporary glioblastoma surgery: results of an institutional protocol combining 5-aminolevulinic acid intraoperative fluorescence imaging and brain mapping. Neurosurgery 2012; 71(5):927–35 [discussion: 935–6].

43. Della Puppa A, De Pellegrin S, d'Avella E, et al. 5-aminolevulinic acid (5-ALA) fluorescence guided surgery of high-grade gliomas in eloquent areas

assisted by functional mapping. Our experience and review of the literature. Acta Neurochir 2013; 155(6):965–72 [discussion: 972].

44. Kamp MA, Felsberg J, Sadat H, et al. 5-ALA-induced fluorescence behavior of reactive tissue changes following glioblastoma treatment with radiation and chemotherapy. Acta Neurochir 2015; 157(2):207–14.

45. Stummer W, Stocker S, Wagner S, et al. Intraoperative detection of malignant gliomas by 5-aminolevulinic acid-induced porphyrin fluorescence. Neurosurgery 1998;42(3):518–25 [discussion: 525–6].

46. Shinoda J, Yano H, Yoshimura S, et al. Fluorescence-guided resection of glioblastoma multiforme by using high-dose fluorescein sodium. Technical note. J Neurosurg 2003;99(3):597–603.

47. Okuda T, Yoshioka H, Kato A. Fluorescence-guided surgery for glioblastoma multiforme using high-dose fluorescein sodium with excitation and barrier filters. J Clin Neurosci 2012;19(12):1719–22.

48. Acerbi F, Broggi M, Eoli M, et al. Is fluorescein-guided technique able to help in resection of high-grade gliomas? Neurosurg Focus 2014; 36(2):E5.

49. Rey-Dios R, Hattab EM, Cohen-Gadol AA. Use of intraoperative fluorescein sodium fluorescence to improve the accuracy of tissue diagnosis during stereotactic needle biopsy of high-grade gliomas. Acta Neurochir 2014;156(6): 1071–5 [discussion: 1075].

50. Diaz RJ, Dios RR, Hattab EM, et al. Study of the biodistribution of fluorescein in glioma-infiltrated mouse brain and histopathological correlation of intraoperative findings in high-grade gliomas resected under fluorescein fluorescence guidance. J Neurosurg 2015;122(6):1360–9.

51. Koc K, Anik I, Cabuk B, et al. Fluorescein sodium-guided surgery in glioblastoma multiforme: a prospective evaluation. Br J Neurosurg 2008;22(1): 99–103.

CHAPTER 15

Minimally Invasive Targeted Therapy for Glioblastoma: Laser Interstitial Thermal Therapy

Danilo Silva, MD[a], Mayur Sharma, MD[a],
Telmo Belsuzarri, MD[b], Gene H. Barnett, MD, MBA[a],*

INTRODUCTION

Laser interstitial thermal therapy (LITT) is a minimally invasive treatment modality for brain tumors and other central nervous system (CNS) disorders, first introduced by Bown[1] in 1983, which has been revived over the last 2 decades because of recent technological advancements in laser technology and MRI thermography.[2,3] At that time, the main limitations of this surgical technique were the inability to monitor or predict the extent of ablation with real-time imaging feedback and the lack of an effective cooling system that could prevent overheating followed by tissue carbonization and optical fiber damage. These pitfalls have now been overcome and LITT is an US Food and Drug Administration–cleared treatment option for ablating CNS tissue such as recurrent glioblastoma,[4] and is emerging as a surgical option for upfront treatment of selected patients with malignant gliomas, brain metastatic disease that failed radiosurgery[5,6] and some forms of epilepsy.[7–9] LITT is ideally suited, but not limited, to patients with tumors located in deep-seated, hard-to-access areas who could develop significant postoperative neurologic deficits after traditional surgical resection leading to poor performance status. The basic biological effect of LITT is thermal damage. Laser near-infrared photons are absorbed by the surrounding tissue, causing excitation and release of thermal energy.[10–13] Ultimately, a cascade of events leads to cell breakdown and coagulative necrosis of the target volume. As clinicians move toward a more individualized approach in cancer care based on the biomolecular profile of different types of tumors, neurosurgeons also offer surgical individualized options for each patient based on their clinical history, performance status, tumor characteristics (size, location), and complication profile of different surgical approaches.

PHYSICAL AND BIOLOGICAL BASIS FOR THE USE OF LASER THERAPY IN THE ABLATION OF GLIOBLASTOMA

LITT exerts its biological effect by inducing thermal damage of the targeted tumor.[14] Laser electromagnetic photons are emitted by the laser source and absorbed by surrounding tissue, causing excitation and release of thermal energy, which is transformed to heat and distributed to nearby structures via convection and conduction.[10–14] The degree of direct heat penetration into surrounding tissue is determined by the properties of the tissue and the wavelength and power density delivered by the laser.[15] Previous studies have shown that the main determinants of laser absorption by tissues are the water and hemoglobin content present.[16] In terms of depth, the greatest degree of tissue penetration, which is several millimeters, is observed with laser radiation at wavelengths in the near-infrared part of the spectrum (1000–1100 nm).[16,17] In addition, the depth of interstitial thermal damage and subsequent necrosis depends on the cooling conditions, power density, and exposure time.[18,19] It is also known that the results obtained after laser interaction with white and gray matter are different. Although white matter displays the lowest level of laser penetration, gray matter

[a] Department of Neurosurgery, The Rose Ella Burkhardt Brain Tumor & Neuro-Oncology Center, Neurological Institute, Cleveland Clinic, Cleveland, OH, USA; [b] Department of Neurosurgery, Hospital Celso Pierro PUC-Campinas, Campinas, SP, Brazil
* Corresponding author. 9500 Euclid Avenue, S73, Cleveland, OH 44195.
E-mail address: barnetg@ccf.org

shows a higher level of laser absorption.[20] Eggert and Blazek[20] were able to show that, within the near-infrared spectral range, glioblastomas and meningioma had the highest degree of laser absorption, whereas low-grade gliomas had optical properties similar to gray matter.[20] LITT triggers a cascade of cellular events that include enzyme induction, denaturation of proteins, cellular membrane breakdown, coagulation necrosis, and blood vessel sclerosis.[16] Two phenomena should ideally be avoided when applying LITT: tissue carbonization and vaporization. Rapid increases in temperature can result in tissue carbonization,[21] preventing adequate laser absorption. Overheating can also cause tissue vaporization, which, if sufficiently severe, could lead to increased intracranial pressure with potentially disastrous consequences.[22] A goal of LITT is to achieve coagulation necrosis of the target volume without provoking carbonization or vaporization of the treated area. Coagulation necrosis occurs at temperatures in the range of 50°C to100°C.[21] Carbonization and vaporization are usually seen at temperatures greater than 100°C.[21]

MRI thermography provides real-time thermal data allowing surgeons to monitor the extent of ablation in an effective and safe manner.[2,3,21] Its principle relies on the temperature-dependent water proton resonance frequency (PRF). PRF image mapping is based on the fact that protons are displaced more efficiently within the magnetic field in the form of free water molecules (H_2O) than in the form of hydrogen bonded water molecules. As thermal energy is delivered during LITT and temperature increases, the number of hydrogen bonds decreases, resulting in an increased number of free H_2O molecules and a lower PRF, which can be visualized with MRI thermometry coupled with advanced computer software in real-time fashion.[23,24]

Three zones of specific histologic changes around the laser probe are observed during LITT.[21] The first zone is the area closest to the tip of the probe and represents the area of greatest tissue damage caused by the highest degree of thermal energy absorption.[21] The second or intermediate zone also undergoes thermal injury. Tissue cells located in the third and most marginal zone, although damaged by thermal energy, are still viable.[21] True coagulation necrosis is observed in the first 2 zones.[21] The NeuroBlate System (Monteris Medical Corporation, Plymouth, MN) displays the 3 zones of thermal damage in the computer software as the thermal-damage-threshold lines (TDT lines), through real-time imaging data acquired by MRI thermography. This distinctive characteristic of the NeuroBlate System

gives surgeons the capability of performing an effective and complete ablation of the tumor by including the target volume in the first 2 zones (TDT lines). Optimal laser ablation is achieved when a sharp border of thermal injury is observed at the brain-tumor interface characterizing a selective procedure with preservation of the normal brain tissue surrounding the tumor.

HISTORICAL CONTEXT AND EVOLUTION OF TECHNOLOGIES USED IN THE MINIMALLY INVASIVE LASER TREATMENT OF GLIOBLASTOMAS

Despite recent advances, surgery of high-grade gliomas remains a challenge, especially in recurrent cases and deep, difficult-to-access regions, where access for aggressive surgical resection is often not possible.[22,25] The median survival with optimal treatment is less than 15 months in glioblastoma and, in cases of recurrent glioblastoma, the overall survival is about 3 to 5 months and treatment options are limited, such as second-line chemotherapy, brachytherapy, and additional surgery.[22,25,26] Additional surgery has increased the overall survival by 8 weeks and often is not an option because of difficult-to-access tumor location in deep or eloquent areas. Focal therapies such as stereotactic radiosurgery and brachytherapy have limited results for recurrent glioblastoma, so the use of these treatments remains controversial. Therefore, with the goal of treating patients with tumors deemed inoperable and/or located in eloquent areas, the use of LITT for recurrent glioblastoma has increased and studies have shown the safety of the procedure.[4]

LITT is a minimally invasive treatment modality for brain tumors, a concept that has existed since the late 1970s, but was first described by Bown[1] in 1983. The use of hyperthermia for the treatment of tumors is based on the selective tumor response during tissue heating.[27] Hahn[27] showed not only that heating has the benefits of thermal ablation but also that some drugs can be enhanced by increased temperatures. Further, after multiple initial attempts, such as ruby, argon, and CO_2 lasers, the most effective neuronal tissue damage was achieved in the near-infrared part of the electromagnetic spectrum.[28] These initial studies have led to specific considerations of the interaction between laser energy and brain tissue and the resultant lesion obtained by the application of laser. Laser emission parameters (wavelength, frequency, and laser mode), specific tissue optical and thermal properties (water and hemoglobin content, thermal conductivity, and specific heat) associated with the intensity and time of exposure determine the desired lesion effect on the exposed tissue, which can be represented by coagulation, hemostasis, cutting, or vaporization.[28] Bown[1] conducted several studies in experimental photocoagulation of gastric ulcers, and, in 1983, the author first described an experiment using a neodymium-doped yttrium-aluminum-garnet (Nd:YAG) laser in a brain tumor model achieving coagulation necrosis without surrounding tissue vaporization. In 1990, Sugiyama and colleagues[30] described the use of LITT for the treatment of brain tumors using a computed tomography stereotactic technique, but, because of the high risk of thermal damage to the surrounding tissue and low efficacy, acceptance was limited.[29,30] At that time, LITT technologies did not gain popularity because of a lack of precision in the thermal energy source, limited ablative volume, and an inability to monitor laser-induced tissue damage in real time.[29] During the past decades, with the advance of MRI technologies, thermal-induced lesions have been monitored by magnetic resonance (MR) thermal imaging, based on PRF. Nowadays, LITT is capable of delivering a controlled, customizable, and precise thermal ablation.[26,28]

Recently, there have also been important technological and design advances in the development of new LITT probes. Initial probes used bare-tip fiberoptic probe designs and, consequently, technical issues related to overheating, tissue carbonization, and fiber damage were noted.[28,29] Nowadays, enclosed fiberoptic probe design with special cooling systems, such as constant fluid (saline or water) or cooled gas (CO_2) mechanisms, allows better results.[29] Classically, thermal energy at the probe tip resulted in ellipsoid lesions along the axis of the fiber. Now, with advances in cooling and probe designs, side-firing laser probes allow asymmetric tissue penetration and better control of laser ablation in cases of complex-shaped tumors.[26,29]

Although survival of patients with newly diagnosed glioblastoma benefits from gross total resection (GTR) compared with chemotherapy and radiation alone, in specific situations GTR is not possible and LITT can be considered as a primary surgical option. In particular, patients with tumors in deep, difficult-to-access locations, low functional status scores, multiple comorbidities, and nonsurgical recurrent glioblastoma can benefit from this minimally invasive therapy.[29]

In addition, several other LITT indications have been reported, such as radiosurgery-resistant brain metastatic disease, epilepsy, and radiation necrosis. Initial technical difficulties have now been overcome and the safety of this technique has been established for future studies and clinical application.[26]

CURRENT EVIDENCE AND TECHNIQUES FOR THE TREATMENT OF GLIOBLASTOMA WITH LASER INTERSTITIAL THERMAL THERAPY (NEUROBLATE SYSTEM)

Primary glial neoplasms account for approximately 28% of all primary brain tumors and 80% of all malignant brain tumors.[31] Of primary glial neoplasms, glioblastoma multiforme (WHO grade IV) accounts for approximately 45% of these tumors.[32] Microneurosurgical resection with the aim of achieving GTR followed by concurrent chemotherapy (temozolomide) and radiation therapy remains the mainstay treatment of newly diagnosed glioblastoma.[33] Despite the best available treatment, the overall prognosis remains poor, with 3-year and 5-year overall survival rates of 16.0% and 9.8%, respectively.[33,34] In addition, median survival and progression-free survival have been reported to be 14.6 months and 6.9 months respectively.[21,33,34] Patients with progressive or recurrent glioblastoma have been shown to have worse outcomes, with a median survival ranging between 6.2 and 9.2 months.[33–35] Various chemotherapeutic options, such as salvage temozolomide, irinotecan, carmustine wafers, cetuximab, or carboplatin alone or in combination with antiangiogenic agents (bevacizumab), have been used in patients with recurrent disease with varied results.[35–41] A recent meta-analysis reported an improved median and progression-free survival with a combination of bevacizumab and irinotecan (compared with bevacizumab alone) in patients with recurrent glioblastoma,[38] but the toxicity and ill effects of this combination on quality of life led to a high discontinuation rate.

Surgical options for patients with recurrent or progressive disease are limited, with controversial data in the literature.[42–49] Young age at diagnosis, good performance status (Karnofsky performance scale [KPS] score at recurrence), and extent of resection at recurrence have been shown to prolong survival in patients with recurrent glioblastoma, irrespective of the extent of resection at initial surgery.[42–47,50] Note that, after adjusting for age, multiple resections have not been shown to be a predictor of overall survival in patients with recurrent glioblastoma. Multiple surgical resections in combination with chemoradiotherapy have been shown to prolong survival in patients with recurrent disease (median survival, 26 months for multiple resections vs 16 months for 2 resections followed by nonsurgical management).[48] Repeat surgical resections for recurrent tumors are usually performed in patients with good performance status and may reflect a selection bias in these studies. Moreover, repeat surgical resections are associated with 18% to 22% incidence of postoperative neurologic deficits.[51,52] Incidence of neurologic deficits has been shown to increase from 4.8% during the first surgical resection, to 12.1% in the second surgery, to 8.2% in the third, and to 11.1% during 4 or more resections for recurrent glioblastoma.[53] Radiosurgery, fractionated radiation therapy, and interstitial brachytherapy have limited roles in these patients.[54,55] Given the risks associated with repeat surgical resections in combination with a paucity of adjunct treatment modalities, LITT is an appealing alternative treatment option in selected patients with recurrent glioblastoma. Also, for patients with recurrent glioblastoma with significant medical comorbidities or those who do not wish to undergo traditional open surgical approaches, LITT can be a reasonable treatment option.

Maximal tumor cytoreduction or GTR is thought to improve outcomes in patients with either newly diagnosed[56–58] or recurrent glioblastoma.[42–45,48] LITT can achieve maximal tumor cytoreduction via photocoagulation of pathologic tissue, similar to the cytoreduction that can be achieved by open surgical techniques. Moreover, LITT is associated with less neurologic morbidity and mortality compared with open surgical techniques, especially for deep-seated or difficult-to-access tumors.[59] Laser interstitial thermotherapy has also been shown to disrupt the blood-brain barrier (BBB) with neovascularization in animal models,[60,61] which may have favorable implications for the effectiveness of early chemotherapy. Given these advantages, LITT can also be a reasonable alternative upfront therapeutic option in carefully selected patients.[59,62]

Laser Interstitial Thermal Therapy for Recurrent Glioblastoma

Several studies have reported the utility of LITT in patients with recurrent glioblastoma.[4,14,25,63–70] Literature documenting the efficacy of LITT in a patient with recurrent glioblastoma dates back to the early 1990s.[68] In 1998, Reimer and colleagues[70] reported the use of LITT in a patient with recurrent gliosarcoma (20 × 35 mm) involving the left precentral gyrus. Tumor progression was noted at 8 months within the ablated zone.[70] Later, Leonardi and colleagues[67] performed 9 LITT procedures in 6 patients with recurrent/residual disease (1 newly diagnosed). The

procedure was performed under local anesthesia using 1064-nm Nd:YAG laser and 0.2-T MRI.[67] Clinical outcome and tumor response rates were not reported in this study, but the investigators noted no correlation between tumor grade and tissue response to thermal therapy. A year later, the investigators reported overall survival and progression-free survival of 9 months and 4 months respectively in 6 patients with recurrent glioblastoma.[66] Good functional status (KPS >70) was maintained for 7.5 months in these patients following LITT.[66] Another report of 2 cases with recurrent glioblastoma (case 1: multifocal disease diagnosed during follow-up and the lesion was treated primarily with LITT. Case 2: true recurrence) reported an overall survival of 13 months (16 months since recurrence) and 15 months (20 months since recurrence) following LITT.[69] A year later, the same investigators reported the utility of LITT in 16 patients (26 LITT procedures) with recurrent glioblastoma and a mean follow-up of 9.1 ± 6.3 months.[14] This study reported a difference in median survival between the first 10 patients and later 6 patients of 5.2 months and 11.2 months, respectively, which the investigators attributed to the time delay between diagnosis of tumor recurrence and LITT (ie, learning curve).[14] There was an overall median survival of 6.9 months following LITT and 9.4 months after first relapse.[14]

Recently, Carpentier and colleagues[63] reported the utility of salvage MR-guided LITT therapy in 4 patients (5 lesions) with recurrent glioblastoma. This study reported a progression-free survival and mean overall survival of 37 days and 10.5 months, respectively. Of note, 2 patients had local recurrence and another 2 had distant recurrence following LITT.[63]

The first human phase I multicenter study evaluating the safety and efficacy of escalating doses of thermal energy using LITT in patients with recurrent glioblastoma was published in 2013.[4] Of 11 patients enrolled in this study at 2 centers (Cleveland Clinic and University Hospital Case Western Reserve Medical Center), 10 underwent LITT and were followed up for a minimum of 6 months or until death. Median overall survival and progression-free survival of 316 days and greater than or equal to 30% at 6 months, respectively, were reported.[4] Median overall survival of 225 days, 198 days, and 434 days following LITT was reported in patients treated using yellow TDT lines, blue TDT lines, and white TDT lines, respectively.[4]

Hawasli and colleagues[64] reported the clinical outcomes in 4 patients who underwent LITT for recurrent glioblastoma. Three of these

4 patients underwent standard treatment (surgery followed by concurrent chemoradiotherapy) and 1 patient had radiation with chemotherapy only. Progression-free survival was reported to be 9.2 months in 1 patient, who underwent a second LITT procedure for recurrence; 8.4 months in the second patient, who had distant recurrence; 7.6 months in the third patient, who was reported to have satellite lesion at recurrence; whereas no recurrence was noted in the fourth patient at 3.2 months of follow-up.[64]

Recently Mohammadi and colleagues[59] investigated the utility of LITT in 24 patients with glioblastoma (out of 34 patients with high-grade gliomas) in difficult-to-access areas in a multicenter retrospective study. Eighteen patients underwent LITT procedures for recurrent high-grade gliomas, whereas 16 patients underwent LITT as an upfront procedure for these tumors; however, the number of patients who underwent an upfront or salvage LITT procedure was not specified in this study.[59] Ninety-one percent of the median tumor volume was covered by blue line and 3 cm was the maximum diameter of tumor treated. Median progressive-free survival ranged between 4.6 months and 9.7 months, based on tumor coverage by TDT lines. Clinical outcome based on upfront or salvage therapy for glioblastoma specifically was not mentioned in this study.[59]

Based on these studies, median overall survival following LITT ranges between 6.9 months and 14.5 months in patients with recurrent glioblastoma compared with between 4 and 6 months in the literature.[33,34] This difference in overall survival may not be attributable to LITT alone and the role of adjunctive therapies cannot be underestimated. However, LITT offers a minimally invasive approach to achieve tumor cytoreduction coupled with possible early opening of the BBB (based on animal studies[60,61]) for adjunct chemotherapies to be effective.[62]

Laser Interstitial Thermal Therapy for Newly Diagnosed or De-novo Glioblastoma

Extent of tumor resection is a strong predictor of overall survival and also has an impact on quality of life in patients with newly diagnosed glioblastoma.[34,56–58,71] There is a subset of patients with newly diagnosed glioblastoma who are either not suitable to undergo traditional open surgical resections because of their associated medical comorbidities, or deeper or eloquent location of the tumor (thalamus basal ganglia, insula), or who choose not to undergo open surgery. In such circumstances, LITT can be a useful alternative treatment modality to achieve adequate cytoreduction

and facilitate adjunct treatment. However, in contrast with LITT for recurrent glioblastoma, efficacy of LITT is less clearly documented in the literature because it is a much newer procedure.

A report documenting the efficacy of LITT in a patient with newly diagnosed high-grade tumor was published in 1992.[68] In 2002, Leonardi and colleagues[66] reported on a 75-year-old patient with deep-seated bifocal glioblastoma, who was treated upfront with LITT, in their series of 6 patients with glioblastoma. However, clinical outcome in patients with newly diagnosed or recurrent disease following LITT was not stratified.[66] Similarly, Mohammadi and colleagues,[59] in their series of 34 patients with deep-seated high-grade gliomas (24 patients with glioblastoma) who underwent either upfront or salvage LITT, did not report the outcome data pertaining specifically to patients with glioblastoma.[59] Jethwa and colleagues[65] reported the utility of LITT in 3 patients with newly diagnosed glioblastoma. Two of these patients were considered high risk by a multidisciplinary oncology team in terms of an open surgical procedure and a third patient had a deep-seated tumor in the left temporal region.[65] One patient with a tumor in the right frontal region required an additional treatment after initial LITT and another patient with tumor in the right frontal region required 2 trajectories (the other 2 had 1 trajectory each).[65] Clinical outcome data were not reported.

Hawasli and colleagues[72] reported the efficacy of LITT in 6 patients (thalamus, n = 4; basal ganglia, n = 1; corpus callosum, n = 1). No recurrence was noted in 4 patients at a mean follow-up of 0.2 months, 10.7 months, 0.1 months, and 0.9 months following LITT with maintenance of good functional status in surviving patients.[72] Progression-free survival was reported to be 2.6 months and 3.2 months following LITT in 2 patients with recurrence. One patient died of fatal CNS infection 0.1 month following LITT and another patient died because of progressive CNS disease at 4.1 months following LITT.[72] Three patients had no disease progression at follow-up of 10.7 months, 0.1 months, and 0.9 months following LITT.[72] Further clinical studies focusing on the efficacy of LITT in patients with newly diagnosed glioblastoma are needed to validate this treatment modality.

Technical Nuances

At present, NeuroBlate System (Monteris Medical Inc, Winnipeg, Canada) and Visualase (Medtronic Inc, Minnesota, MN) are the two commercially available systems for LITT in patients with brain tumors in the United States.

At our center we use the NeuroBlate System for laser ablation. The procedure is typically performed under general anesthesia in an intraoperative MRI suite (IMRIS, Winnipeg, Canada). Following anesthesia induction, the patient's head is placed and secured in an operative position using a DORO head clamp (pro med instruments GmbH, Freiburg, Germany) and MRI scans (magnetization-prepared rapid acquisition gradient-echo with contrast and/or T2 volume) are obtained using scalp-applied fiducials. These images are then fused with preoperative MRI planning sequences for registration purposes. The patient's head location is then registered with image space using the iPlan Curve navigation system (Brainlab AG, Munich, Germany). The site of skin incision is determined using the Varioguide system (Brainlab AG, Munich, Germany) and the bone is drilled with a twist drill. Stereotactic placement of an anchoring head bolt (4.5-mm outer diameter) is then performed using image guidance. A laser probe (either side firing or diffuse tip) is then inserted through the head bolt and connected to the robotic probe driver. M•Vision software is then used for planning and treatment at a workstation. This software integrates with the intraoperative MRI suite and uses a pulsed diode laser (Nd:YAG; range, 1046 nm; output, 12 W) to ablate the pathologic tissue.[26] Gaseous CO_2 is used to cool the tip of the fiberoptic probe to avoid tissue vaporization as well as to enhance conformal treatment contours.[25,26] Laser ablation is monitored in real time using MR thermometry and TDT lines are generated on the M•Vision workstation, which can be viewed throughout the procedure. Once satisfactory tumor ablation is achieved (tumor covered by blue TDT line [43°C for at least 10 minutes]),[25,26,59] the procedure is concluded by explanting the bolts and suturing the skin incision. Multiple and larger lesions (up to 40–50 cm^3 in volume) can be treated in a single setting. However, for larger tumors, multiple trajectories are required and consideration must be given to the ability to safely accommodate postablation edema.

SUMMARY

Glioblastoma is a malignant brain tumor with an overall poor prognosis. Maximal safe resection followed by concurrent chemoradiation therapy has been the standard of care in patients with glioblastoma. LITT is a stereotactic, minimally invasive technique that is gaining acceptance with advances in stereotactic and neuroimaging techniques. For patients with deep-seated tumors or multiple medical comorbidities, or for those who do not wish to undergo open surgical resection, LITT may be an effective treatment option. The minimally invasive nature of this therapy, coupled with cytoreduction and opening of BBB, offers a distinct advantage compared with standard open surgical approaches in such patients. At present, there is moderate evidence supporting the safety and efficacy of LITT in selected patients with recurrent glioblastoma. For newly diagnosed glioblastoma, there is still a paucity of clinical studies supporting the role of LITT. Future prospective studies will better define the role of LITT in patients with newly diagnosed or recurrent glioblastoma.

REFERENCES

1. Bown SG. Phototherapy in tumors. World J Surg 1983;7(6):700–9.
2. Kahn T, Bettag M, Ulrich F, et al. MRI-guided laser-induced interstitial thermotherapy of cerebral neoplasms. J Comput Assist Tomogr 1994;18(4):519–32.
3. Morrison PR, Jolesz FA, Charous D, et al. MRI of laser-induced interstitial thermal injury in an in vivo animal liver model with histologic correlation. J Magn Reson Imaging 1998;8(1):57–63.
4. Sloan AE, Ahluwalia MS, Valerio-Pascua J, et al. Results of the NeuroBlate System first-in-humans Phase I clinical trial for recurrent glioblastoma: clinical article. J Neurosurg 2013;118(6):1202–19.
5. Carpentier A, McNichols RJ, Stafford RJ, et al. Laser thermal therapy: real-time MRI-guided and computer-controlled procedures for metastatic brain tumors. Lasers Surg Med 2011; 43(10):943–50.
6. Rao MS, Hargreaves EL, Khan AJ, et al. Magnetic resonance-guided laser ablation improves local control for postradiosurgery recurrence and/or radiation necrosis. Neurosurgery 2014;74(6):658–67 [discussion: 667].
7. Kang JY, Wu C, Tracy J, et al. Laser interstitial thermal therapy for medically intractable mesial temporal lobe epilepsy. Epilepsia 2016;57(2):325–34.
8. Buckley R, Estronza-Ojeda S, Ojemann JG. Laser ablation in pediatric epilepsy. Neurosurg Clin N Am 2016;27(1):69–78.
9. Gross RE, Willie JT, Drane DL. The role of stereotactic laser amygdalohippocampotomy in mesial temporal lobe epilepsy. Neurosurg Clin N Am 2016; 27(1):37–50.
10. Stafford RJ, Fuentes D, Elliott AA, et al. Laser-induced thermal therapy for tumor ablation. Crit Rev Biomed Eng 2010;38(1):79–100.
11. Stafford RJ, Shetty A, Elliott AM, et al. Magnetic resonance guided, focal laser induced interstitial

thermal therapy in a canine prostate model. J Urol 2010;184(4):1514–20.

12. Ahrar K, Gowda A, Javadi S, et al. Preclinical assessment of a 980-nm diode laser ablation system in a large animal tumor model. J Vasc Interv Radiol 2010;21(4):555–61.

13. Fuentes D, Feng Y, Elliott A, et al. Adaptive real-time bioheat transfer models for computer-driven MR-guided laser induced thermal therapy. IEEE Trans Biomed Eng 2010;57(5):1024–30.

14. Schwarzmaier HJ, Eickmeyer F, von Tempelhoff W, et al. MR-guided laser-induced interstitial thermotherapy of recurrent glioblastoma multiforme: preliminary results in 16 patients. Eur J Radiol 2006; 59(2):208–15.

15. Higuchi N, Bleier AR, Jolesz FA, et al. Magnetic resonance imaging of the acute effects of interstitial neodymium:YAG laser irradiation on tissues. Invest Radiol 1992;27(10):814–21.

16. Mensel B, Weigel C, Hosten N. Laser-induced thermotherapy. Recent Results Cancer Res 2006;167:69–75.

17. Yaroslavsky AN, Schulze PC, Yaroslavsky IV, et al. Optical properties of selected native and coagulated human brain tissues in vitro in the visible and near infrared spectral range. Phys Med Biol 2002;47(12):2059–73.

18. Svaasand LO. Photodynamic and photohyperthermic response of malignant tumors. Med Phys 1985;12(4):455–61.

19. Svaasand LO, Ellingsen R. Optical properties of human brain. Photochem Photobiol 1983;38(3): 293–9.

20. Eggert HR, Blazek V. Optical properties of human brain tissue, meninges, and brain tumors in the spectral range of 200 to 900 nm. Neurosurgery 1987;21(4):459–64.

21. Norred SE, Johnson JA. Magnetic resonance-guided laser induced thermal therapy for glioblastoma multiforme: a review. Biomed Res Int 2014; 2014:761312.

22. Rahmathulla G, Recinos PF, Kamian K, et al. MRI-guided laser interstitial thermal therapy in neuro-oncology: a review of its current clinical applications. Oncology 2014;87(2):67–82.

23. McNichols RJ, Gowda A, Kangasniemi M, et al. MR thermometry-based feedback control of laser interstitial thermal therapy at 980 nm. Lasers Surg Med 2004;34(1):48–55.

24. Rieke V, Butts Pauly K. MR thermometry. J Magn Reson Imaging 2008;27(2):376–90.

25. Mohammadi AM, Schroeder JL. Laser interstitial thermal therapy in treatment of brain tumors–the NeuroBlate System. Expert Rev Med Devices 2014;11(2):109–19.

26. Missios S, Bekelis K, Barnett GH. Renaissance of laser interstitial thermal ablation. Neurosurg Focus 2015;38(3):E13.

27. Hahn GM. Potential for therapy of drugs and hyperthermia. Cancer Res 1979;39(6 Pt 2):2264–8.

28. Devaux BC, Roux FX. Experimental and clinical standards, and evolution of lasers in neurosurgery. Acta Neurochir 1996;138(10):1135–47.

29. Medvid R, Ruiz A, Komotar RJ, et al. Current applications of MRI-guided laser interstitial thermal therapy in the treatment of brain neoplasms and epilepsy: a radiologic and neurosurgical overview. AJNR Am J Neuroradiol 2015;36(11): 1998–2006.

30. Sugiyama K, Sakai T, Fujishima I, et al. Stereotactic interstitial laser-hyperthermia using Nd-YAG laser. Stereotact Funct Neurosurg 1990;54-55:501–5.

31. Ostrom QT, Gittleman H, Farah P, et al. CBTRUS statistical report: primary brain and central nervous system tumors diagnosed in the United States in 2006-2010. Neuro Oncol 2013;15(Suppl 2):ii1–56.

32. Ostrom QT, Bauchet L, Davis FG, et al. The epidemiology of glioma in adults: a "state of the science" review. Neuro Oncol 2014;16(7):896–913.

33. Stupp R, Hegi ME, Mason WP, et al. Effects of radiotherapy with concomitant and adjuvant temozolomide versus radiotherapy alone on survival in glioblastoma in a randomised phase III study: 5-year analysis of the EORTC-NCIC trial. Lancet Oncol 2009;10(5):459–66.

34. Stupp R, Mason WP, van den Bent MJ, et al. Radiotherapy plus concomitant and adjuvant temozolomide for glioblastoma. N Engl J Med 2005; 352(10):987–96.

35. Friedman HS, Prados MD, Wen PY, et al. Bevacizumab alone and in combination with irinotecan in recurrent glioblastoma. J Clin Oncol 2009;27(28): 4733–40.

36. Hart MG, Grant R, Garside R, et al. Chemotherapy wafers for high grade glioma. Cochrane Database Syst Rev 2011;(3):CD007294.

37. Brem H, Piantadosi S, Burger PC, et al. Placebo-controlled trial of safety and efficacy of intraoperative controlled delivery by biodegradable polymers of chemotherapy for recurrent gliomas. The Polymer-brain Tumor Treatment Group. Lancet (London) 1995;345(8956):1008–12.

38. Zhang G, Huang S, Wang Z. A meta-analysis of bevacizumab alone and in combination with irinotecan in the treatment of patients with recurrent glioblastoma multiforme. J Clin Neurosci 2012;19(12): 1636–40.

39. Hasselbalch B, Lassen U, Hansen S, et al. Cetuximab, bevacizumab, and irinotecan for patients with primary glioblastoma and progression after radiation therapy and temozolomide: a phase II trial. Neuro Oncol 2010;12(5):508–16.

40. Moller S, Grunnet K, Hansen S, et al. A phase II trial with bevacizumab and irinotecan for patients with primary brain tumors and progression after

standard therapy. Acta Oncol (Stockholm, Sweden) 2012;51(6):797–804.

41. Chen C, Xu T, Lu Y, et al. The efficacy of temozolomide for recurrent glioblastoma multiforme. Eur J Neurol 2013;20(2):223–30.

42. Bloch O, Han SJ, Cha S, et al. Impact of extent of resection for recurrent glioblastoma on overall survival: clinical article. J Neurosurg 2012;117(6): 1032–8.

43. Oppenlander ME, Wolf AB, Snyder LA, et al. An extent of resection threshold for recurrent glioblastoma and its risk for neurological morbidity. J Neurosurg 2014;120(4):846–53.

44. Hervey-Jumper SL, Berger MS. Reoperation for recurrent high-grade glioma: a current perspective of the literature. Neurosurgery 2014;75(5):491–9 [discussion: 498–9].

45. Chaichana KL, Zadnik P, Weingart JD, et al. Multiple resections for patients with glioblastoma: prolonging survival. J Neurosurg 2013;118(4):812–20.

46. Barbagallo GM, Jenkinson MD, Brodbelt AR. 'Recurrent' glioblastoma multiforme, when should we reoperate? Br J Neurosurg 2008;22(3):452–5.

47. Ortega A, Sarmiento JM, Ly D, et al. Multiple resections and survival of recurrent glioblastoma patients in the temozolomide era. J Clin Neurosci 2016;24: 105–11.

48. Hong B, Wiese B, Bremer M, et al. Multiple microsurgical resections for repeated recurrence of glioblastoma multiforme. Am J Clin Oncol 2013;36(3): 261–8.

49. Sughrue ME, Sheean T, Bonney PA, et al. Aggressive repeat surgery for focally recurrent primary glioblastoma: outcomes and theoretical framework. Neurosurg Focus 2015;38(3):E11.

50. Barker FG 2nd, Chang SM, Gutin PH, et al. Survival and functional status after resection of recurrent glioblastoma multiforme. Neurosurgery 1998;42(4): 709–20 [discussion: 720–3].

51. Chang SM, Parney IF, McDermott M, et al. Perioperative complications and neurological outcomes of first and second craniotomies among patients enrolled in the Glioma Outcome Project. J Neurosurg 2003;98(6): 1175–81.

52. Moiyadi AV, Shetty PM. Surgery for recurrent malignant gliomas: feasibility and perioperative outcomes. Neurol India 2012;60(2):185–90.

53. Hoover JM, Nwojo M, Puffer R, et al. Surgical outcomes in recurrent glioma: clinical article. J Neurosurg 2013;118(6):1224–31.

54. Tsao MN, Mehta MP, Whelan TJ, et al. The American Society for Therapeutic Radiology and Oncology (ASTRO) evidence-based review of the role of radiosurgery for malignant glioma. Int J Radiat Oncol Biol Phys 2005;63(1):47–55.

55. Chan TA, Weingart JD, Parisi M, et al. Treatment of recurrent glioblastoma multiforme with GliaSite

brachytherapy. Int J Radiat Oncol Biol Phys 2005; 62(4):1133–9.

56. Grabowski MM, Recinos PF, Nowacki AS, et al. Residual tumor volume versus extent of resection: predictors of survival after surgery for glioblastoma. J Neurosurg 2014;121(5):1115–23.

57. Sanai N, Polley MY, McDermott MW, et al. An extent of resection threshold for newly diagnosed glioblastomas. J Neurosurg 2011;115(1):3–8.

58. Lacroix M, Abi-Said D, Fourney DR, et al. A multivariate analysis of 416 patients with glioblastoma multiforme: prognosis, extent of resection, and survival. J Neurosurg 2001;95(2):190–8.

59. Mohammadi AM, Hawasli AH, Rodriguez A, et al. The role of laser interstitial thermal therapy in enhancing progression-free survival of difficult-to-access high-grade gliomas: a multicenter study. Cancer Med 2014;3(4):971–9.

60. Sabel M, Rommel F, Kondakci M, et al. Locoregional opening of the rodent blood-brain barrier for paclitaxel using Nd:YAG laser-induced thermo therapy: a new concept of adjuvant glioma therapy? Lasers Surg Med 2003;33(2):75–80.

61. Nakagawa M, Matsumoto K, Higashi H, et al. Acute effects of interstitial hyperthermia on normal monkey brain–magnetic resonance imaging appearance and effects on blood-brain barrier. Neurol Med Chir 1994;34(10):668–75.

62. Hawasli AH, Kim AH, Dunn GP, et al. Stereotactic laser ablation of high-grade gliomas. Neurosurg Focus 2014;37(6):E1.

63. Carpentier A, Chauvet D, Reina V, et al. MR-guided laser-induced thermal therapy (LITT) for recurrent glioblastomas. Lasers Surg Med 2012; 44(5):361–8.

64. Hawasli AH, Bagade S, Shimony JS, et al. Magnetic resonance imaging-guided focused laser interstitial thermal therapy for intracranial lesions: single-institution series. Neurosurgery 2013;73(6): 1007–17.

65. Jethwa PR, Barrese JC, Gowda A, et al. Magnetic resonance thermometry-guided laser-induced thermal therapy for intracranial neoplasms: initial experience. Neurosurgery 2012;71(1 Suppl Operative): 133–44, 144–5.

66. Leonardi MA, Lumenta CB. Stereotactic guided laser-induced interstitial thermotherapy (SLITT) in gliomas with intraoperative morphologic monitoring in an open MR: clinical experience. Minim Invasive Neurosurg 2002;45(4):201–7.

67. Leonardi MA, Lumenta CB, Gumprecht HK, et al. Stereotactic guided laser-induced interstitial thermotherapy (SLITT) in gliomas with intraoperative morphologic monitoring in an open MR-unit. Minim Invasive Neurosurg 2001;44(1): 37–42.

68. Sakai T, Fujishima I, Sugiyama K, et al. Interstitial laserthermia in neurosurgery. J Clin Laser Med Surg 1992;10(1):37–40.

69. Schwarzmaier HJ, Eickmeyer F, von Tempelhoff W, et al. MR-guided laser irradiation of recurrent glioblastomas. J Magn Reson Imaging 2005;22(6): 799–803.

70. Reimer P, Bremer C, Horch C, et al. MR-monitored LITT as a palliative concept in patients with high grade gliomas: preliminary clinical experience. J Magn Reson Imaging 1998;8(1):240–4.

71. Brown PD, Maurer MJ, Rummans TA, et al. A prospective study of quality of life in adults with newly diagnosed high-grade gliomas: the impact of the extent of resection on quality of life and survival. Neurosurgery 2005;57(3):495–504 [discussion: 495–504].

72. Hawasli AH, Ray WZ, Murphy RK, et al. Magnetic resonance imaging-guided focused laser interstitial thermal therapy for subinsular metastatic adenocarcinoma: technical case report. Neurosurgery 2012; 70(2 Suppl Operative):332–7 [discussion: 338].

CHAPTER 16

Local Drug Delivery in the Treatment of Glioblastoma

Kalil G. Abdullah, MD[a,b], Jason A. Burdick, PhD[b,*]

The prognosis following diagnosis of glioblastoma remains poor. Historically, there have been many notable attempts to use local drug delivery to treat glioblastoma, including convection-enhanced delivery (CED), direct tumor injection, and the use of to deliver chemotherapeutics.[1–3] The use of polymer wafers resulted in the only US Food and Drug Administration (FDA)–approved intracranial drug implant for treatment of recurrent and de novo glioblastoma, Gliadel.[4] Over a period of several decades, the delivery of the chemotherapeutic 1,3-bis(2-chloroethyl)-1-nitrosourea (BCNU) from biodegradable polyanhydride polymeric wafers was developed and tested for efficacy and safety, culminating in the wafer's approval for recurrent glioblastoma in 1996 and de novo glioblastoma in 2003. To date, this polymeric delivery vehicle is the most extensively tested and also one of the few drug-eluting systems created for intracranial drug delivery. This chapter reviews the scientific challenges and evolution of local compounds for glioblastoma, including BCNU wafers, CED, direct injection, and hydrogel-based delivery.

BACKGROUND TO INTRACRANIAL DRUG DELIVERY

The impetus for local drug delivery is fundamentally based on the ability to bypass the blood-brain barrier (BBB). The BBB is composed of endothelial cells in brain capillaries forming nearly impenetrable tight junctions (zonula occludens), with limited to almost no detectable pathways for transendothelial transport of molecules of greater than 200 Da. Beyond a physical barrier, the BBB also forms a metabolic gate, inactivating passive compounds via intracellular and extracellular enzymes. Elsewhere in this publication, techniques and modalities specialized for bypassing the BBB for more efficacious systemic administration of drugs are described. More specifically, this chapter addresses the tools, materials, and techniques used in the direct bypass of the BBB by local, intracranial drug delivery.

The implantation of drug-eluting biomaterials within the brain is limited by several factors. The first and most important is that any implantable material must maintain a highly favorable safety profile. All implantable devices within the brain parenchyma are subject to interaction between the device and brain tissue and must be (1) completely biocompatible without eliciting a biological reaction, (2) unable to migrate and cause mechanical damage to the ventricular system or anatomic structures, and (3) limited in its ability to cause severe side effects from leakage of the dissolving or migrating compound.

A major barrier to the implementation of local and topical drugs for the treatment of glioblastoma is the cellular infiltrative nature of the disease, which extends beyond where a resection may take place surgically, or where a topical agent can be applied. Local drug delivery can provide controlled, sustained release of the compound, or can enhance the permeability of the BBB in some cases to promote uptake of the therapeutic, but does not change the underlying pathophysiologic nature of diffuse cellular infiltration.

CONVECTION-ENHANCED DELIVERY

On the basis that intratumoral drug administration is limited by poor diffusion of drugs through brain interstitium, CED promotes improved diffusion and distribution of small and large molecules via establishment and maintenance of a pressure gradient during interstitial infusion.[5,6] This

[a] Department of Neurosurgery, Perelman School of Medicine, Hospital of the University of Pennsylvania, 3400 Spruce Street, Philadelphia, PA 19104, USA; [b] Department of Bioengineering, University of Pennsylvania, 3400 Spruce Street, Philadelphia, PA 19104, USA
* Corresponding author.
E-mail address: burdick2@seas.upenn.edu

improvement is accomplished by administering a controlled pressure differential via interstitial infusate. Practically, this is accomplished by stereotactically placing a cannula or microcatheter near to or around the tumor cavity through a burr hole in the skull. This catheter is connected to a mechanized pumping device that creates a pressure gradient through a constant infusion rate, concentration, and duration of administration. The system has several advantages. The first is that it allows bypass of the BBB, and allows larger molecules to be administered within whatever volume of parenchyma is being perfused by CED. This ability may manifest on the order of kilodaltons or greater, compared with the 200 Da that are able to permeate the BBB without convection. The distribution of infusates can also be targeted, and they are generally thought to be more homogeneously distributed than with other delivery approaches. Further, the effective diffusion distance from initial microcatheter placement can be as much as 3 cm, compared with the several millimeters that can be achieved via continuous local infusion without CED, or with topical drug placement without convection. The downsides to CED are that smaller, hydrophilic molecules are more likely to leak out into the interstitial tissue from the central nervous system vasculature and into the systemic circulation (**Fig. 16.1**).

The clinical use of CED has been wide-ranging. In addition to conventional chemotherapeutics, the delivery of a variety of toxins, antibodies, and vectors has been attempted. The best clinical evidence regarding the use of CED is the phase III PRECISE trial.[7] CED of cintredekin besudotox (a recombinant chimeric cytotoxin of human interleukin-13 fused to a mutated form of *Pseudomonas* exotoxin that kills tumor cells expressing the interleukin 13 receptor overexpressed by malignant glioma cell lines) was compared with Gliadel wafers in patients with their first recurrence of glioblastoma. A total of 296 patients were enrolled at 2 centers and were randomized to either CED of the toxin or Gliadel wafers. The overall survival from time of randomization was the primary end point. Median overall survival was 9.1 months for CED and 8.8 months for Gliadel wafers ($P = .476$). In addition to being nonsuperior, the pulmonary embolism rate was higher in the CED group (8% vs 1%). As described,[3] the study may have been flawed by an inadequate percentage of catheter placements being performed per protocol specifications and stringent requirements for showing survival benefit. It should also be noted that there was an improvement in progression-free survival (17.7 weeks for CED vs 11.4 weeks for Gliadel wafer) but this was considered post hoc and not a primary or secondary end point by the study investigators.

In past few years, additional agents, such as liposomes and nanoparticles, have been the focus of preclinical investigation with CED. Advances in catheter placement and technique, as well as visualization of convection with real-time imaging, are improving preclinical promise, and both phase I and phase II trials are underway and may progress to phase 3 over the next few years.

DRUG-ELUTING WAFERS

The Gliadel wafer (carmustine wafer [CW]) is by far the most well established and well studied of the local drug-eluting systems for intracranial delivery, and the only FDA-approved compound therapy for use in glioblastoma apart from temozolomide and bevacizumab. The development of this product originated from work by Robert Langer and Judah Folkman in the 1970s on the

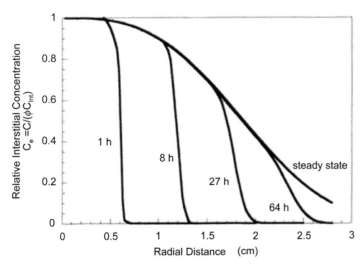

Fig. 16.1 Theoretic profile of diffusion distances of a 180-kDa macromolecule within nonbinding brain tissue with convection-enhanced delivery. (*From* Lonser RR, Sarntinoranont M, Morrison PF, et al. Convection-enhanced delivery to the central nervous system. J Neurosurg 2015;122:670; with permission.)

use of polymers for sustained release of proteins and macromolecules.[8] The biocompatibility of these delivery systems was then tested and evaluated throughout the 1980s for both safety and efficacy in preclinical models by Henry Brem and his team at Johns Hopkins Hospital.[9] As described by Brem and Gabikian,[4] the CW (BCNU) was integrated into a controlled delivery polymer (poly[bis(p-carboxyphenoxy) propane with sebacic acid) for controlled release. As a chemotherapeutic, BCNU functions as an alkylating agent to inhibit the synthesis of DNA, RNA, and other proteins. Its efficacy during systemic distribution is hampered by severe toxicities that include bone marrow suppression and cytotoxic effects on end-organ systems. The integration of BCNU into a controlled-delivery polymer both circumvented the BBB and allowed sustained release of high concentrations of BCNU directly into the tumor resection cavity, with sustained release that was found 2 weeks or longer after implantation.[4]

After successful animal studies, a phase I to II trial of 21 patients with recurrent glioblastoma was performed with CW treatment in 1981, which showed successful release of BCNU with no adverse effects to the study population.[10] This study was followed in 1995 by a randomized, placebo-controlled prospective study of CW in recurrent glioblastoma. A total of 222 patients in 27 medical centers were randomized to either receive functioning CW or placebo wafers. The median survival of the 110 patients who received CW was 31 weeks versus 23 weeks for the 112 patients who received a placebo. During the study there were no clinically noted adverse events attributable to the CW.[11] Long-term follow-up data of this patient population were published in 2003, which included additional patients with de novo glioblastoma and reported a sustained

survival benefit of 13.9 months for patients receiving the CW and 11.6 months in the placebo group. However, at that time adverse events attributable to CW were significantly greater when accounting for cerebrospinal fluid leaks and intracranial hypertension. As a result of these studies, and after FDA review, the CWs now known as Gliadel gained FDA approval for recurrent glioblastoma in 1996, and de novo glioblastoma in 2003[12] (**Fig. 16.2**).

The use of Gliadel wafers (**Fig. 16.3**) has been controversial because the statistically significant increase in survival of 2.3 months (similar to temozolomide) must be offset by potential toxicity and cost. For example, there is a risk of surgical site infection, CSF leak, and potentially brain swelling.[13] These risks can be averted by meticulous attention to dural closure, judicious use of steroids.

There have also been significant concerns regarding increased rates of infection with Gliadel implantation, which was originally reported at less than 5% but has subsequently been reported at up to 30%.[13] Several recent meta-analyses have examined survival outcomes and safety after implantation of Gliadel wafers.[14–16] Chowdhary and colleagues[14] reviewed 60 publications including 3162 cases of Gliadel implantation and 1736 controls. For de novo glioblastoma, the 1-year median overall survival was 16.4 months with Gliadel and 13.1 months without. In recurrent glioblastoma, the median survival was 9.7 months with Gliadel and 8.6 months without. Both of these findings reached statistical significance, but Gliadel wafer usage was linked to complications such as surgical site infection, hydrocephalus, cyst formation, hematomas, and wound dehiscence.[15] The overall complication rate in patients with newly diagnosed glioblastoma was as high as 42.7%,[15] however this was a review of the literature with uncontrolled

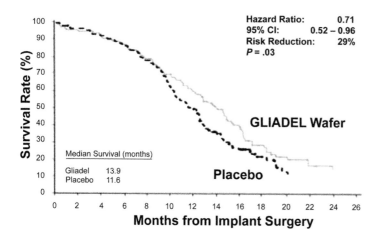

Hazard Ratio: 0.71
95% CI: 0.52 – 0.96
Risk Reduction: 29%
P = .03

Median Survival (months)
Gliadel 13.9
Placebo 11.6

Fig. 16.2 Overall survival in patients receiving CW and radiation, or placebo and radiation. CI, confidence interval. (*From* Westphal M, Hilt DC, Bortey E, et al. A phase 3 trial of local chemotherapy with biodegradable carmustine (BCNU) wafers (Gliadel wafers) in patients with primary malignant glioma. Neuro Oncol 2003;5:72; with permission.)

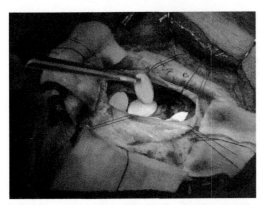

Fig. 16.3 Gliadel wafer being implanted. (*Courtesy of* Arbor Pharmaceuticals, LLC, Atlanta, GA; with permission.)

series, and the morbidity of radiation, chemotherapy, as well as surgery itself should be taken into account. Based on the results of randomized controlled trials,[11] Gliadel wafers are FDA-approved for both newly diagnosed and recurrent glioblastoma.

The biomechanical foundations for some of these complications may be related to the properties of the delivery system. Rigid polymers such as the polyanhydrides used in Gliadel are prone to microshearing activity as they move within the brain cavity after implantation.[17] This microshearing is posited to result in micromotion and vasogenic edema over time, which can be clinically relevant.[15,16] Further, their use must be limited to areas that do not directly border the ventricular system because they may migrate and result in obstructive hydrocephalus. In addition, as they dissolve, their

contents could release in a nonlinear manner depending on intracranial conditions, leaving behind degradation products (an inert polymer and dissolved chemotherapeutic in liquid form). The development and implementation of Gliadel as a therapy for glioblastoma remains a landmark achievement for clinical and translational science and neurosurgery, but recent advances in material science may improve on the concept of sustained-release materials for the treatment of glioblastoma.

RECENT ADVANCES

Discoveries in material science over the past decades have brought forward a range of biomaterials that possess substantial biocompatibility and tunable release profiles when used for drug administration.[18] One class of biomaterials, known as hydrogels, are three-dimensional, cross-linked networks of hydrophilic polymers. Depending on their constitution, they may be completely biocompatible and biodegradable because their high water content and physiochemical characteristics are similar to those of the tissue extracellular matrix.[18] One example that is widely used in biomedical applications is a contact lens. The consistency of these compounds is similar to a soft but firm gel capable of adhering to a physical structure on contact, and they are capable of delivering encapsulated therapeutics through combinations of hydrogel degradation and drug diffusion from the secondary network (**Fig. 16.4**).

Thus far, experimentation with thermal gel depots has shown promising results in animal models.[19–21] In addition to these biodegradable

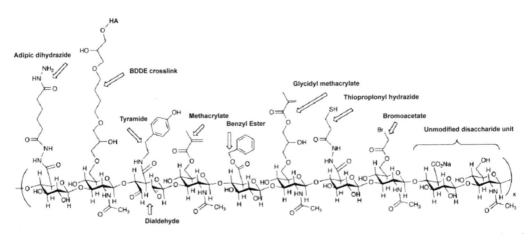

Fig. 16.4 Structure of hypothetical hyaluronic acid molecule showing a range of modifications to disaccharide repeat units that are possible through chemical synthesis. BDDE, 1,4-butanediol diglycidyl ether. (*From* Burdick JA, Prestwich GD. Hyaluronic acid hydrogels for biomedical applications. Adv Mater 2011;23(12):H1-43; with permission.)

options, microelectrical mechanical systems, local gene therapy, and focused ultrasonography have also shown promise in preclinical studies.[22,23]

SUMMARY

Operative intervention and surgical debulking of glioblastoma remain the mainstay of treatment in de novo, and in many cases recurrent, glioblastoma. This necessary intrusion into the central nervous system provides a logical extension toward the application of topical treatment strategies. There has been substantial progress in the creation of both delivery mechanisms via CED and in the creation of a controlled-release substrate manifested by the Gliadel wafer. Given the brisk pace of scientific advance in the realms of bioengineering, nanotechnology, and material science, the ability for less toxic, more efficacious local and topical delivery of drugs to the central nervous system is a possibility in the near future.

REFERENCES

1. Lonser RR, Sarntinoranont M, Morrison PF, et al. Convection-enhanced delivery to the central nervous system. J Neurosurg 2015;122:697–706.
2. Mehta AI, Linninger A, Lesniak MS, et al. Current status of intratumoral therapy for glioblastoma. J Neurooncol 2015;125:1–7.
3. Vogelbaum MA, Aghi MK. Convection-enhanced delivery for the treatment of glioblastoma. Neuro Oncol 2015;17(Suppl 2):ii3–8.
4. Brem H, Gabikian P. Biodegradable polymer implants to treat brain tumors. J Control Release 2001;74:63–7.
5. Bobo RH, Laske DW, Akbasak A, et al. Convection-enhanced delivery of macromolecules in the brain. Proc Natl Acad Sci U S A 1994;91:2076–80.
6. Morrison PF. Principles of clinical pharmacology. In: Atkinson AJ Jr, Huang SM, Lertora JJL, editors. San Diego (CA): Academic Press; 2001. p. 117–38.
7. Kunwar S, Chang S, Westphal M, et al. Phase III randomized trial of CED of IL13-PE38QQR vs Gliadel wafers for recurrent glioblastoma. Neuro Oncol 2010;12:871–81.
8. Langer R, Folkman J. Polymers for the sustained release of proteins and other macromolecules. Nature 1976;263:797–800.
9. Langer R, Brem H, Tapper D. Biocompatibility of polymeric delivery systems for macromolecules. J Biomed Mater Res 1981;15:267–77.
10. Brem H, Mahaley MS Jr, Vick NA, et al. Interstitial chemotherapy with drug polymer implants for the treatment of recurrent gliomas. J Neurosurg 1991;74:441–6.
11. Brem H, Piantadosi S, Burger PC, et al. Placebo-controlled trial of safety and efficacy of intraoperative controlled delivery by biodegradable polymers of chemotherapy for recurrent gliomas. The Polymer-brain Tumor Treatment Group. Lancet 1995;345:1008–12.
12. Westphal M, Hilt DC, Bortey E, et al. A phase 3 trial of local chemotherapy with biodegradable carmustine (BCNU) wafers (Gliadel wafers) in patients with primary malignant glioma. Neuro Oncol 2003;5:79–88.
13. McGovern PC, Lautenbach E, Brennan PJ, et al. Risk factors for postcraniotomy surgical site infection after 1,3-bis (2-chloroethyl)-1-nitrosourea (Gliadel) wafer placement. Clin Infect Dis 2003;36:759–65.
14. Chowdhary SA, Ryken T, Newton HB. Survival outcomes and safety of carmustine wafers in the treatment of high-grade gliomas: a meta-analysis. J Neurooncol 2015;122:367–82.
15. Bregy A, Shah AH, Diaz MV, et al. The role of Gliadel wafers in the treatment of high-grade gliomas. Expert Rev Anticancer Ther 2013;13:1453–61.
16. Xing WK, Shao C, Qi ZY, et al. The role of Gliadel wafers in the treatment of newly diagnosed GBM: a meta-analysis. Drug Des Devel Ther 2015;9: 3341–8.
17. Fleming AB, Saltzman WM. Pharmacokinetics of the carmustine implant. Clin Pharmacokinet 2002;41: 403–19.
18. Buwalda SJ, Boere KW, Dijkstra PJ, et al. Hydrogels in a historical perspective: from simple networks to smart materials. J Control Release 2014; 190:254–73.
19. Vellimana AK, Recinos VR, Hwang L, et al. Combination of paclitaxel thermal gel depot with temozolomide and radiotherapy significantly prolongs survival in an experimental rodent glioma model. J Neurooncol 2013;111:229–36.
20. Tyler B, Fowers KD, Li KW, et al. A thermal gel depot for local delivery of paclitaxel to treat experimental brain tumors in rats. J Neurosurg 2010;113:210–7.
21. Fourniols T, Randolph LD, Staub A, et al. Temozolomide-loaded photopolymerizable PEG-DMA-based hydrogel for the treatment of glioblastoma. J Control Release 2015;210:95–104.
22. Masi BC, Tyler BM, Bow H, et al. Intracranial MEMS based temozolomide delivery in a 9L rat gliosarcoma model. Biomaterials 2012;33:5768–75.
23. Aryal M, Arvanitis CD, Alexander PM, et al. Ultrasound-mediated blood-brain barrier disruption for targeted drug delivery in the central nervous system. Adv Drug Deliv Rev 2014;72:94–109.

CHAPTER 17

Tumor-Treating Electric Fields for Glioblastoma

Kenneth D. Swanson, PhD[a], Edwin Lok, MS[a], Eric T. Wong, MD[a,b,*]

HISTORICAL CONTEXT OF ELECTRIC FIELD TREATMENT

The application of physical energy from various parts of the electromagnetic spectrum is common in glioblastoma treatment. The most widely used involves energies from the higher end of the spectrum in exahertz (the 10^{18}-Hz range), in which ionizing radiation is used to treat various types of malignancies, including glioblastoma (**Fig. 17.1**). Therapeutic radiation can be diffuse, as in whole-brain and involved-field radiotherapy, or highly conformal, as in stereotactic radiosurgery (SRS), and the biological responses to these different types of radiation are different, as modeled by the linear-quadratic dose-effect relationship.[1–3] At the lower end of the spectrum, in the gigahertz or 10^9-Hz microwave range, laser interstitial thermal therapy (LITT) is being used for the thermocoagulation of brain tumors and the treatment of radiation necrosis.[4–6] MRI technology now allows the real-time visualization of temperature changes during LITT treatment of a target lesion. In addition, at an even lower part of the electromagnetic spectrum, in the kilohertz or 10^3-Hz range, alternating electric field therapy or tumor-treating electric fields (TTFields) are now an established treatment for glioblastoma.[7] This chapter provides a summary of the cell biology and physical science effects of TTFields on tumor cells and tumors in the brain, as well as a historical perspective of the clinical studies conducted in the glioblastoma population.

BIOLOGICAL BASIS AND PHYSICAL SCIENCE SUPPORTING THE USE OF TUMOR-TREATING ELECTRIC FIELDS

Cell Biology Effects of Tumor-treating Fields

Early *in vitro* studies showed that cells exposed to TTFields underwent violent membrane blebbing during mitosis, thought to be a result of the disruption of alpha/beta tubulin assembly in mitotic spindles.[8,9] More detailed analysis revealed that these cells seem to transit normally through metaphase, showing normal rates of cyclin B destruction and metaphase exit at times consistent with the expected entry into anaphase.[10] However, anaphase and cytokinesis were perturbed, leading to aberrant mitotic exit. Mitosis is dominated by a myriad of processes that must be regulated spatially and temporally in order to ensure even distribution of parental genomic DNA into the resulting daughter cells. Most of the regulatory events during mitosis control functions that are involved in the migration and alignment of chromosomes, as well as the timing of the contraction of the cytokinetic furrow following chromosome separation. Given the timing of the TTField-induced cellular disruption during mitosis, they likely exert their effect on intracellular proteins that are necessary during late metaphase or anaphase and that bear high electric charges on which the TTFields can act. It is not clear whether these TTField effects are caused by their combined activities on multiple proteins or whether they arise from the perturbation of a single protein that serves a critical function. In order to serve as a TTField target,

[a] Brain Tumor Center & Neuro-Oncology Unit, Department of Neurology, Beth Israel Deaconess Medical Center, Harvard Medical School, 330 Brookline Avenue, Boston, MA 02215, USA; [b] Department of Physics, University of Massachusetts in Lowell, One University Avenue, Lowell, MA, USA
* Corresponding author. Brain Tumor Center & Neuro-Oncology Unit, Beth Israel Deaconess Medical Center, 330 Brookline Avenue, Boston, MA 02215.
E-mail address: ewong@bidmc.harvard.edu

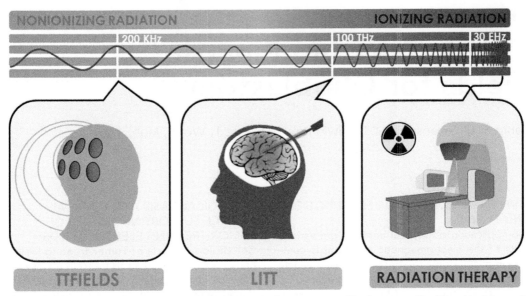

Fig. 17.1 Application of the electromagnetic spectrum in the treatment of brain tumors. Traditional ionizing radiation has a frequency in the exahertz, or 10^{18} Hz, range, whereas laser-induced thermal therapy uses microwaves in the gigahertz, or 10^9 Hz, range to induce thermocoagulation. Tumor-treating electric fields use the lower end of the electromagnetic spectrum in the kilohertz, or 10^3 Hz, range. LITT, laser interstitial thermal therapy; TTFields, tumor-treating fields. (*Courtesy of* Kisa Zhang, BS, Boston, MA.)

proteins must possess a sufficiently high dipole moment in order for the alternating electric fields generated by the TTField therapy device to perturb its function in mitosis.

By examining the published dipole moment database of different proteins, the authors found that the heterotrimeric protein complex composed of septin 2, 6, and 7 possesses a dipole moment of 2711 Debyes (or 10^{-18} statC·cm SI equivalent), which is 5 standard deviations greater than the median value derived from an analysis of more than 14,000 intracellular proteins.[10,11]

Importantly, this septin complex performs important functions during both metaphase and anaphase and its disruption by short hairpin RNA-mediated depletion resulted in blebbing during mitosis similar to that seen in TTField-treated cells.[12] TTFields are able to perturb normal septin localization during mitosis and cell spreading, which strongly suggests that TTFields physically interact with this complex and exert their effects on mitotic cells by preventing the proper localization of this septin-containing complex to proper sites of action during mitosis (**Fig. 17.2**).

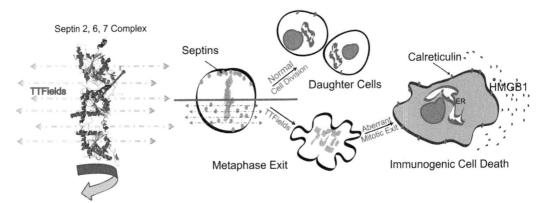

Fig. 17.2 Interaction between TTFields and tumor cells undergoing mitosis. TTFields induce an electromechanical force on the septin 2, 6, and 7 complex that has an extremely large dipole moment of 2711 Debyes. This movement results in mitotic catastrophe and aberrant mitotic exit, leading to an increased cell surface expression of the endoplasmic reticulum chaperonin calreticulin and the secretion of HMGB1, which acts as a danger signal when released from cells, both of which are essential for immunogenic cell death.

The TTField-induced catastrophe during anaphase results in a failure to complete division that results in a G_0/G_1 arrest and p53-dependent apoptosis. Therefore, TTFields are likely to exert an effect on multiple proteins and the resulting cumulative perturbation may be necessary to drive the observed mitotic catastrophe.

Postmitotic cells that are treated with TTFields and aberrantly exit mitosis develop aneuploidy, and these aneuploid cells are in general resistant to apoptosis, a process that is known to trigger an immunosuppressive response in the host.[13,14] However, TTFields also cause cytoplasmic stress and additional signs of immunogenic cell death, including high mobility group box 1 (HMGB1) secretion into the extracellular space, calreticulin upregulation on the cell surface, and annexin V binding.[15,16] These findings suggest that TTFields may increase the immunogenicity of tumor cells *in vivo*. When highly metastatic VX-2 tumors were injected into the kidney capsules of rabbits and were treated with TTFields for 7 days after their establishment, metastases to the lungs were markedly reduced compared with nontreated animals. Recovered lung metastases also revealed a significant increase in infiltration of immune cells within the tumors.[17,18] An interpretation of these results is that TTFields acted to sensitize the animals against metastatic spread and that the increased leukocytic infiltrates reflected an increased requirement for the immunosuppressive stroma for their establishment and maintenance. As discussed later, patients treated with the immunosuppressive steroidal antiinflammatory drug dexamethasone seem not to respond to TTField treatments and those with higher levels of CD3+, CD4+, and CD8+ lymphocytes are more likely to have a better outcome on this therapy.[19] Collectively, these data strongly support an immunologic basis for the antitumor response from TTField treatment.

Physical Properties of Tumor-treating Fields and Electric Field Distribution Within the Brain

The physical effects of TTFields are governed by the fundamental physics of Gauss' law, Ohm's law, the continuity equation, and Coulomb's law.[20] In addition, several factors, including a medium's electrical conductivity (a measure of the ability to pass charges) and relative permittivity (a measure of the ability to hold charges), can affect the electric field distribution within the brain tissue. Because each tissue type is unique, the intracranial structures must therefore be characterized based on their conductivity and permittivity values. The highly heterogeneous consistency and geometry of the brain therefore distort the intracranial electric fields as induced by an external source. Electric fields are generally defined by instantaneous changes in electric potential. These changes in electric potential result in electromotive disruption of mitotic structures and are therefore the basis for the therapeutic benefit of TTFields.[9,10] TTField therapy for glioblastoma is delivered by 2 pairs of transducer arrays positioned orthogonally on the shaved scalp, adhered by a thin layer of conductive gel that provides good conductivity (**Fig. 17.3**).[20,21] TTFields are generated by a battery-powered alternating current generator, operating at 200 kHz with maximum voltage alternating from +50 to −50 V.

To obtain a comprehensive model of the electric field's distribution in the brain, computer modeling can be performed using coregistered patient DICOM (Digital Imaging and Communications in Medicine) data sets from T1-weighed postgadolinium, T2, and MPRAGE (Magnetization-Prepared Rapid Acquisition with Gradient Echo) MRI. Previously, Lok and colleagues[22] showed a heterogeneous distribution of electric fields in the brain, and the regions adjacent to the ventricular horns had a particularly high electric field intensity (**Fig. 17.4**). This high field intensity is likely caused by the higher electric conductivity of cerebrospinal fluid than the surrounding tissues, which behaves like the terminal of a capacitor, with the surrounding tissues functioning like a dielectric between conductive terminals. Since a dielectric medium generally retains charge, the rate at which the medium is able to collect and retain the charge is defined by its conductivity and relative permittivity. At 200 kHz, the effect of permittivity is overwhelmed by the conductivity of the medium (**Fig. 17.5**).[23] Furthermore, each medium has a unique capacitive reactance characteristic of the medium's conductivity, and the rate at which the medium is able to collect and retain charges is frequency dependent. At high frequencies, the medium only has limited time to collect a finite amount of charges and retain them before the field collapses as the polarity changes direction, thereby discharging the initially retained charges before repeating the process.

Because cerebrospinal fluid has a low permittivity value compared with its surrounding tissues, it is a poor dielectric medium and thus charges migrate through the fluid layer at a much faster rate with minimal charge retention. This property explains why most of the cerebrospinal fluid has very low electric field intensity. But this is not true at the interface between cerebrospinal fluid and its adjacent brain tissue. For a perfect solid

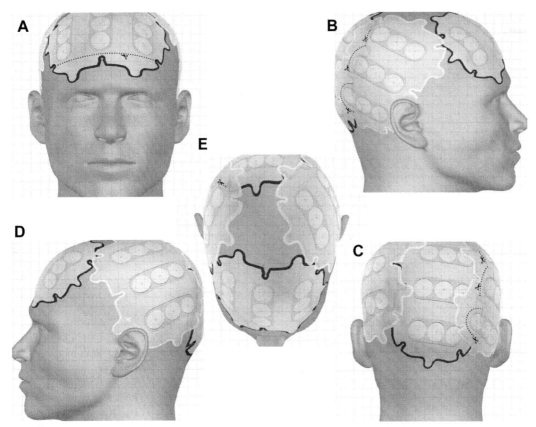

Fig. 17.3 Transducer array placement for TTField therapy. TTFields are delivered by 2 pairs of transducer arrays placed orthogonally (*A–E*) on the shaved scalp. The arrays are connected to a battery-operated current generator, operating at 200 kHz with peak-to-peak voltage from +50 to −50 V.

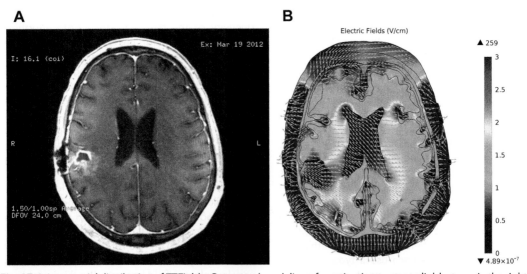

Fig. 17.4 Intracranial distribution of TTFields. Computed modeling of a patient's recurrent glioblastoma in the right parietal brain (*A*) revealed inhomogeneous electric field distribution within the intracranial space (*B*). High field strength was seen at the ventricular horns and the medial aspect of the tumor facing the lateral ventricle.

A

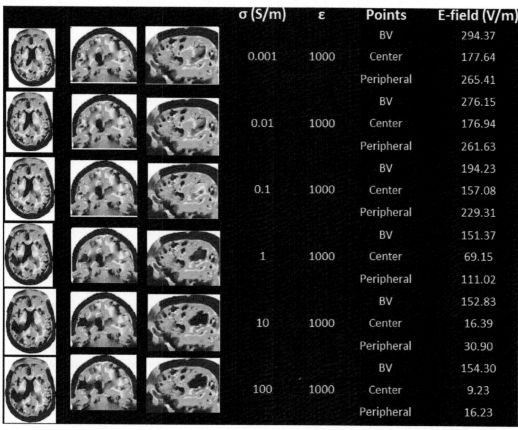

σ (S/m)	ε	Points	E-field (V/m)
		BV	294.37
0.001	1000	Center	177.64
		Peripheral	265.41
		BV	276.15
0.01	1000	Center	176.94
		Peripheral	261.63
		BV	194.23
0.1	1000	Center	157.08
		Peripheral	229.31
		BV	151.37
1	1000	Center	69.15
		Peripheral	111.02
		BV	152.83
10	1000	Center	16.39
		Peripheral	30.90
		BV	154.30
100	1000	Center	9.23
		Peripheral	16.23

B

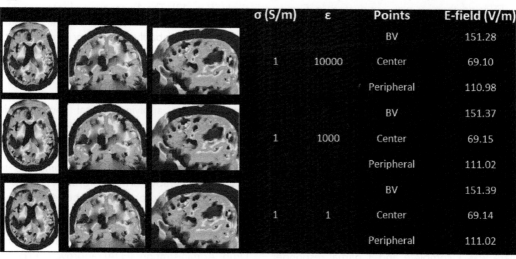

σ (S/m)	ε	Points	E-field (V/m)
		BV	151.28
1	10000	Center	69.10
		Peripheral	110.98
		BV	151.37
1	1000	Center	69.15
		Peripheral	111.02
		BV	151.39
1	1	Center	69.14
		Peripheral	111.02

Fig. 17.5 Sensitivity analysis of the electric field distribution in the gross tumor volume (GTV) as a function of conductivity or permittivity. (A) The electric field intensity of the GTV and the surrounding tissues decreased as the conductivity increased from 0.001 to 100 S/m. (B) However, the electric field intensity and distribution did not change significantly as permittivity varied from 1 to 10,000. BV, bilateral ventricles.

conductor, the electric field within it is zero, and the charges are uniformly distributed on the surface of the conductor. However, cerebrospinal fluid is neither a perfect conductor nor a dielectric. When charges are positioned across a parallel flat surface, repulsive forces are generated and the charges dissipate away from each other. However, on surfaces with very steep geometric gradients (ie, sharp corners), the repulsive forces are greatly increased because the charge density is much higher within a smaller surface area. Therefore, it is expected that the ventricular horns have a significantly higher electric field intensity than the rest of the cerebrospinal fluid space as a result of the bunching effect of charge distribution in a region with an irregularly sharp geometry.

The electric properties of gliomas can also vary among patients depending on their tumor composition. Tumors with larger necrotic cores are likely to have higher field intensities in the gross tumor volume because of the capacitive reactance, as explained earlier. In contrast, tumors with smaller or no necrotic core are likely to have lower field intensities at the center of the volume because of absence of an adjacent conductive medium to act as an electric current source. This property may become clinically relevant due to the increased requirement for time of exposure to TTFields as the outer layers of the gross tumor volume are treated by lower field intensities.

EVIDENCE FOR THE USE OF TUMOR-TREATING ELECTRIC FIELDS IN THE TREATMENT OF RECURRENT AND *DE NOVO* GLIOBLASTOMAS
First-in-Human Tumor-Treating Fields Therapy for Glioblastoma

The first-in-human pilot trial for safety and efficacy of TTFields therapy was conducted in Europe from 2004 to 2005 and enrolled 10 patients with recurrent glioblastoma.[8] The most common adverse event was contact dermatitis, which occurred in 9 patients and was thought to be a result of hydrogel-induced irritation on the scalp. Two patients experienced partial seizures that were related to their tumors. No toxicity on blood count or chemistry was seen, except for increased liver enzyme levels in those taking anticonvulsants. The median overall survival (mOS) of the 10 patients was 14.4 months. The time to tumor progression was 6.0 months and the 1-year overall survival (OS) rate was 67.5%, which compared favorably with the historical data of 5.8 months for mOS, 2.1 months for median progression-free survival (mPFS), and 21% for 1-year OS.[8,24] There was 1 complete and 1 partial responder who were alive at 84 and 87 months, respectively, from treatment initiation.[25] Importantly, the intensity of electric fields as directly measured in 1 patient was validated to be within 10% of the values estimated by computer modeling of the electric field distribution within the brain.[8]

A concurrent pilot study was conducted from 2005 to 2007 that enrolled 10 patients with newly diagnosed glioblastoma.[25] TTFields were added to adjuvant temozolomide after initial standard-of-care radiotherapy and concomitant daily temozolomide.[26] The mPFS was 35.8 months and mOS was greater than 39 months, which compared favorably with the mPFS of 6.9 months and mOS of 14.6 months from the data in the phase III trial.[25,26] The only adverse event noted in the pilot cohort was scalp dermatitis, and that could be ameliorated by topical corticosteroids and periodic shifting of transducer arrays.[25] There were 2 long-term survivors who lived 84 and 64 months from their initial diagnoses.[25]

Tumor-Treating Fields for Recurrent Glioblastoma

The phase III pivotal trial of TTFields for recurrent glioblastoma was conducted from 2006 to 2009 and the primary end point was OS (NCT00379470).[27] In the intent-to-treat population, the median OS was 6.6 months for subjects treated with TTFields versus 6.0 months for those who received best physician's choice (BPC) chemotherapy, with a hazard ratio of 0.86 ($P = .27$) (Fig. 17.6). About 31% of the BPC chemotherapy cohort received bevacizumab alone or in combination with chemotherapy. The mPFS was 2.2 and 2.1 months respectively for TTFields and BPC chemotherapy treatment, with a hazard ratio of 0.81 ($P = .16$). The progression-free survival (PFS) at 6 months was 21.4% and 15.1%, respectively ($P = .13$). The 1-year survival rate was 20% in both cohorts. The outcome of the trial indicated that TTFields probably had efficacy comparable to chemotherapy and bevacizumab.

Grade 1 or 2 scalp irritations were the most common adverse events associated with the device. Shifting the arrays slightly during array exchange and applying topical corticosteroid can minimize this irritation.[28] There were far less hematological toxicity, appetite loss, constipation, diarrhea, fatigue, nausea, vomiting, and pain associated with the device when compared to BPC chemotherapy. Furthermore, analysis showed that device-treated patients had better cognitive and emotional functions. Based on the comparable efficacy results and absence of serious TTField-associated toxicities, the US Food and Drug Administration (FDA) approved TTFields therapy on April 8, 2011 for the treatment of recurrent glioblastoma.

The discrepancy in the OS rates between the results of the phase III trial and the robust outcome from the first-in-human pilot study prompted a series of *post hoc* analyses of the trial data. The first analysis centered on responders. This analysis showed that 5 of 14 responders treated with

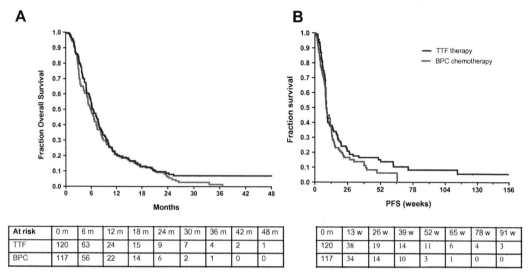

Fig. 17.6 Intent-to-treat Kaplan-Meier OS and PFS curves in the pivotal trial for patients with recurrent glioblastoma comparing TTField therapy with BPC chemotherapy. (A) The median OS was 6.6 months for patients treated with TTFields versus 6.0 months for those received BPC chemotherapy, with a hazard ratio of 0.86 (P = .27). (B) The median PFS was 2.2 and 2.1 months respectively for TTFields and BPC chemotherapy treatment, with a hazard ratio of 0.81 (P = .16). TTF, TTFields.

TTField monotherapy had prior low-grade histology, whereas none of the 7 responders treated with BPC chemotherapy did.[29] Second, the analysis revealed significantly less dexamethasone use in responders when compared to nonresponders.[29] Responders in the TTField monotherapy group received a median dexamethasone dose of 1.0 mg/d while nonresponders received 5.2 mg/d. A similar difference was also noted in the median cumulative dexamethasone dose of 7.1 mg for responders compared to 261.7 mg for nonresponders. In the chemotherapy cohort, the median dexamethasone dose used was 1.2 mg/d for responders while it was 6.0 mg/d for nonresponders. However, the median cumulative dexamethasone dose was not significantly different: 348.5 mg for responders versus 242.3 mg for nonresponders. These data suggest that TTFields efficacy may be influenced by concurrent dexamethasone use, which is a clinically modifiable factor. This finding prompted an in-depth analysis of the dexamethasone effect in the entire trial population.

Applying an unsupervised modified binary search algorithm that stratified the TTField monotherapy arm of the phase III trial based on the dexamethasone dosage that provided the greatest statistical difference in survival revealed that subjects who used greater than 4.1 mg/d of dexamethasone had a markedly shortened median OS of 4.8 months compared with those who received less than or equal to 4.1 mg/d, who had a median OS of 11.0 months (**Fig. 17.7**).[19] Subjects in the chemotherapy arm were observed to have a

similar, but less robust, dichotomization and those who used greater than 4.1 mg/d and less than or equal to 4.1 mg/d of dexamethasone had a median OS of 6.0 and 8.9 months, respectively. This difference in OS based on dexamethasone dose was unrelated to tumor size but was most likely caused by interference with patient immune effector function. A single-institution validation cohort of patients treated with TTField therapy, using their CD3+, CD4+, and CD8+ T lymphocyte levels as a marker of immune competency, suggested the importance of immune competence to TTField therapy. Importantly, a dexamethasone dosage of greater than 4.0 mg/d was also a poor prognostic factor in newly diagnosed patients who completed radiotherapy,[30] supporting the conclusion that dexamethasone can interfere with treatment. With successive increases in dexamethasone dosage, both cohorts reached an inflection point near 8.0 mg/d, after which the rate of survival decreased slowly. Taken together, dexamethasone exerts a generalized and profound interference on the efficacy of both TTFields and chemotherapeutic treatment against glioblastoma. Therefore, dexamethasone use should be aggressively minimized.[19,31]

Use of Tumor-Treating Fields Therapy in Clinical Practice

The post–FDA-approval usage of TTField therapy in routine clinical practice may differ from that in the registration trial, primarily because clinical trial data may not always be representative of

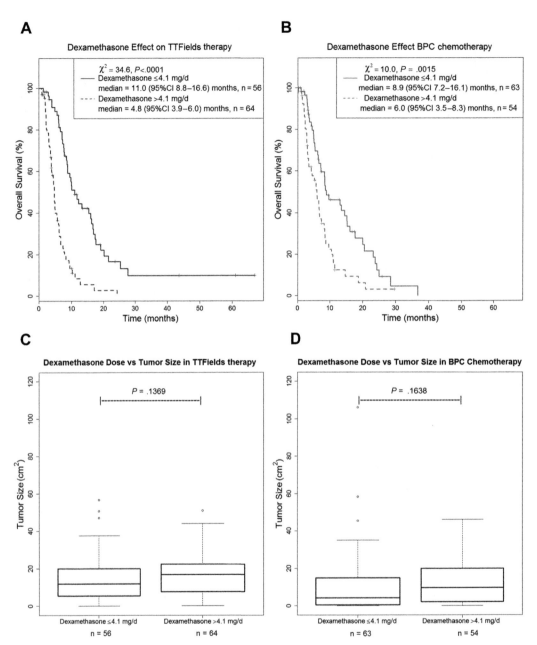

Fig. 17.7 Kaplan-Meier OS and tumor size with respect to dexamethasone requirement of less than or equal to 4.1 mg/d versus greater than 4.1 mg/d from subjects enrolled in the phase III trial comparing TTField therapy with BPC chemotherapy. (A) Subjects enrolled in the TTField treatment arm taking dexamethasone less than or equal to 4.1 mg/d (*solid blue*) versus greater than 4.1 mg/d (*dashed blue*), which was determined by an unsupervised binary partitioning algorithm. Subjects who used less than or equal to 4.1 mg/d of dexamethasone (n = 56) had a median OS of 11.0 months (95% confidence interval [CI], 8.8–16.6) compared with those who used greater than 4.1 mg/d (n = 64), who had a median OS of 4.8 months (95% CI, 3.9–6.0) (χ^2 = 34.6; P<.0001). (B) Subjects enrolled in the BPC chemotherapy arm taking dexamethasone less than or equal to 4.1 mg/d (*solid red*) versus greater than 4.1 mg/d (*dashed red*), which was determined by the same unsupervised binary partitioning algorithm. Subjects who used less than or equal to 4.1 mg/d of dexamethasone (n = 63) had a median OS of 8.9 months (95% CI, 7.2–16.1) compared with those who used greater than 4.1 mg/d (n = 54), who had a median OS of 6.0 months (95% CI, 3.5–8.3; χ^2 = 10.0; P = .0015). (C) Box-and-whisker plot of bidimensional tumor size in the TTField therapy cohort that received dexamethasone less than or equal to 4.1 mg/d versus greater than 4.1 mg/d. Subjects who took dexamethasone less than or equal to 4.1 mg/d (n = 56) had a median tumor size of 11.9 cm² (range, 0.0–56.7 cm²) compared with those who used greater than 4.1 mg/d (n = 64), who had a

treatment outcome in routine clinical practice environments. Reasons for this discrepancy may arise from the prespecified clinical characteristics that trial subjects must possess that real-world patients may not have. As a result, trial subjects typically have healthier neurologic functions, better performance status, and fewer medical comorbidities, all of which may enable trial subjects to benefit more from the new treatment. Furthermore, the FDA must strike a fine balance between providing the public rapid access to new treatments for deadly diseases and requiring comprehensive data and protracted reviews on their benefits and risks. This action sometimes results in the reversal of prior accelerated approval decisions. Therefore, these issues prompted the development of the Patient Registry Data Set (PRiDe) to capture data on TTField usage among patients in the routine clinical practice environment.

PRiDe consisted of 457 patients from 91 treatment centers in the United States. Patients treated in PRiDe had a median OS of 9.6 months compared with 6.6 months in the TTField monotherapy arm in the registration trial.[27,32] The 1-year OS rate was also longer at 44% compared with 20%, respectively.[27,32] The difference in survival characteristics is most likely caused by the higher proportion of patients treated with TTFields at first recurrence in PRiDe (33%) than in the registration trial (9%). Treatment at an earlier timepoint in the disease process may provide a higher efficacy than treatment at a later timepoint. Absence of prior bevacizumab usage was also favorable.[32] Nevertheless, the heterogeneity in the adjunctive treatments used in conjunction with TTField therapy in PRiDe that was not adequately captured, which included cytotoxic chemotherapy, bevacizumab, or even alternative medicine, is an important caveat that makes it statistically noncomparative with the TTField monotherapy arm in the phase III trial.

Efficacy of Tumor-Treating Fields Therapy for Newly Diagnosed Glioblastoma

A phase III randomized open-label study of TTField therapy was conducted in 700 patients with newly diagnosed glioblastoma between 2009 and 2014 (NCT00916409). After their initial radiotherapy and concomitant daily temozolomide, subjects were randomized in a 2:1 fashion to receive either TTFields plus maintenance temozolomide or maintenance temozolomide alone.[33] The primary end point was PFS. In a prespecified interim analysis of the first 315 subjects after a minimum follow-up of 18 months, the intent-to-treat cohort that received TTFields plus temozolomide had a longer PFS than the cohort treated with temozolomide alone: median 7.1 versus 4.0 months (hazard ratio = 0.62; 95% confidence interval [CI], 0.43–0.89; log rank P = .0014) (Fig. 17.8). The median OS also favors the TTFields plus temozolomide group, at 19.6 versus 16.6 months respectively (hazard ratio = 0.74; 95% CI, 0.56–0.98; log rank P = .034), as well as the per protocol population that completed more than 1 cycle of treatment, at 20.5 versus 15.6 months respectively (hazard ratio = 0.64; 95% CI, 0.42–0.98; log rank P = .004).

The trial population experienced no unexpected adverse events.[33] Grade 3 and 4 hematological toxicities between the TTFields plus temozolomide and temozolomide alone cohorts (12% vs 9%), gastrointestinal disorders (5% vs 2%), and convulsions (7% vs 7%) were not significantly different. Only scalp reaction was more commonly seen in those who received TTFields plus temozolomide. Based on the favorable efficacy and toxicity data, the US FDA granted approval on October 5, 2015 to use TTFields in conjunction with maintenance temozolomide in the adjuvant setting for patients with newly diagnosed glioblastoma.

SUMMARY

Human clinical trial testing of TTField efficacy was started in neuro-oncology, initially for the treatment of recurrent glioblastoma (NCT00379470) and later in newly diagnosed glioblastoma (NCT00916409).[27,33] This route of development for a new anticancer therapy is highly unusual because treatments in neuro-oncology were traditionally adopted from established therapies from other disease sites, when the accompanying preclinical scientific data on the mechanisms of action had been firmly established. Nevertheless, the 2 pivotal trials conducted in glioblastoma have

---

median tumor size of 16.8 cm^2 (range, 0.3–51.0 cm^2). (P = .1369). (D) Box-and-whisker plot of bidimensional tumor size in the BPC chemotherapy cohort that received dexamethasone less than or equal to 4.1 mg/d versus greater than 4.1 mg/d. Subjects who took dexamethasone less than or equal to 4.1 mg/d (n = 63) had a median tumor size of 4.2 cm^2 (range, 0.0–11.2 cm^2) compared with those who used greater than 4.1 mg/d (n = 54), who had a median tumor size of 9.6 cm^2 (range, 0.0–46.0 cm^2) (P = .1638).

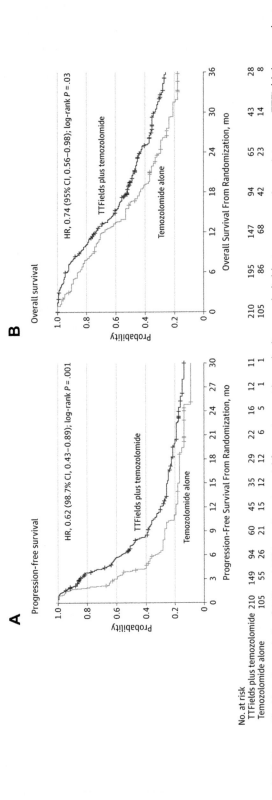

Fig. 17.8 Prespecified interim analysis of PFS and OS in registration trial for patients with newly diagnosed glioblastoma comparing maintenance TTField therapy plus temozolomide versus temozolomide alone. Kaplan-Meier comparison of the two cohorts showed (A) a median PFS of 7.1 versus 4.0 months respectively, with a hazard ratio of 0.62 (P = .0014), and (B) a median OS of 19.6 versus 16.6 months respectively, with a hazard ratio of 0.74 (P = .034).

helped to established TTFields as a *bona fide* anti-cancer treatment and its efficacy is being actively investigated in glioblastoma as well as other malignancies both within and outside the central nervous system.

To improve the efficacy of TTFields treatment of recurrent glioblastomas, there is a strong rationale for combining it with SRS. Large-fraction radiotherapy might potentiate immune-mediated antitumor activity.[34,35] The addition of TTFields after SRS may further potentiate this effect because exposed tumor cells show cell surface expression of calreticulin and secretion of HMGB1, both of which are required to generate immunogenic cell death.[15,36,37] Furthermore, a *post hoc* analysis of the phase III trial for recurrent glioblastoma showed that the application of TTFields among subjects who had progressed on bevacizumab (n = 23) resulted in a longer mOS of 6.0 months compared with a mOS of 3.3 months (n = 21) in those treated with BPC chemotherapy (hazard ratio = 0.43; 95% CI, 0.22–0.85; χ^2 P = .06).[38] In addition, the favorable intracranial safety profile of TTFields and bevacizumab suggests that the combination will most likely have an acceptable level of toxicity.[38,39] There is a planned Radiation Therapy Oncology Group foundation study on TTFields and bevacizumab in patients with recurrent glioblastoma who have progressed while on bevacizumab.

Several investigator-initiated combination trials are being conducted using (1) TTFields in combination with bevacizumab and carmustine in patients with glioblastoma at first relapse (NCT02348255), (2) TTFields with bevacizumab and hypofractionated stereotactic radiotherapy for bevacizumab-naive patients with recurrent glioblastoma (NCT01925573), and (3) TTFields in combination with temozolomide and bevacizumab for patients with newly diagnosed glioblastoma in the maintenance phase of treatment, after initial radiotherapy with concomitant temozolomide and bevacizumab (NCT02343549). In addition, a study has been designed to find genomic signatures of recurrent glioblastoma that may correlate with response to TTFields (NCT0194576). Collectively, these planned and ongoing studies indicate the current state of interest in combining TTFields with other established modalities of treatment for glioblastoma.

REFERENCES

1. Wang JZ, Huang Z, Lo SS, et al. A generalized linear-quadratic model for radiosurgery, stereotactic body radiation therapy, and high-dose rate brachytherapy. Sci Transl Med 2010;2(39):39ra48.

2. Barendsen GW. Dose fractionation, dose rate and iso-effect relationships for normal tissue responses. Int J Radiat Oncol Biol Phys 1982;8(11):1981–97.

3. Dale RG. The application of the linear-quadratic dose-effect equation to fractionated and protracted radiotherapy. Br J Radiol 1985;58(690):515–28.

4. Rahmathulla G, Recinos PF, Valerio JE, et al. Laser interstitial thermal therapy for focal cerebral radiation necrosis: a case report and literature review. Stereotact Funct Neurosurg 2012;90(3):192–200.

5. Kahn T, Bettag M, Ulrich F, et al. MRI-guided laser-induced interstitial thermotherapy of cerebral neoplasms. J Comput Assist Tomogr 1994;18(4):519–32.

6. Rahmathulla G, Recinos PF, Kamian K, et al. MRI-guided laser interstitial thermal therapy in neuro-oncology: a review of its current clinical applications. Oncology 2014;87(2):67–82.

7. Fonkem E, Wong ET. NovoTTF-100A: a new treatment modality for recurrent glioblastoma. Expert Rev Neurother 2012;12(8):895–9.

8. Kirson ED, Dbaly V, Tovarys F, et al. Alternating electric fields arrest cell proliferation in animal tumor models and human brain tumors. Proc Natl Acad Sci U S A 2007;104(24):10152–7.

9. Kirson ED, Gurvich Z, Schneiderman R, et al. Disruption of cancer cell replication by alternating electric fields. Cancer Res 2004;64(9):3288–95.

10. Gera N, Yang A, Holtzman TS, et al. Tumor treating fields perturb the localization of septins and cause aberrant mitotic exit. PLoS One 2015;10(5):e0125269.

11. Felder CE, Prilusky J, Silman I, et al. A server and database for dipole moments of proteins. Nucleic Acids Res 2007;35(Web Server Issue):W512–21.

12. Gilden JK, Peck S, Chen YC, et al. The septin cytoskeleton facilitates membrane retraction during motility and blebbing. J Cell Biol 2012;196(1):103–14.

13. Castedo M, Coquelle A, Vitale I, et al. Selective resistance of tetraploid cancer cells against DNA damage-induced apoptosis. Ann N Y Acad Sci 2006;1090:35–49.

14. Voll RE, Herrmann M, Roth EA, et al. Immunosuppressive effects of apoptotic cells. Nature 1997;390(6658):350–1.

15. Lee SX, Wong ET, Swanson KD. Disruption of cell division within anaphase by tumor treating electric fields (TTFields) leads to immunogenic cell death. Neuro Oncol 2013;15:iii66–7.

16. Chaput N, De Botton S, Obeid M, et al. Molecular determinants of immunogenic cell death: surface exposure of calreticulin makes the difference. J Mol Med (Berl) 2007;85(10):1069–76.

17. Kirson ED, Schneiderman RS, Dbaly V, et al. Chemotherapeutic treatment efficacy and sensitivity are increased by adjuvant alternating electric fields (TTFields). BMC Med Phys 2009;9:1.

18. Kirson ED, Giladi M, Gurvich Z, et al. Alternating electric fields (TTFields) inhibit metastatic spread

of solid tumors to the lungs. Clin Exp Metastasis 2009;26(7):633–40.

19. Wong ET, Lok E, Gautam S, et al. Dexamethasone exerts profound immunologic interference on treatment efficacy for recurrent glioblastoma. Br J Cancer 2015;113(11):1642.

20. Lok E, Swanson KD, Wong ET. Tumor treating fields therapy device for glioblastoma: physics and clinical practice considerations. Expert Rev Med Devices 2015;12(6):717–26.

21. Mcadams ET, Jossinet J, Lackermeier A, et al. Factors affecting electrode-gel-skin interface impedance in electrical impedance tomography. Med Biol Eng Comput 1996;34(6):397–408.

22. Lok E, Hua V, Wong ET. Computed modeling of alternating electric fields therapy for recurrent glioblastoma. Cancer Med 2015;4(11):1697–9.

23. Ramos A, Morgan H, Green NG, et al. AC electrokinetics: a review of forces in microelectrode structures. J Phys D Appl Phys 1998;31:2338–53.

24. Wong ET, Hess KR, Gleason MJ, et al. Outcomes and prognostic factors in recurrent glioma patients enrolled onto phase II clinical trials. J Clin Oncol 1999;17(8):2572–8.

25. Rulseh AM, Keller J, Klener J, et al. Long-term survival of patients suffering from glioblastoma multiforme treated with tumor-treating fields. World J Surg Oncol 2012;10:220.

26. Stupp R, Mason WP, Van Den Bent MJ, et al. Radiotherapy plus concomitant and adjuvant temozolomide for glioblastoma. N Engl J Med 2005; 352(10):987–96.

27. Stupp R, Wong ET, Kanner AA, et al. NovoTTF-100A versus physician's choice chemotherapy in recurrent glioblastoma: a randomised phase III trial of a novel treatment modality. Eur J Cancer 2012;48(14):2192–202.

28. Lacouture ME, Davis ME, Elzinga G, et al. Characterization and management of dermatologic adverse events with the NovoTTF-100A System, a novel anti-mitotic electric field device for the treatment of recurrent glioblastoma. Semin Oncol 2014; 41(Suppl 4):S1–14.

29. Wong ET, Lok E, Swanson KD, et al. Response assessment of NovoTTF-100A versus best physician's choice chemotherapy in recurrent glioblastoma. Cancer Med 2014;3(3):592–602.

30. Back MF, Eng ELL, Ng WH, et al. Improved median survival for glioblastoma multiforme following introduction of adjuvant temozolomide chemotherapy. Ann Acad Med Singapore 2007;36(5):338–42.

31. Wong ET, Swanson KD. Response to: Comment on 'Dexamethasone exerts profound immunologic interference on treatment efficacy for recurrent glioblastoma'. Br J Cancer 2015;113(11):1633–4.

32. Mrugala MM, Engelhard HH, Dinh Tran D, et al. Clinical practice experience with NovoTTF-100A system for glioblastoma: the Patient Registry Dataset (PRiDe). Semin Oncol 2014;41(Suppl 6): S4–13.

33. Stupp R, Taillibert S, Kanner AA, et al. Maintenance therapy with tumor-treating fields plus temozolomide vs temozolomide alone for glioblastoma: a randomized clinical trial. JAMA 2015;314(23):2535–43.

34. Postow MA, Callahan MK, Barker CA, et al. Immunologic correlates of the abscopal effect in a patient with melanoma. N Engl J Med 2012; 366(10):925–31.

35. Dewan MZ, Galloway AE, Kawashima N, et al. Fractionated but not single-dose radiotherapy induces an immune-mediated abscopal effect when combined with anti-CTLA-4 antibody. Clin Cancer Res 2009;15(17):5379–88.

36. Kepp O, Senovilla L, Vitale I, et al. Consensus guidelines for the detection of immunogenic cell death. Oncoimmunology 2014;3(9):e955691.

37. Kepp O, Tesniere A, Schlemmer F, et al. Immunogenic cell death modalities and their impact on cancer treatment. Apoptosis 2009;14(4):364–75.

38. Kanner AA, Wong ET, Villano JL, et al. Post hoc analyses of intention-to-treat population in phase III comparison of NovoTTF-100A system versus best physician's choice chemotherapy. Semin Oncol 2014;41(Suppl 6):S25–34.

39. Zuniga RM, Torcuator R, Jain R, et al. Efficacy, safety and patterns of response and recurrence in patients with recurrent high-grade gliomas treated with bevacizumab plus irinotecan. J Neurooncol 2009;91(3): 329–36.

ACKNOWLEDGMENTS

The authors acknowledge and thank Kisa Zhang for her artwork in **Fig. 17.1**.

CHAPTER 18

Brain Plasticity and Reorganization Before, During, and After Glioma Resection

Hugues Duffau, MD, PhD[a,b,*]

INTRODUCTION

The traditional principle in neuro-oncology is to study the tumor first, with little consideration regarding the host; that is, the brain. Nevertheless, to define the optimal therapeutic management for each patient bearing a diffuse glioma (DG), the concept of oncofunctional balance must be taken into account. Although understanding of the natural history of the disease is crucial, this is not enough. The adaptive reaction of the central nervous system (CNS) induced by the glioma growth and spread should also be investigated. Dynamic interactions between the glioma and the CNS may allow neuroplasticity phenomena, resulting in the compensation of glial tumor progression and in the preservation of quality of life until the limits of plastic potential are reached, thus leading to seizures and/or neurologic deficits.[1,2]

This chapter analyzes mechanisms underpinning brain plasticity, based on original insights from cerebral mapping and functional outcomes in patients who have had awake surgery for DG. The aim is to switch from a localizationist model to a hodopical framework of neural processing. Such a connectomal account of brain organization results in tailoring an adapted therapeutic strategy according to the dynamic relationships between DG course and adaptational cerebral functional remapping at the individual level.[3]

NEURAL PLASTICITY
Historical Note

For more than 1 century, 2 different concepts of CNS functioning were suggested. First, the theory of equipotentiality hypothesized that the whole brain, or at least 1 complete hemisphere, was involved in the practice of a functional task. By contrast, in the theory of localizationism (based on phrenology), each part of the brain was supposed to correspond with a specific function. Progressively, an intermediate view emerged, namely a brain organized (1) in highly specialized functional areas, called eloquent regions (eg, the rolandic, Broca, and Wernicke areas), for which any lesion generates major permanent neurologic deficits; and (2) in noneloquent regions, with no functional consequences when damaged. Therefore, the dogma of a static CNS organization, with the inability to compensate for any damage involving the eloquent regions, was settled for a long time. Nevertheless, thanks to regular observations of functional improvement after injuries of structures considered as critical, this principle of a rigid CNS was called into question. If there is a lesion of neural tissue, the brain can reallocate the remaining physiologic resources to maintain a satisfactory level of function in a cognitively and socially demanding environment. Thus, many investigations were performed, initially in vitro and in animals, then more recently in

Conflicts of Interest: None.
Funding Sources: None.
[a] Department of Neurosurgery, Gui de Chauliac Hospital, Montpellier University Medical Center, 80 Avenue Augustin Fliche, Montpellier 34295, France; [b] U1051 Laboratory, National Institute for Health and Medical Research (INSERM), Team "Brain Plasticity, Stem Cells and Glial Tumors", Institute for Neurosciences of Montpellier, Montpellier University Medical Center, 80 Avenue Augustin Fliche, Montpellier 34091, France
* Department of Neurosurgery, Gui de Chauliac Hospital, Montpellier University Medical Center, 80 Avenue Augustin Fliche, Montpellier 34295, France.
E-mail address: h-duffau@chu-montpellier.fr

humans, in order to study the mechanisms underlying these compensatory phenomena: the concept of neuroplasticity was developed.[4] Advances in functional mapping and neuroimaging techniques have dramatically changed the classic modular model for a new dynamic and distributed perspective of CNS organization, able to reorganize itself both during everyday life (learning) and after a pathologic event such as a DG. However, although there are a few literature reports on cases of functional recovery or adaptation in various neurologic contexts, the most persuasive body of evidence for the brain's lesion-induced plasticity comes from neurosurgery in general and from the resection of DG in particular.[5]

Definition and Mechanisms

Neuroplasticity is a continuous processing allowing short-term, medium-term, and long-term remodeling of the neuronosynaptic organization, with the aim of optimizing the functioning of neural networks during phylogenesis, ontogeny, and physiologic learning, and following brain injury. At a microscopic scale, pathophysiologic mechanisms underlying plasticity are mainly represented by synaptic efficacy modulations, unmasking of latent connections, phenotypic modifications, synchrony changes, and neurogenesis. At a macroscopic scale, diaschisis, functional redundancies, cross-modal plasticity with sensory substitution, and morphologic changes are involved. The behavioral consequences of these phenomena have been investigated, in particular the ability to recover after cerebral damage (postlesional plasticity), and the underlying patterns of functional remapping have been analyzed.[6] Neural plasticity can be conceived only in a dynamic account of CNS organization; the brain is an ensemble of complex networks that form, reshape, and flush information dynamically.[7] Thus, reorganization could occur, based on the existence of multiple and overlapping redundancies organized hierarchically. These findings have shown that neuronal aggregates, beside or outlying a lesion, can increasingly adopt the function of the damaged area and switch their own activation pattern to substitute the lesioned structure while facilitating functional recovery.[6]

In this context, the concept of the brain connectome has recently emerged. This concept captures the characteristics of spatially distributed dynamic neural processes at multiple spatial and temporal scales.[8] The new science of brain connectomics is contributing to both theoretic and computational models of the brain as a complex system, and experimentally to new indices and metrics (eg, nodes, hubs, efficiency, modularity)

in order to characterize and scale the functional organization of the healthy and diseased CNS.[9] However, in pathology, neural plasticity is possible only if the subcortical connectivity is preserved, to allow spatial communication and temporal synchronization among large interconnected networks, according to the principle of hodotopy.[10,11] Although distinct patterns of subcortical plasticity were identified, namely unmasking of perilesional latent networks, recruitment of accessory pathways, introduction of additional relays within neuron-synaptic circuits, and involvement of parallel long-distance association pathways, the real capacity to build a new structural connectivity (so-called rewiring) leading to functional recovery have not yet been shown in humans.[12]

THE TIME COURSE OF DISEASES AND CENTRAL NERVOUS SYSTEM RESHAPING

In contrast with acute lesions such as stroke or traumatic cerebral injury, DG is a progressively growing tumor that invades the CNS over weeks/months (high-grade gliomas) or even over years (low-grade gliomas). For example, this slow time course explains why patients with low-grade gliomas usually have no or only mild functional deficits, despite the frequent involvement of eloquent structures,[13] because these lesions induce progressive functional brain reshaping. In high-grade gliomas, because of their more rapid growth, neurologic deficits are more frequent at the time of diagnosis. However, because of facilitated access to neuroimaging, many patients with anaplastic glioma or glioblastoma now show only slight or moderate neurologic deficits at the time of diagnosis, supporting some degree of neural reorganization. Therefore, neuroplasticity cannot be fully understood without considering the temporal pattern of the cerebral injury.[4] In stroke, even if many patients improve within the months following damage, only around 25% of patients totally recover, whereas more than 90% of patients with diffuse low-grade glioma (DLGG) (same location as stroke) have a normal neurologic examination.[14]

Using a neurocomputational model based on the training of a series of parallel distributed processing neural network models, a recent study simulated acute versus slow-growing injuries.[15] A very different pattern emerged in the simulation of DG compared with the simulation of stroke, with slow decay of the links within the same subnetwork leading to minimal performance decline, in agreement with the patient literature. Moreover, at the end of the decay regimen, the entire affected hidden layer could be removed on the simulation with no effect on performance, which closely matches the lack of major impairment from DG resection. This finding is likely caused by abrupt stroke causing rapid neuronal death, whereas DG initially spares neuronal tissue and thus gives time for cerebral remapping. Thus, the functional status at the time of diagnosis might be a good reflection of the natural history of the disease.

PREOPERATIVE FUNCTIONAL REALLOCATION IN PATIENTS WITH DIFFUSE GLIOMA

Concerning the neural foundations of functional compensation in DG before any treatment, the patterns of reorganization may differ between patients. Preoperative functional neuroimaging has shown that 4 kinds of preoperative functional redistribution are possible in patients without any deficit[1]: (1) function still persists within DG, thus there is a very limited chance to perform a fair resection; (2) eloquent areas are redistributed around the tumor, thus there is a reasonable chance to perform at least a near-total resection despite a likely immediate transient deficit and subsequent recovery; (3) a preoperative compensation by remote areas within the lesional hemisphere has occurred; (4) areas are recruited in the contralateral hemisphere and, in the 2 last patterns, the chances to achieve a total resection are very high, with only a slight and transient worsening. These different patterns can be associated. Therefore, in DG involving eloquent areas, plasticity mechanisms seem to be based on a hierarchically organized model; that is, first there is intrinsic reorganization within injured areas (index of favorable outcome); second, when this reshaping is not sufficient, other regions implicated in the functional network are recruited, in the ipsilateral hemisphere (close or even remote to the tumoral site) and then in the contralateral hemisphere if necessary.[3,16,17]

To sum up, as recently supported by magneto-encephalography study, a focal DG disturbs the functional and effective connectivity within the whole brain, and not only in restricted areas around the tumor.[18] These network dysfunctions are related to cognitive processing in patients with DG.[19] When objective neuropsychological and health-related quality-of-life assessments have been performed, visuospatial, memory, attention, planning, learning, emotional, motivational, and behavioral deficits have regularly been observed in patients with glioma.[20] These results show that brain plastic potential has limitations, which should be studied at the individual level. Because surgical treatment itself may induce changes in large-scale functional connectivity,[21] such knowledge of individual patterns of remapping should be taken into account in order to tailor personalized therapeutic management in patients with DG.

INTRAOPERATIVE PLASTICITY IN DIFFUSE GLIOMA SURGERY

Intrasurgical Electrostimulation Mapping

During surgery for DG, especially in eloquent areas, it has become common clinical practice to awaken patients in order to assess the functional role of restricted cerebral regions. Surgeons can maximize the extent of resection, and thereby improve the overall survival, without generating functional impairments, thanks to the individual mapping and preservation of critical structures.[22] Therefore, resection is not performed according to purely anatomic and oncological limits, but up to functional boundaries.[23] Patients perform several sensorimotor, language, cognitive, and emotional tasks while the surgeon temporarily interacts with discrete areas within the gray and white matter around the tumor, using direct electrostimulation mapping (DEM). If the patients stops to perform the task or produces an incorrect response, the surgeon avoids removing the stimulated site.[24,25] DEM transiently interacts locally with a small cortical or axonal site but also nonlocally, because focal perturbation disrupts the whole subnetwork sustaining a given function.[26,27] Thus, DEM represents a unique opportunity to identify with great accuracy and reproducibility, in vivo in humans, the structures that are crucial for brain functions both at cortical and subcortical (white matter and deep gray nuclei) levels[11] (**Figs. 18.1** and **18.2**).

Task Selection for Intrasurgical Cognitive Mapping

Optimal selection of the tasks used during intraoperative mapping is essential to preserve a normal life.[28] For example, language mapping can be used to identify possible crucial epicenters in the right, nondominant, hemisphere in left-handers or ambidextrous patients (and even in some right-handers) if language disturbances are detected on the preoperative cognitive assessment, even in cases of left-lateralization on functional MRI.[29] The aim is to map the neural circuits underpinning the different but interactive subfunctions, which should be preserved intraoperatively, by serving as boundaries of resection. DEM allows the mapping of many functions, such as movement

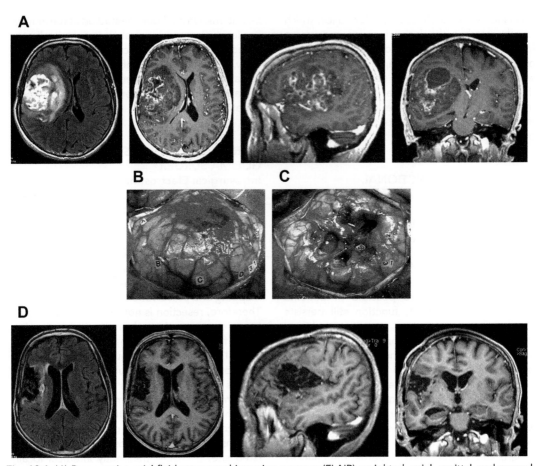

Fig. 18.1 (*A*) Preoperative axial fluid-attenuated inversion recovery (FLAIR)–weighted, axial, sagittal, and coronal enhanced T1-weighted MRI in a 54-year-old right-handed woman who experienced seizures, showing a high-grade glioma involving the right central region. The preoperative neurologic examination revealed a slight left central palsy, with no cognitive disorders. (*B*) Intraoperative view before resection. The anterior part of the right hemisphere is on the left and its posterior part is on the right. Letter tags correspond with the projection on the cortical surface of the tumor limits identified using ultrasonography. Number tags show areas of positive DEM in the precentral gyrus, as follows: (1) primary motor cortex of the tongue; (2) primary somatosensory cortex of the face; (3) primary motor cortex of the face. (*C*) Intraoperative view after resection, performed up to eloquent structures, both at cortical and subcortical levels. DEM of white matter tracts allowed the detection of the pyramidal tract in the depth (tag 50, used as deep functional limit of surgical resection). (*D*) Postoperative axial FLAIR-weighted, axial, sagittal, and coronal enhanced T1-weighted MRI, showing a complete resection of the enhancement and a subtotal removal of the FLAIR hypersignal. After administration of chemotherapy and radiotherapy, the patient resumed a normal familial, social, and professional life, with no functional deficits (2 years of follow-up).

(including control of bimanual coordination)[30]; somatosensory function[31]; visual function[32]; auditory-vestibular function[33]; spatial awareness[34]; language, including spontaneous speech and counting, object naming, verbal comprehension, writing, reading, syntax, bilingualism, switching from one language to another (see Ref.[35] for a recent model of anatomofunctional connectivity of language based on DEM); higher-order functions such as calculation, memory, attention, cognitive control, cross-modal judgement, nonverbal comprehension[11,36–38]; mentalizing; and consciousness.[39–42]

Acute Functional Remapping During Diffuse Glioma Surgery

First, intraoperative stimulation mapping before resection can confirm the functional reshaping induced by DG, as supposed using preoperative functional neuroimaging.[1,3] Nonetheless, recent studies comparing preoperative functional MRI with intraoperative DEM have shown a low reliability of neuroimaging, in particular for high-grade gliomas, with a sensitivity of only 37.1% and a specificity of only 83.4% for language mapping, showing that this technique is not reliable enough for it to be used in clinical practice.[43]

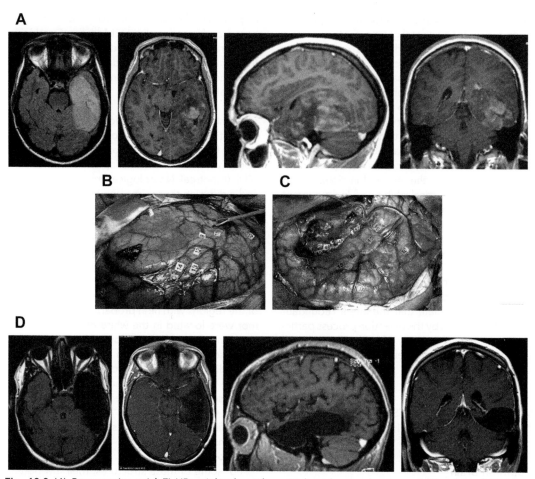

Fig. 18.2 (*A*) Preoperative axial FLAIR-weighted, axial, sagittal, and coronal enhanced T1-weighted MRI in a 42-year-old right-handed woman who experienced some language disorders (missing words), showing a high-grade glioma involving the left temporal region. The preoperative neurologic examination revealed naming and reading disturbances. (*B*) Intraoperative view before resection. The anterior part of the left hemisphere is on the right and its posterior part is on the left. Letter tags correspond with the projection on the cortical surface of the tumor limits, identified using ultrasonography. Number tags show areas of positive DEM in the precentral gyrus, as follows: (10) ventral premotor cortex (eliciting complete anarthria when stimulated); (11–15) naming sites (within the superior temporal gyrus) generating anomia or semantic paraphasia during stimulation. (*C*) Intraoperative view after resection, performed up to eloquent structures, both at cortical and subcortical levels. DEM of white matter tracts allowed the detection of the subcortical pathways, as follows: (47) inferior fronto-occipital fascicle (generating semantic paraphasia when stimulated); (46) optic radiations (eliciting visual field deficit during stimulation); (48) posterior part of the inferior longitudinal fascicle (inducing reading disturbances when stimulated); (49) temporal part of the arcuate fascicle (generating phonological paraphasia during DEM). All of these subcortical pathways have been used as deep functional limits of surgical resection. (*D*) Postoperative axial FLAIR-weighted, axial, sagittal, and coronal enhanced T1-weighted MRI, showing a complete resection of the glioma. After administration of chemotherapy and radiotherapy, the patient resumed a normal familial, social, and professional life, with no functional deficits (7 years of follow-up).

Regarding intrasurgical plasticity, a remarkable observation concerns the existence of acute functional remapping triggered by the resection itself and taking place within 30 to 60 minutes of beginning the surgery. This type of acute reorganization has been well documented in the sensorimotor system. In several patients harboring a frontal lesion, although stimulation of the precentral gyrus induced motor responses only at the level of a limited number of cortical sites before resection, an acute unmasking of redundant motor sites located within the same precentral gyrus, and eliciting the same movements as the previous adjacent sites when stimulated, was observed immediately following lesion removal.[44] Acute unmasking of redundant somatosensory sites was also regularly observed within the retrocentral gyrus in patients operated on for a parietal glioma. Furthermore, it was equally possible to detect a redistribution within a larger network involving the whole rolandic region; that is, with unmasking of functional homologues located in the precentral gyrus for the first cortical representation and in the retrocentral gyrus for its redundancy (or vice versa).[45] The most likely hypothesis suggests that a local increase of cortical excitability allows an acute unmasking of latent functional redundancies (ie, multiple cortical representations of the same function), via a decrease of intracortical inhibition.[6] In agreement with this idea, animal models have shown that focal brain damages induce large zones of enhanced cortical excitability in both the lesioned and the intact hemispheres.[46] Likewise, human studies have provided evidence that the level of intracortical inhibition is reduced in the damaged hemisphere in patients with stroke.[47] Therefore, it is tempting to speculate that the latent redundant networks revealed by the resection process participate in functional recovery. This idea fits well with the importance of adjacent reorganizations for behavioral recuperation.

WHITE MATTER TRACTS AS THE LIMIT OF NEURAL PLASTICITY: THE CONCEPT OF HODOTOPY

Subcortical Connectivity and the Minimal Common Brain

Although the plastic potential is high at the cortical level, subcortical plasticity is low, implying that axonal connectivity should be surgically preserved to allow postoperative compensation.[5,10–12] By combining cortical function and axonal connectivity, an updated model of CNS processing was proposed, moving from the localizationist model to a hodotopical framework. In pathology, a topological mechanism (from the Greek topos, meaning place) refers to a dysfunction of the cortex (deficit, hyperfunction, or a combination of both), whereas a hodological mechanism (hodos, meaning road or path) refers to dysfunction related to connecting pathways (disconnection, hyperconnection, or a combination of both).[48,49] Thus, clinicians should take into account the complex functioning of a large-scale distributed corticosubcortical network to understand its physiology as well as the functional consequences of a lesion in this circuit, with possible different deficits depending on the location and the extent of the damage (eg, purely cortical, or purely subcortical, or both).

Recently, probabilistic atlases of postsurgical residue and of functional plasticity were computed in patients who underwent resection for a DG based on intraoperative DEM.[10,50,51] Combining the intrasurgical functional data with postoperative anatomic imaging provided both a greater understanding of the functional limits of surgical removal, and new insights into neuroplasticity. These atlases provided a general framework to establish anatomofunctional correlations by computing for each brain voxel its probability to be left, because of its functional role, on the postoperative MRI. Their overlap with the cortical MNI (Montreal Neurological Institute) template and a diffusion tensor imaging tractography atlas offered a unique tool to analyze the potentialities and the limitations of interindividual variability and plasticity, both for cortical areas and axonal pathways. These atlases highlighted the crucial role of the axonal pathways in postlesional reorganization. A low probability of residual tumors on the cortical surface was observed, whereas most of the regions with high probability of residual tumor were located in the white matter. Thus, the functions subserved by long-range projection and association fibers seem to be less subject to interindividual variability and reorganization than cortical sites (except in primary unimodal areas in a small set of neural hubs). Because these pathways define the surgical deep limits, and because DGs infiltrate these tracts,[52] subcortical connectivity constitutes the main obstacle to radical resection.[10,50,51]

For some of these structures, their low potential of remodeling could be explained because they act as input or output areas: input sites convey, or are the first relay of, information entering the brain, whereas output sites are the last relay or the fiber tracts sending information outside the brain. These areas include the primary motor and somatosensory areas, the corticospinal and thalamocortical tracts, and the optic radiations (ie, the projection fibers). These areas are mainly unimodal and organized serially. The absence of a parallel alternative pathway explains the impossibility of restoring their function after any damage.[12] For all other areas, their nonresectability should be analyzed within a network perspective. High-order cognitive processes are mediated by short-range and long-range networks, with cortical epicenters connected by U-shaped fibers, associative and commissural pathways, and a particular network topology (like the small word one) is required to allow proper synchronization between several distant areas.[53] As mentioned, a local lesion can disturb a whole network, which in turn could ultimately hamper the function sustained by this network. For example, beyond the posterior part of the left superior temporal gyrus, subcortical structures like the inferior fronto-occipital fascicle (IFOF) and arcuate fascicle (AF) are nonresectable because their lesions would cause such major changes in the network that the dynamic plastic potential would be overwhelmed.[11] Note that areas such as the left posterosuperior temporal gyrus are considered as hubs in revisited models of cognition.[54,55] These functional epicenters allow a plurimodal integration of multiple data coming from the unimodal areas. This integration may lead to conceptualization, performed at the level of a wide network that includes the hubs. These hubs are interconnected by subcortical pathways, themselves crucial for brain function; for example, the AF, which enables a direct communication between the posterior temporal and frontal plurimodal regions. The reproducibility of these results, despite the interindividual anatomofunctional variability and plastic mechanisms, may suggest the existence of a minimal common brain, necessary for the basic cognitive functions, even if it is not likely to be sufficient for more complex functions such as multiprocessing.[10] This hypothesis is in good agreement with recent biomathematical models analyzing the effect of a simulated focal lesion on the whole-brain network topology.[56] For these areas, even biological plasticity would fail in the long term to repair the connectivity required to rebuild an effective network topology, hence a functional circuit.[12]

In summary, these atlases shed new light on the topological organization of CNS, may be useful in predicting the likelihood of recovery (as a function of lesion topology), and thus give an objective preoperative estimation of the expected extent of resection for DG resected under intraoperative DEM. This rationale assists neurosurgeons in decisions regarding surgical resection and may contribute to the elaboration of a therapeutic consensus for DG.[50]

Anatomofunctional Subcortical Connectivity Subserving Neural Functions

Neurosurgeons should therefore improve their knowledge of white matter circuitry. As mentioned earlier, because DG migrates along the main projection, commissural, and long-distance association bundles,[52] the optimal therapeutic approach cannot be defined without understanding the organization of individual neural networks. Cognitive neurosciences are closely related to neurooncology, because the use of DEM also provides new insights into the circuits mediating cognitive and behavioral functions.

For example, beyond the corticospinal (pyramidal) and thalamocortical (somatosensory) tracts,

the functional connectivity underpinning movement planning and execution also includes the negative motor network, partly subserved by the frontostriatal tract.[30,57] The visuospatial network is subserved not only by the optic radiations[32] but also by the inferior longitudinal fascicle (ILF), which is critical for visual recognition,[58] and part II of the superior longitudinal fascicle (SLF), which is crucial for spatial cognition, especially in the right hemisphere.[34] Language is mediated by dorsal and ventral pathways. Schematically, the medial part of dorsal stream (AF) subserves phonological and repetition processing,[35,59] and the lateral part of the SLF subserves speech articulation, and also represents the limiting factor of plastic potential of the left ventral premotor cortex.[60] The ventral stream, mainly underlain by the IFOF (direct ventral route), subserves language semantics,[61,62] whereas the ILF (indirect ventral route) is involved in lexical retrieval and reading.[63] Concerning the network sustaining mentalizing (theory of mind), which is crucial for emotion and social cognition, intraoperative DEM combined with preoperative and postoperative behavioral examinations showed that this function is made possible by parallel functioning of 2 subsystems: accuracy of identification (mirror system; ie, the ability to appreciate other people's emotions) and attribution of mental states (high-level inferential mentalizing) are subserved by the AF/SLF complex and the cingulum, respectively.[39,40]

To sum up, the vision of the neural basis of cognition begins to shift. For a long time, cognitive functions were conceived in associationist terms of centers and pathways, the general assumption being that information is processed in localized cortical regions with the serial passage of information between areas through white matter tracts. In the hodotopical account, brain functions are conceived as resulting from parallel delocalized processing performed by distributed groups of connected neurons rather that individual centers. In contrast with serial models in which 1 process must be finished before the information accedes to another level of processing, these new models of independent networks state that different processing can be performed simultaneously with interactive feedbacks. In this connectomal view, neurologic function comes from the synchronization between different epicenters, working in phase during a given task, and explaining why the same hub may take part in several functions depending on the other cortical areas with which it is temporarily connected at any time. Brain processing therefore should not be conceived as the sum of several subfunctions. Rather, cerebral function results from the integration and potentiation of parallel (although partially overlapped) subnetworks.[11]

To illustrate this multimodal model of brain networking, DEM showed the existence of an amodal executive system (including prefrontal cortex, anterior cingulum, and caudate nucleus) involved in the cognitive control of more dedicated subcircuits; for instance, the subnetwork underlying language switching in multilingual people (itself constituted by a wide corticosubcortical network comprising posterotemporal areas, supramarginal and angular gyri, inferior frontal gyrus, and SLF).[64] Similar reasoning can be applied to the multimodal (verbal and nonverbal) working memory and attentional functions, which seem to be supported by distinct subparts of the SLF, according to the data provided by axonal DEM combined with perioperative neurocognitive assessments.[59,65] Simultaneous recruitment of these subnetworks in addition to the distinct circuits specifically involved in language and visuospatial cognition are necessary if a person performs a sustained double task (eg, combination speech and line bisection test every 4 seconds throughout the resection) as regularly asked of awake patients during electrostimulation to increase the reliability of functional mapping, each axonal DEM being able to disrupt a specific subfunction with no consequences for the others.[11] The next step is to explore interaction between corticosubcortical circuits involved in different types of consciousness, such as noetic consciousness (the awareness of knowing and understanding the world and the self, while being aware of such an awareness)[38] and consciousness of the external environment.[41,42]

THE IMPLICATIONS OF NEUROPLASTICITY FOR DIFFUSE GLIOMA SURGERY

Maximal surgical resection is the first option in DG, whatever the grade, because it increases the overall survival, at least if a subtotal resection is achieved.[66–68] Consequently, the preoperative estimation of the extent of resection should be reliable. As mentioned, such a prediction directly depends on the involvement (or not) of subcortical pathways that cannot be functionally compensated, and it leads to the selection of surgery as a first treatment or, in contrast, to the proposal of a single biopsy followed by chemotherapy/radiotherapy, especially in patients with severe neurologic deficit not attributable to mass effect.[50] In patients without deficit on a standard neurologic examination, neuropsychological assessment is also required in the investigation of the individual plastic potential. If the patient has already experienced significant cognitive disorder, this means that the limits of neuroplasticity have been reached, preventing functional compensation. Such parameters should be incorporated in the surgical strategy in patients with DG in order to (1) extend the indications of resection in eloquent structures traditionally considered as inoperable; (2) maximize the extent of glioma removal, by performing the resection up to functional boundaries; and (3) preserve or even improve the quality of life.[22,23]

Owing to the phenomena of preoperative and intraoperative neuroplasticity, it is possible to remove DG with minimal morbidity while invading eloquent structures such as the rolandic area, Broca area, Wernicke area, or the insula[69–73] (see **Figs. 18.1** and **18.2**). Beyond the role of DEM in fundamental research, intraoperative electrical mapping and the hodotopical view of cerebral processing have dramatically improved the results of surgical neuro-oncology. In a recent meta-analysis of more than 8000 patients with glioma, DEM was found to be a well-tolerated procedure that identifies cortical and subcortical structures that are crucial for brain function, allowing surgery to be performed in eloquent areas previously considered unresectable (such as the Broca area or Wernicke area).[74] In addition, this approach reduces the risk of permanent postoperative neurologic deficits to less than 4%, even when operating in these crucial structures, and enables resections to be made according to functional limits, without a margin, thereby optimizing tumor removal and increasing overall survival. As a consequence, universal implementation of intraoperative DEM as standard of care for glioma surgery has been proposed.[74]

Nonetheless, when the tumor invades regions that are still crucial for a function, only incomplete DG resection can be performed. Recent findings from serial mapping have led to the proposal for a multistage surgical approach.[5,75] Following resection, the whole network can self-reorganize, explaining the good functional status within the weeks after surgery. Early and intensive postoperative functional rehabilitation plays a major role in optimizing the neurologic and cognitive recovery.[76] By performing serial investigations based on preoperative and postoperative functional neuroimaging following surgery in patients with DG with a complete recovery, a recruitment of perilesional areas and/or remote regions within the ipsilesional hemisphere and/or a recruitment of contralateral structures was observed.[75] Longitudinal changes in cerebellar and thalamic spontaneous neuronal activity have recently been shown using resting-state functional MRI.[77] Thus, a second surgery was proposed using intraoperative DEM, with the goal of validating the mechanisms of brain reorganization suggested but not proved by functional neuroimaging performed before the additional resection.[78] In a recent series of low-grade gliomas (at least at the time of the first surgery, because 58% had progressed to high-grade glioma when the second surgery was achieved), 74% of resections were complete or subtotal after reoperation, despite no additional serious neurologic deficit, and there was even an improvement in 16% of cases.[79] Seizures were reduced or disappeared in 82% of patients with epilepsy before the second operation. The median time between the two operations was 4.1 years, and all patients were still alive with a median follow-up of 6.6 years. Therefore, these original data showed that, thanks to mechanisms of neuroplasticity, patients with DG involving eloquent areas can be reoperated with a minimal morbidity and an increase of the extent of resection.[79] This multistage surgical approach can also be incorporated within a dynamic multimodal therapeutic management, in particular including chemotherapy, when a wide reresection is not possible for functional reasons.[78] Neoadjuvant chemotherapy was recently advocated in both low-grade glioma[80] and high-grade glioma,[81] to induce tumor shrinkage before an operation or a reoperation, but also possibly to facilitate functional redistribution.[82] By contrast, recent studies have shown that cerebral irradiation compromises neural architecture, especially by inducing significant reduction in dendritic complexity, synaptic protein levels, spine density, and morphology, such that a decrease in synaptic plasticity presents a risk of limiting the potential for brain reorganization.[83]

SUMMARY: NEUROPLASTICITY AND THE CONCEPT OF ONCOFUNCTIONAL BALANCE

The cognitive neurosciences represent a useful addition to neuro-oncology by providing new opportunities to elaborate therapeutic strategies, and thus to improve both quality of life and median survival. It is time to switch from a modular to a hodotopical (delocalized) and dynamic model of CNS processing. The combination of serial perioperative functional neuroimaging and intraoperative DEM has resulted in new individual and integrative models of functioning of neuronosynaptic circuits. Such networking models allow a better assessment of the dynamic potential of spatiotemporal reorganization of the parallel and interactive networks, namely the mechanisms of neuroplasticity, but

also a better understanding of its limitations, mainly represented by the subcortical connectivity.[11,51] In this framework, surgical resection of DG in areas classically considered as inoperable is possible while preserving brain functions. Therefore, based on this new concept of a hodotopical and plastic brain, the next surgical goal in DG will be to move toward personalized serial therapeutic management. The aim is to weigh the value of the extent of resection versus the neurologic worsening that could be voluntarily generated by a radical resection; that is, to study the oncofunctional balance at the individual level.[84] The benefit/risk ratio of different strategies of resection should be considered, according to the brain structures invaded and their plastic potential. The goal is to increase both the quantity of life and the time with a normal quality of life, based on strong interactions between the tumor course, brain reorganization, and a multistage surgical approach adapted to each patient over time: this makes possible the concept of functional surgical neuro-oncology.[85] In the era of evidence-based medicine, it is crucial not to forget individual-based medicine, taking into account the considerable interindividual anatomofunctional variability of the brain.[86]

REFERENCES

1. Duffau H. Lessons from brain mapping in surgery for low-grade glioma: insights into associations between tumour and brain plasticity. Lancet Neurol 2005;4:476–86.
2. Szalisznyo K, Silverstein DN, Duffau H, et al. Pathological neural attractor dynamics in slowly growing gliomas supports an optimal time frame for white matter plasticity. PLoS One 2013;8:e69798.
3. Duffau H. Brain plasticity and tumors. Adv Tech Stand Neurosurg 2008;3:3–33.
4. Desmurget M, Bonnetblanc F, Duffau H. Contrasting acute and slow growing lesions: a new door to brain plasticity. Brain 2007;130:898–914.
5. Duffau H. The huge plastic potential of adult brain and the role of connectomics: new insights provided by serial mappings in glioma surgery. Cortex 2014;58:325–37.
6. Duffau H. Brain plasticity: from pathophysiological mechanisms to therapeutic applications. J Clin Neurosci 2006;13:885–97.
7. Werner G. Brain dynamics across levels of organization. J Physiol Paris 2007;101:273–9.
8. Sporns O, Tononi G, Kötter R. The human connectome: a structural description of the human brain. PLoS Comput Biol 2005;1:e42.
9. Basset DS, Bullmore ET. Human brain networks in health and disease. Curr Opin Neurol 2009;22:340–7.

10. Ius T, Angelini E, Thiebaut de Schotten M, et al. Evidence for potentials and limitations of brain plasticity using an atlas of functional resectability of WHO grade II gliomas: towards a "minimal common brain". Neuroimage 2011;56:992–1000.

11. Duffau H. Stimulation mapping of white matter tracts to study brain functional connectivity. Nat Rev Neurol 2015;11:255–65.

12. Duffau H. Does post-lesional subcortical plasticity exist in the human brain? Neurosci Res 2009;65:131–5.

13. Duffau H. Diffuse low grade glioma in adults: natural history, interaction with the brain, and new individualized therapeutic strategies. London: Springer; 2013.

14. Varona JF, Bermejo F, Guerra JM, et al. Long-term prognosis of ischemic stroke in young adults. Study of 272 cases. J Neurol 2004;251:1507–14.

15. Keidel JL, Welbourne SR, Lambon Ralph MA. Solving the paradox of the equipotential and modular brain: a neurocomputational model of stroke vs. slow-growing glioma. Neuropsychologia 2010;48:1716–24.

16. Duffau H. Brain mapping: from neural basis of cognition to surgical applications. New York: Springer Wien; 2011.

17. Duffau H. Diffuse low-grade gliomas and neuroplasticity. Diagn Interv Imaging 2014;95:945–55.

18. Bartolomei F, Bosma I, Klein M, et al. How do brain tumors alter functional connectivity? A magnetoencephalography study. Ann Neurol 2006;59:128–38.

19. Bosma I, Douw L, Bartolomei F, et al. Synchronized brain activity and neurocognitive function in patients with low-grade glioma: a magnetoencephalography study. Neuro Oncol 2008;10:734–44.

20. Klein M, Duffau H, De Witt Hamer PC. Cognition and resective surgery for diffuse infiltrative glioma: an overview. J Neurooncol 2012;108:309–18.

21. Douw L, Baayen JC, Bosma I, et al. Treatment-related changes in functional connectivity in brain tumor patients: a magnetoencephalography study. Exp Neurol 2008;212:285–90.

22. Duffau H. The challenge to remove diffuse low-grade gliomas while preserving brain functions. Acta Neurochir (Wien) 2012;154:569–74.

23. Duffau H. Resecting diffuse low-grade gliomas to the boundaries of brain functions: a new concept in surgical neuro-oncology. J Neurosurg Sci 2015;69:361–71.

24. Duffau H. Contribution of cortical and subcortical electrostimulation in brain glioma surgery: methodological and functional considerations. Neurophysiol Clin 2007;37:373–82.

25. Duffau H. A new concept of diffuse (low-grade) glioma surgery. Adv Tech Stand Neurosurg 2012;38:3–27.

26. Mandonnet E, Winkler P, Duffau H. Direct electrical stimulation as an input gate into brain functional networks: principles, advantages and limitations. Acta Neurochir 2010;152:185–93.

27. Vincent M, Rossel O, Hayashibe M, et al. The difference between electrical microstimulation and direct electrical stimulation - towards new opportunities for innovative functional brain mapping? Rev Neurosci 2016;27(3):231–58.

28. Fernández Coello A, Moritz-Gasser S, Martino J, et al. Selection of intraoperative tasks for awake mapping based on relationships between tumor location and functional networks. J Neurosurg 2013;119:1380–94.

29. Vassal M, Le Bars E, Moritz-Gasser S, et al. Crossed aphasia elicited by intraoperative cortical and subcortical stimulation in awake patients. J Neurosurg 2010;113:1251–8.

30. Rech F, Herbet G, Moritz-Gasser S, et al. Disruption of bimanual movement by unilateral subcortical stimulation. Hum Brain Mapp 2014;35:3439–45.

31. Duffau H, Capelle L. Récupération fonctionnelle après résection de gliomes infiltrant l'aire somatosensorielle primaire (SI): étude par stimulations électriques per-opératoires. Neurochirurgie 2001;47:534–41.

32. Gras-Combes G, Moritz-Gasser S, Herbet G, et al. Intraoperative subcortical electrical mapping of optic radiations in awake surgery for glioma involving visual pathways. J Neurosurg 2012;117:466–73.

33. Spena G, Gatignol P, Capelle L, et al. Superior longitudinal fasciculus subserves vestibular network in humans. Neuroreport 2006;17:1403–6.

34. Thiebaut de Schotten M, Urbanski M, Duffau H, et al. Direct evidence for a parietal-frontal pathway subserving spatial awareness in humans. Science 2005;309:2226–8.

35. Duffau H, Moritz-Gasser S, Mandonnet E. A re-examination of neural basis of language processing: proposal of a dynamic hodotopical model from data provided by brain stimulation mapping during picture naming. Brain Lang 2014;131:1–10.

36. Duffau H, Denvil D, Lopes M, et al. Intraoperative mapping of the cortical areas involved in multiplication and subtraction: an electrostimulation study in a patient with a left parietal glioma. J Neurol Neurosurg Psychiatry 2002;73:733–8.

37. Plaza M, Gatignol P, Cohen H, et al. A discrete area within the left dorsolateral prefrontal cortex involved in visual-verbal incongruence judgment. Cereb Cortex 2008;18:1253–9.

38. Moritz-Gasser S, Herbet G, Duffau H. Mapping the connectivity underlying multimodal (verbal and non-verbal) semantic processing: a brain electrostimulation study. Neuropsychologia 2013;51:1814–22.

39. Herbet G, Lafargue G, Moritz-Gasser S, et al. Interfering with the neural activity of mirror-related frontal areas impairs mentalistic inferences. Brain Struct Funct 2015;220:2159–69.

40. Herbet G, Lafargue G, Bonnetblanc F, et al. Inferring a dual-stream model of mentalizing from associative white matter fiber disconnection. Brain 2014; 137:944–59.

41. Herbet G, Lafargue G, de Champfleur NM, et al. Disrupting posterior cingulate connectivity disconnects consciousness from the external environment. Neuropsychologia 2014;56:239–44.

42. Herbet G, Lafargue G, Duffau H. The dorsal cingulate cortex as a critical gateway in the network supporting conscious awareness. Brain 2016;139(Pt 4):e23.

43. Kuchcinski G, Mellerio C, Pallud J, et al. Three-tesla functional MR language mapping: comparison with direct cortical stimulation in gliomas. Neurology 2015;84:560–8.

44. Duffau H. Acute functional reorganisation of the human motor cortex during resection of central lesions: a study using intraoperative brain mapping. J Neurol Neurosurg Psychiatry 2001;70:506–13.

45. Duffau H, Sichez JP, Lehéricy S. Intraoperative unmasking of brain redundant motor sites during resection of a precentral angioma. Evidence using direct cortical stimulations. Ann Neurol 2000;47:132–5.

46. Buchkremer-Ratzmann I, August M, Hagemann G, et al. Electrophysiological transcortical diaschisis after cortical photothrombosis in rat brain. Stroke 1996;27:1105–9.

47. Cicinelli P, Pasqualetti P, Zaccagnini M, et al. Interhemispheric asymmetries of motor cortex excitability in the postacute stroke stage: a paired-pulse transcranial magnetic stimulation study. Stroke 2003;34:2653–8.

48. De Benedictis A, Duffau H. Brain hodotopy: from esoteric concept to practical surgical applications. Neurosurgery 2011;68:1709–23.

49. Ffytche DH, Catani M. Beyond localization: from hodology to function. Philos Trans R Soc Lond B Biol Sci 2005;360:767–79.

50. Mandonnet E, Jbabdi S, Taillandier L, et al. Preoperative estimation of residual volume for WHO grade II glioma resected with intraoperative functional mapping. Neuro Oncol 2007;9:63–9.

51. Herbet G, Maheu M, Costi E, et al. Mapping the neuroplastic potential in brain-damaged patients. Brain 2016;139(Pt 3):829–44.

52. Mandonnet E, Capelle L, Duffau H. Extension of paralimbic low grade gliomas: toward an anatomical classification based on white matter invasion patterns. J Neurooncol 2006;78:179–85.

53. Stam CJ. Characterization of anatomical and functional connectivity in the brain: a complex networks perspective. Int J Psychophysiol 2010;77:186–94.

54. Hickok G, Poeppel D. The cortical organization of speech processing. Nat Rev Neurosci 2007;8:393–402.

55. Ueno T, Saito S, Rogers TT, et al. Lichtheim 2: synthesizing aphasia and the neural basis of language in a neurocomputational model of the dual dorsal-ventral language pathways. Neuron 2011;72:385–96.

56. Alstott J, Breakspear M, Hagmann P, et al. Modeling the impact of lesions in the human brain. PLoS Comput Biol 2009;5:e1000408.

57. Kinoshita M, De Champfleur NM, Deverdun J, et al. Role of fronto-striatal tract and frontal aslant tract in movement and speech: an axonal mapping study. Brain Struct Funct 2015;220:3399–412.

58. Fernández Coello A, Duvaux S, De Benedictis A, et al. Involvement of the right inferior longitudinal fascicle in visual hemiagnosia: a brain stimulation mapping study. J Neurosurg 2013;118:202–5.

59. Moritz-Gasser S, Duffau H. The anatomo-functional connectivity of word repetition: insights provided by awake brain tumor surgery. Front Hum Neurosci 2013;7:405.

60. Van Geemen K, Herbet G, Moritz-Gasser S, et al. Limited plastic potential of the left ventral premotor cortex in speech articulation: evidence from intraoperative awake mapping in glioma patients. Hum Brain Mapp 2014;35:1587–96.

61. Duffau H, Gatignol P, Mandonnet E, et al. New insights into the anatomo-functional connectivity of the semantic system: a study using cortico-subcortical stimulations. Brain 2005;128:797–810.

62. Duffau H, Herbet G, Moritz-Gasser S. Toward a pluri-component, multimodal, and dynamic organization of the ventral semantic stream in humans: lessons from stimulation mapping in awake patients. Front Syst Neurosci 2013;7:44.

63. Zemmoura I, Herbet G, Moritz-Gasser S, et al. New insights into the neural network mediating reading processes provided by cortico-subcortical electrical mapping. Hum Brain Mapp 2015;36:2215–30.

64. Moritz-Gasser S, Duffau H. Evidence of a large-scale network underlying language switching: a brain stimulation study. J Neurosurg 2009;111:729–32.

65. Charras P, Herbet G, Deverdun J, et al. Functional reorganization of the attentional networks in low-grade glioma patients: a longitudinal study. Cortex 2014;63:27–41.

66. Capelle L, Fontaine D, Mandonnet E, et al. Spontaneous and therapeutic prognostic factors in adult hemispheric World Health Organization grade II gliomas: a series of 1097 cases. J Neurosurg 2013;118:1157–68.

67. Keles GE, Chang EF, Lamborn KR, et al. Volumetric extent of resection and residual contrast enhancement on initial surgery as predictors of outcome in adult patients with hemispheric anaplastic astrocytoma. J Neurosurg 2006;105:34–40.

68. Sanai N, Polley MY, McDermott MW, et al. An extent of resection threshold for newly diagnosed glioblastomas. J Neurosurg 2011;115:3–8.

69. Schucht P, Ghareeb F, Duffau H. Surgery for low-grade glioma infiltrating the central cerebral region: location as a predictive factor for neurological deficit, epileptological outcome, and quality of life. J Neurosurg 2013;119:318–23.

70. Benzagmout M, Gatignol P, Duffau H. Resection of WHO Health Organization grade II gliomas involving Broca's area: methodological and functional considerations. Neurosurgery 2007;61:741–52.

71. Plaza M, Gatignol P, Leroy M, et al. Speaking without Broca's area after tumor resection. Neurocase 2009;9:1–17.

72. Sarubbo S, Le Bars E, Moritz-Gasser S, et al. Complete recovery after surgical resection of left Wernicke's area in awake patient: a brain stimulation and functional MRI study. Neurosurg Rev 2012;35:287–92.

73. Duffau H. A personal consecutive series of surgically treated 51 cases of insular WHO Grade II glioma: advances and limitations. J Neurosurg 2009;110:696–708.

74. De Witt Hamer PC, Robles SG, Zwinderman AH, et al. Impact of intraoperative stimulation brain mapping on glioma surgery outcome: a meta-analysis. J Clin Oncol 2012;30:2559–65.

75. Gil Robles S, Gatignol P, Lehéricy S, et al. Long-term brain plasticity allowing multiple-stages surgical approach for WHO grade II gliomas in eloquent areas: a combined study using longitudinal functional MRI and intraoperative electrical stimulation. J Neurosurg 2008;109:615–24.

76. Herbet G, Moritz-Gasser S. Functional rehabilitation in patients with diffuse low-grade gliomas. In: Duffau H, editor. Diffuse low grade glioma in adults: natural history, interaction with the brain, and new individualized therapeutic strategies. London: Springer; 2013. p. 463–73.

77. Boyer A, Deverdun J, Duffau H, et al. Longitudinal changes in cerebellar and thalamic spontaneous neuronal activity after wide-awake surgery of brain tumors: a resting-state fMRI study. Cerebellum 2016;15(4):451–65.

78. Duffau H, Taillandier L. New concepts in the management of diffuse low-grade glioma: proposal of a multistage and individualized therapeutic approach. Neuro Oncol 2015;17:332–42.

79. Martino J, Taillandier L, Moritz-Gasser S, et al. Re-operation is a safe and effective therapeutic strategy in recurrent WHO grade II gliomas within eloquent areas. Acta Neurochir (Wien) 2009;151:427–36.

80. Blonski M, Pallud J, Gozé C, et al. Neoadjuvant chemotherapy may optimize the extent of resection of World Health Organization grade II gliomas: a case series of 17 patients. J Neurooncol 2013;113:267–75.

81. Voloschin AD, Louis DN, Cosgrove GR, et al. Neoadjuvant temozolomide followed by complete resection of a 1p- and 19q-deleted anaplastic oligoastrocytoma: case study. Neuro Oncol 2005;7:97–100.

82. Blonski M, Taillandier L, Herbet G, et al. Combination of neoadjuvant chemotherapy followed by surgical resection as a new strategy for WHO grade II gliomas: a study of cognitive status and quality of life. J Neurooncol 2012;106:353–66.

83. Parihar VK, Limoli CL. Cranial irradiation compromises neuronal architecture in the hippocampus. Proc Natl Acad Sci U S A 2013;110:12822–7.

84. Duffau H, Mandonnet E. The "onco-functional balance" in surgery for diffuse low-grade glioma: integrating the extent of resection with quality of life. Acta Neurochir (Wien) 2013;155:951–7.

85. Duffau H. Surgery of low-grade gliomas: towards a "functional neurooncology". Curr Opin Oncol 2009;21:543–9.

86. Duffau H. A two-level model of interindividual anatomo-functional variability of the brain and its implications for neurosurgery. Cortex 2016. [Epub ahead of print].

CHAPTER 19

General Principles of Immunotherapy for Glioblastoma

Andrew I. Yang, MD, MS[a], Marcela V. Maus, MD, PhD[b],
Donald M. O'Rourke, MD[a],*

BACKGROUND

Despite trimodal therapy consisting of maximal safe resection and adjuvant partial radiotherapy with concurrent and subsequent temozolomide, glioblastoma (GBM) has a dismal prognosis, with a median survival of 14.6 months and an overall survival of only 9.8% at 5 years.[1]

Further contributing to therapeutic challenge is the intertumoral and intratumoral heterogeneity of GBM.[2] The strongest predictor for response to temozolomide according to Stupp and colleagues[1] was methylation of the MGMT (O6-alkylguanine DNA alkyltransferase) promotor. However, intratumoral heterogeneity in MGMT methylation status has been noted,[3,4] perhaps explaining the positive response to temozolomide in some patients with unmethylated GBMs. Furthermore, a small population of glioma cancer cells, postulated to be stem-like cells that are able to self-renew and produce diverse daughter cells, have been shown to be chemoresistant and radioresistant,[5–7] leading to inevitable tumor recurrence.

In this context, there has been considerable interest in an alternate approach to cancer therapy to further prolong survival and perhaps even offer a cure, namely by harnessing the unique specificity of the immune system. The central nervous system (CNS) has classically been considered immunologically less active, based on early experiments showing prolonged survival of skin grafts within the CNS compared with other sites.[8] This notion has historically been furthered by reports of isolation from the immune system imposed by the blood-brain barrier (BBB), absence of CNS lymphatic drainage, and immune incompetence of native antigen-presenting cells (APCs). In contrast, active immune responses in the CNS are common clinical entities, such as in multiple sclerosis or Alzheimer disease.

Recent developments argue against the dogma of the CNS as an immunologically isolated site. The BBB is disrupted by tissue injury and inflammation, notably in the setting of malignant gliomas, allowing entry of immune cells into the CNS.[9] Even in the absence of BBB disruption, peripheral immune cells can circumvent the BBB using trafficking signals.[10] Moreover, CNS T cells and antigens drain into cervical lymphatics via the subarachnoid space, along the olfactory nerve, and across the cribriform plate.[11,12] In addition, the resident macrophages of the CNS, microglia, can express major histocompatibility complex (MHC) class II antigens and induce differentiation of naive T cells.[13]

The association between infection and remission of cancer (the infection-remission coincidence) has been noted in the literature for more than a hundred years.[14] More recently, a retrospective, single-center, cohort study has reported a 2-fold survival benefit in patients with GBM who developed postoperative bacterial infections.[15] In addition, an inverse relationship between atopic disease and gliomas has also been observed in numerous reports (as reviewed in Ref.[16]). The US Food and Drug Administration (FDA) approval of the antigen-specific agent sipuleucel-T for prostate cancer in 2010, and an immune checkpoint inhibitor ipilimumab for

[a] Department of Neurosurgery, Perelman School of Medicine, University of Pennsylvania, HUP - 3 Silverstein, 3400 Spruce Street, Philadelphia, PA 19104, USA; [b] Cancer Center, Massachusetts General Hospital, Harvard Medical School, Room 7.219, Building 149, Thirteenth Street, Charlestown, Boston, MA 02129, USA
* Corresponding author.
E-mail address: donald.orourke@uphs.upenn.edu

metastatic melanoma in 2011, among others, has led to the emergence of cancer immunotherapy into the clinical mainstream. These developments, in addition to the dismal prognosis of patients with GBM with standard therapy, have sparked interest in the potential of harnessed immunotherapy for brain tumors.

Cancer immunotherapy can be broadly defined as therapy based on the immune system's ability to target and kill tumor cells. It can be classified by mechanism into immunomodulatory, passive, and active immunotherapy. Immunomodulatory therapy involves administration of interleukins, cytokines, and chemokines to enhance the antitumor activity of native effector cells. A phase III trial in recurrent GBMs is currently underway that involves inactivation of checkpoint mediators CTLA-4 (cytotoxic T-lymphocyte-associated protein 4) and PD-1 (programmed cell death protein 1).[17] Passive immunotherapy historically refers to administration of antibodies to target tumor antigens (eg, antibodies against the HER2 [human epidermal growth factor receptor 2]/neu receptor in breast cancer), and is currently undergoing resurgence in the form of transfer of ex vivo expanded effectors cells. In addition, active immunotherapy depends on activation of the patient's immune system with so-called tumor vaccines, a term that encompasses a variety of products. Examples of phase III trials of active immunotherapy in GBM include one based on dendritic cells (DCs) (NCT00045968), and another based on peptides (NCT01480479), the latter of which has recently been discontinued.

PEPTIDE TARGETING

Considerable effort has been invested in the peptide vaccine rindopepimut (also called cdx-110) targeting the tumor antigen epidermal growth factor receptor variant III (EGFRvIII). Rindopepimut is a peptide that spans the mutation site of EGFRvIII, conjugated to the immunogenic carrier protein keyhole limpet hemocyanin. Peptide vaccines have the advantage of being simple to manufacture compared with vaccines that require harvesting tumor or serum samples from patients. Three phase II trials of rindopepimut conducted on patients with newly diagnosed, EGFRvIII-positive GBM have shown promising results, with reports of overall survival of 24 to 26 months (Fig. 19.1). Most tumors showing progression no longer expressed EGFRvIII. According to the immunoediting hypothesis,[18] this finding suggests that rindopepimut was effective in eradicating its target cell population via immunologic pressure. A phase II trial in recurrent GBM showed a survival advantage of 11.6 versus 9.3 months with the addition of rindopepimut to bevacizumab.[19] In spite of these early successes, a phase III trial of rindopepimut for newly diagnosed GBM[20] has recently been discontinued with an interim analysis showing equivalent overall survival in the treatment group (20.4 months) versus control (21.1 months).[21] These results emphasize that further work is needed to refine the peptide vaccine approach for EGFRvIII.

EGFRvIII is expressed on the cell surfaces in approximately 30% of all human GBMs,[22–24] representing the most common epidermal growth

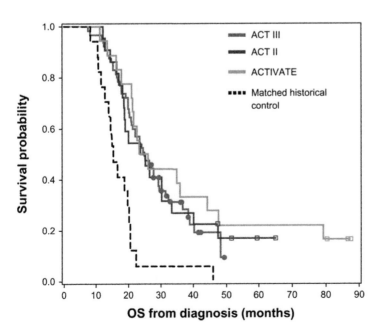

Fig. 19.1 Kaplan-Meier curves of overall survival of newly diagnosed patients with GBM receiving the peptide EGFRvIII vaccine in each of the 3 phase II studies. ACT, adoptive cellular therapy; OS, overall survival. (From Babu R, Adamson DC. Rindopepimut: an evidence-based review of its therapeutic potential in the treatment of EGFRvIII-positive glioblastoma. Core Evid 2012;7:98; with permission.)

factor receptor (EGFR) mutation. More recently, this has been confirmed by custom next-generation sequencing–based assay on RNA from tissue specimens.[25] EGFRvIII is known to enhance tumor invasiveness,[26] cell motility,[27] and chemoradioresistance,[28,29] and is independently associated with a poorer prognosis.[30] Because this mutation promotes tumorigenesis, it likely represents a driver mutation unique to cancer cells, and indeed it has shown specificity for tumor cells.[31] Moreover, EGFRvIII has also been shown to be expressed in a subpopulation of GBM cells that share properties of cancer stem cells.[32]

Peptides have also been targeted through the use of tumor-derived heat shock proteins (HSP). HSPs function in antigen carriage and in the targeting and activation of APCs, including DCs, which then leads to priming of the immune system's effector cells. This family of proteins is upregulated by cellular stressors; for example, heat, hypoxia, infection, and malignant transformation. Only HSPs derived from tumor cells, and when complexed to tumor antigens, are capable of inducing antitumor immunity.[33] Hence, HSP vaccines require HSPs complexed to antigen peptides (HSP-protein complexes), procured from the patient's tumor.

Most HSP vaccine trials have been based on prophages (also called HSP-96 protein complex), using a tumor-lysate approach. HSP-96 has notable substrates implicated in tumorigenesis, including EGFRvIII, platelet-derived growth factor receptor (PDGFR), FAK, AKT, p53, and phosphatidylinositol 3 kinase (PI3K). In a phase II trial for recurrent GBM, median overall survival was 90.2% at 6 months, and 29.3% at 12 months.[34] Another trial in newly diagnosed GBMs showed a median overall survival of 23.8 months.[35] A phase II trial of prophages in combination with bevacizumab for recurrent GBMs is currently underway (NCT01814813).

VIRAL VACCINES

Tumor vaccines based on viruses have also been widely studied, in which viruses are used as vectors for either in vitro or in vivo gene transfer, with the goal of expressing a protein that kills cells directly (so-called suicide gene therapy) or activating the immune system to kill the target cells (**Fig. 19.2**).[36] Viruses are particularly effective vectors because they are often tropic to certain cells. The most investigated suicide gene is that encoding type I herpes simplex virus thymidine kinase (HSV1-TK), which monophosphorylates the antiviral drug ganciclovir. The

monophosphorylated ganciclovir is then converted by the host cell into triphosphate ganciclovir, and is subsequently used in DNA synthesis. Triphosphate ganciclovir blocks chain elongation, halting cell division.

Initially, retroviral vectors were used to transduce the HSV1-TK system into brain tumors.[37] Because retroviral RNA must be converted into DNA before replication in the host cell, this vector was specific to proliferating cells actively synthesizing DNA. However, because most tumor cells are mitotically arrested, most cells were not transduced by retroviruses during HSV1-TK/ganciclovir therapy. Subsequent studies used adenoviral vectors, which allow transfer of genes into both dividing and nondividing cells, but this enhanced efficacy came at the expense of tumor specificity, and hence safety.[38]

ONCOLYTIC VIRAL THERAPY

Oncolytic viral therapy enables tumor-selective conditional viral replication, leading to local self-amplification in which lytic cell destruction and release of viral progeny maintain propagation of viral attacks throughout the tumor. The herpes simplex virus (HSV) shows natural neurotropism, and is clinically known to cause necrotizing encephalitis. Genetically engineered HSV, in which the machinery for DNA viral replication has been attenuated, allowed the conditional replication of viruses selectively in dividing cells.[39]

Adenoviruses have also been used in oncolytic therapy. Adenoviral gene products of E1A and E1B normally interact with host cellular control, allowing viral replication in host cells. Proteins from the E1A gene trigger cells to enter the S phase by inhibiting cellular retinoblastoma (pRb); E1B-encoded proteins suppress apoptosis by inactivating cellular p53.

Conditional replication in tumor cells has been made possible by deletion of these genes, as these tumor suppressor proteins are often dysregulated in malignant gliomas.[40] The E1B-deleted adenovirus (ONYX-015) has been studied in a phase I trial.[41] Although there were no significant toxicities, it did not have therapeutic efficacy. Notably, the ONYX-015 trial involved peritumoral injection of the oncolytic virus into brain tissue following fresh resection. The E2B-deleted adenovirus (Delta-24) has shown tumor selectivity,[42] and has been further engineered to target tumor-associated receptors (eg, integrins) on the surface of cancer cells (Delta-24-RGD; also called DNX-2401).[43] A phase I study of intratumoral and peritumoral injections of Delta-24-RGD for recurrent GBMs is currently underway.[44]

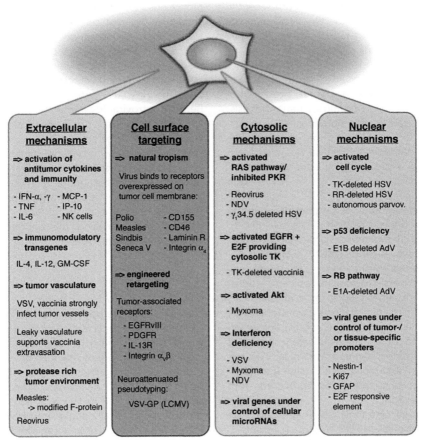

Fig. 19.2 Timeline of viral vaccine development for GBMs. AdV, adenovirus; GFAP, glial fibrillary acidic protein; GM-CSF, granulocyte-macrophage colony-stimulating factor; HSV, herpes simplex virus; IFN, interferon; IL, interleukin; IP, interferon-γ-inducible protein 10; LCMV, lymphocytic choriomeningitis virus; MCP-1, monocyte chemoattractant protein-1; NDV, newcastle disease virus; NK, natural killer; PKR, protein kinase R; TK, thymidine kinase; TNF, tumor necrosis factor; VSV, lymphocytic choriomeningitis virus; VSV-GP, lymphocytic choriomeningitis virus-glycoprotein. (*From* Wollmann G, Ozduman K, van den Pol AN. Oncolytic virus therapy for glioblastoma multiforme: concepts and candidates. Cancer J 2012;18(1):72; with permission.)

Polioviruses, clinically known to target motor neurons that can lead to poliomyelitis, show natural tropism to CE155 receptors overexpressed on tumor cell surfaces,[45] and have shown lytic growth in glioma cells.[46] Neurotoxicity of the poliovirus is mediated by its internal ribosome entry gene site.[46] An attenuated polio recombinant was engineered by replacing this element with its counterpart from the rhinovirus. A phase I trial is currently underway for recurrent GBMs, using a single intratumoral convection-enhanced delivery of the engineered poliovirus before tumor resection.[47]

Oncolytic viral therapy has the potential to combine multiple modes of action, including infection of endothelial cells leading to vascular collapse, direct viral destruction of infected tumor cells, and induction of innate and adaptive immune responses leading to destruction of both infected and neighboring tumor cells.[48]

DENDRITIC CELL VACCINES

A widely studied form of vaccine therapy is based on DCs. In contrast with tumor cells, which are poor APCs, DCs are considered professional APCs. Administration of tumor antigen–loaded DCs therefore represents an attractive strategy to generate tumor-specific effector cells. The first DC vaccine introduced was sipuleucel-T for prostate cancer, which was approved by the FDA in 2010. DC vaccines are developed from the patient's peripheral blood monocytes, which are differentiated into DCs in vitro, then pulsed with antigens (**Fig. 19.3**). Note that DC vaccines rely on endogenous T cells, which may limit its treatment effect because of the immunosuppressive nature of GBMs.[49]

DC vaccines have been developed targeting EGFRvIII. In a phase I trial for newly diagnosed GBMs,[50] immune response was confirmed

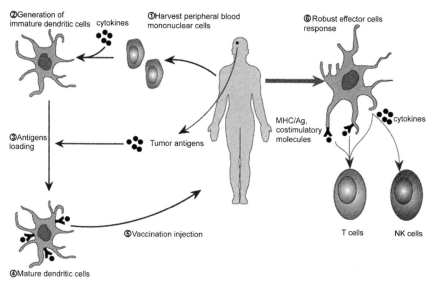

②Generation of immature dendritic cells cytokines

①Harvest peripheral blood mononuclear cells

⑥Robust effector cells response

③Antigens loading

Tumor antigens

MHC/Ag, costimulatory molecules

cytokines

④Mature dendritic cells

⑤Vaccination injection

T cells   NK cells

Fig. 19.3 Clinical application of DC vaccines. Ag, antigen. (*From* Wang Xiaowen TC. A Systemic review of clinical trials on dendritic-cells based vaccine against malignant glioma. J Carcinog Mutagen 2015;6(2):2; with permission.)

with proliferation of antigen-specific T cells in vitro, and with delayed-type hypersensitivity responses in vivo. There were no significant adverse effects.

Polyvalent DC vaccines, in which numerous tumor antigen epitopes are targeted, have also been reported to be safe in numerous studies, in spite of the theoretically increased risk of selection for autoreactive T cells. The ICT-107 vaccine was developed with autologous DCs pulsed with 6 tumor antigens overexpressed specifically in the cancer stem cell population (MAGE-1 [melanoma antigen-1], HER-2 [human epidermal growth factor receptor 2], AIM-2 [immunoselected melanoma-2], TRP-2 [tyrosinase-related protein-2], gp100 [glycoprotein 100], interleukin [IL]-13Rα2).[51] Median overall survival was promising at 38.4 months. A randomized phase II trial is currently under analysis.[52]

In another polyvalent DC vaccine, DC-Vax-L,[53] DCs were pulsed with tumor lysates prepared from resection specimens. Adverse effects were likewise not significant. Median overall survival rates in patients with either newly diagnosed or recurrent GBMs were also favorable relative to historical controls, at 31.4 months since the date of initial surgical diagnosis. A phase III trial of DC-Vax-L is currently underway.[54]

ADOPTIVE CELLULAR THERAPY AND CHIMERIC ANTIGEN RECEPTOR T CELLS

More recently there has been much interest in adoptive cellular therapy (ACT), which entails the administration of autologous or allogeneic antitumor lymphocytes. It is typically preceded by lymphodepletion in order to eliminate T-regulatory cells and native lymphocytes that compete for homeostatic cytokines, thereby providing an optimal environment for the transferred cells. Lymphocytes with the desired antitumor properties are selected and expanded ex vivo, and then infused into patients (**Fig. 19.4**).

Human ACT was first studied in melanomas, for which it required the identification of naturally occurring tumor-infiltrating lymphocytes (TILs) with high affinity for tumor antigens. Autologous TILs were harvested from resected melanoma specimens, expanded in vitro with IL-2, and then reinfused into patients.[55] In conjunction with a lymphodepleting regimen, TIL therapy led to objective responses in 50% to 70% of patients. Objective response in these patients correlated with persistence of the infused cells in vivo. Notably, administration of TILs was shown to lead to regressions at multiple metastatic sites, including the brain.[56]

TILs not only require surgery to procure tumor specimens but also cannot be reliably generated in all patients. This finding led to the development of genetically modified T cells, in which high-affinity T-cell receptors (TCRs) are introduced via viral gene transfer vectors into the patient's lymphocytes, generating T-cell clones with high affinity for the target tumor antigen. These TCRs have been generated by immunizing human leukocyte antigen (HLA) transgenic mice with the desired antigen peptide[57] or with phage display

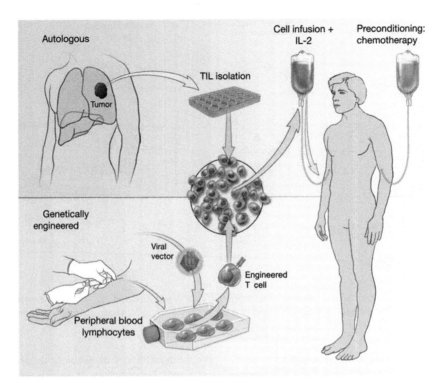

Fig. 19.4 Clinical application of ACT. TIL, tumor-infiltrating lymphocytes. (*From* Park TS, Rosenberg SA, Morgan RA. Treating cancer with genetically engineered T cells. Trends Biotechnol 2011;29(11):551; with permission.)

technology.[58] TCR-engineered T cells replicate the specificity of the parental clone for the tumor antigen.

One drawback of TCR therapy is that it imposes MHC class restriction to one HLA type, limiting therapeutic applicability to patients expressing that particular HLA type. Furthermore, TCR-engineered T cells cannot kill tumor cells that evade the immune system via downmodulation of MHC class I expression.[59] To address these limitations, T cells expressing chimeric antigen receptors (CARs) have been engineered. CARs consist of the tumor antigen–binding extracellular domain of a single-chain variable fragment antibody in place of the MHC-restricted TCR. These antigen-specific extracellular domains are then coupled to the nonspecific intracellular signaling domains of TCRs. CARs can be engineered with a much greater number of tumor antigen antibodies than the number of known antitumor TCRs. Notably, although TCRs can recognize both intracellular and extracellular peptide antigens, CARs require antigens to be present extracellularly. Moreover, CARs have the ability to target peptides, carbohydrates, and glycolipids.

CAR T-cell therapy (CAR-T therapy) directed to CD19 has been shown to lead to durable remissions in B-cell malignancies.[60] However, in solid tumors, lack of a surface antigen specific to cancer cells has been a limiting factor. On-target, off-tumor expression of the target antigen or cross reactivity to self-antigens has the potential to lead to significant toxicities.[61] This is particular relevant for CAR T cells because they have not undergone thymic selection.

CAR-T therapy and other ACTs fundamentally contrast with immunotherapeutics in which endogenous T-cell responses are induced (eg, peptide or DC vaccines), which are constrained by the native repertoire of T cells (ie, by tumor antigens that are processed by HLA for presentation at the cell surface). CAR-T therapy overcomes this limitation, potentially having efficacy against tumors with acquired defects in antigen processing and presentation. At present there are 2 phase I/II trials of CAR-T therapy for EGFRvIII-positive GBMs.[62] One is directed at recurrent GBM, and uses a retrovirus encoding the EGFRvIII CAR for transduction, in addition to costimulatory domains CD28 and 4-1BB (NCT01454596). The other was designed for recurrent or newly diagnosed GBM, and uses lentivirus with a 4-1BB costimulatory domain (NCT02209376). Preliminary data from the latter trial on 9 patients with multifocal, recurrent disease are promising, without any evidence of off-tumor toxicity. Five of the patients who underwent resection postinfusion showed infiltration of the CAR T cells, and, in some cases, loss of the EGFRvIII target antigen (ie, immunoediting).[63] Newly diagnosed GBMs will not be enrolled in NCT02209376.

Phase I trials of CAR-T therapy targeting other GBM antigens (ie, HER2 [NCT01109095] and IL-13Rα2 [NCT02208362]) are also underway for GBM not responsive to front-line therapy and recurrent GBMs. The former trial is notable for use of HER2 CAR T cells that are also specific for cytomegalovirus (CMV), a common virus present in most of the adult human population. CMV has not only been shown to be tropic to GBM cells,[64] but also implicated in its tumorigenesis in conjunction with glioma cancer stem cells.[65] The latter trial uses intratumoral or intracavitary catheters to deliver IL-13Rα2 CAR T cells, with preliminary data showing their infiltration into the tumor region and a decrease in tumor cells expressing IL-13Rα2 (not published).

LIMITATIONS AND CHALLENGES OF CANCER IMMUNOTHERAPY

In spite of the rapid pace of development in CAR-T therapy, there remain considerable challenges, many of which can be generalized to all forms of cancer immunotherapeutics.

Malignant gliomas are known to exert an immunosuppressive effect via alterations in either systemic or local immune responses.[66,67] In particular, the tumor microenvironment is infiltrated with immunosuppressive factors that hinder migration, survival, and effector functionality of T cells. Potential strategies to target immunosuppressive pathways are numerous: CAR T cells engineered to release cytokines, enhancing their antitumor activity; coadjuvant therapy such as supplemental oxygen to improve T-cell survival in the hypoxic tumor microenvironment. Moreover, markers of the tumor microenvironment, such as tumor-derived cytokines, can be used to improve the target precision of CAR-T therapy.

Immunologic escape, in which some tumor cells escape elimination from targeted immune responses, give rise to new cancer cells, and ultimately lead to recurrence,[68] represents a major barrier to the efficacy of CAR-T therapy. For example, in the case of EGFRvIII peptide vaccine therapy, 82% of patients with recurrence had lost EGFRvIII expression,[69] suggesting that targeting multiple antigens may be necessary. Recent proof-of-concept preclinical studies have shown the efficacy of CAR T cells that are bispecific to 2 distinct tumor antigens.[70] Supra-additive antitumor activity when both antigens are encountered has also been shown to be possible.[71]

More generally, there is a developing interest in combination therapy to enhance tumor response to CAR-T therapy. For example, combination with inhibitors of checkpoint receptors and ligands, which are overexpressed in the immunosuppressive tumor microenvironment, can aid in the trafficking of immune cells to the target.[72] Furthermore, combination with chemotherapy agents, either as lymphodepleting agents or as immunogenic modulators that sensitize tumors to CAR T cells, is under study. In preclinical studies of EGFRvIII CAR-T therapy, efficacy was highest when coadministered with temozolomide.[62] Furthermore, there is also preclinical evidence that radiation can enhance antigen presentation in tumor cells,[73] furthering the notion of synergistic combinations of immunotherapeutics with current standard of care.

The challenges in developing CAR-T therapy for mainstream medicine are the highly personalized nature of the therapy, and the expertise and logistics required in the handling, manufacturing, and administration of the cells. Cellular therapies are thus more difficult to commercialize compared with off-the-shelf drugs. In some ways, CAR-T therapy is more of a service than a drug, and experience with precedents such as sipuleucel-T will prove invaluable.

An important area of development entails noninvasive means to evaluate for genetic alterations (eg, EGFRvIII). At present this requires invasive methods (either brain biopsy or surgical resection) to procure tissue specimens for genetic and histopathologic analysis. With the wide application of not only anatomic MRI but also physiologic MRI in clinical medicine, an imaging biomarker for specific mutations has significant implications: selection of patients for preoperative debulking with targeted therapeutics; reduction of sampling error in light of tumoral heterogeneity with image-guided biopsies; characterization of residual tumor or recurrences in assessing patient eligibility or monitoring response to targeted therapies. Recent work has focused on MR perfusion-weighted imaging, given that tumoral angiogenesis and increased neovascularity are mediated in part by EGFRvIII expression. Preliminary evidence points to maximum relative tumor blood volume[23] and relative peak height[74] as potential biomarkers of EGFRvIII expression.

In addition, there are methodological hurdles in the design of clinical trials in cancer immunotherapy, and in metrics of success. In more than 500 patients with malignant glioma treated with DC vaccine therapy, objective responses based on radiological findings have been low, at 15.6%.[75] The dissociation between tumor burden and patient survival in immunotherapeutics is well recognized, in that the immediate clinical response to immunotherapy is the modulation of immune processes. Hence, outcomes measures such as the Response Evaluation Criteria in Solid Tumors or World Health Organization criteria, which were designed for cytotoxic agents, may not be appropriate.[76] The Immunotherapy Response Assessment in Neuro-oncology working group has redefined responses and disease progression based on the evolving understanding of immunotherapy kinetics and mechanism.[77] Ultimately, until the advent of a standardized biomarker, patient overall survival will be the definitive measure of therapeutic benefit.

REFERENCES

1. Stupp R, Hegi ME, Mason WP, et al. Effects of radiotherapy with concomitant and adjuvant temozolomide versus radiotherapy alone on survival in glioblastoma in a randomised phase III study: 5-year analysis of the EORTC-NCIC trial. Lancet Oncol 2009;10(5):459–66.
2. Sturm D, Bender S, Jones DTW, et al. Paediatric and adult glioblastoma: multiform (epi)genomic culprits emerge. Nat Rev Cancer 2014;14(2):92–107.
3. Hamilton MG, Roldán G, Magliocco A, et al. Determination of the methylation status of MGMT in different regions within glioblastoma multiforme. J Neurooncol 2011;102(2):255–60.
4. Natsume A, Kondo Y, Ito M, et al. Epigenetic aberrations and therapeutic implications in gliomas. Cancer Sci 2010;101(6):1331–6.
5. Chen J, Li Y, Yu T-S, et al. A restricted cell population propagates glioblastoma growth after chemotherapy. Nature 2012;488(7412):522–6.
6. Bao S, Wu Q, McLendon RE, et al. Glioma stem cells promote radioresistance by preferential activation of the DNA damage response. Nature 2006; 444(7120):756–60.
7. Liu G, Yuan X, Zeng Z, et al. Analysis of gene expression and chemoresistance of CD133+ cancer stem cells in glioblastoma. Mol Cancer 2006;5:67.
8. Medawar PB. Immunity to homologous grafted skin; the fate of skin homografts transplanted to the brain, to subcutaneous tissue, and to the anterior chamber of the eye. Br J Exp Pathol 1948;29(1):58–69.
9. Prins RM, Shu CJ, Radu CG, et al. Anti-tumor activity and trafficking of self, tumor-specific T cells against tumors located in the brain. Cancer Immunol Immunother 2008;57(9):1279–89.
10. Ransohoff RM, Kivisäkk P, Kidd G. Three or more routes for leukocyte migration into the central nervous system. Nat Rev Immunol 2003;3(7):569–81.
11. Cserr HF, Harling-Berg CJ, Knopf PM. Drainage of brain extracellular fluid into blood and deep cervical lymph and its immunological significance. Brain Pathol Zurich Switz 1992;2(4):269–76.
12. Goldmann J, Kwidzinski E, Brandt C, et al. T cells traffic from brain to cervical lymph nodes via the cribroid plate and the nasal mucosa. J Leukoc Biol 2006;80(4):797–801.
13. Carson MJ, Sutcliffe JG, Campbell IL. Microglia stimulate naive T-cell differentiation without stimulating T-cell proliferation. J Neurosci Res 1999; 55(1):127–34.
14. Hobohm U. Fever and cancer in perspective. Cancer Immunol Immunother 2001;50(8):391–6.
15. De Bonis P, Albanese A, Lofrese G, et al. Postoperative infection may influence survival in patients with glioblastoma: simply a myth? Neurosurgery 2011; 69(4):864–8 [discussion: 868–9].
16. Linos E, Raine T, Alonso A, et al. Atopy and risk of brain tumors: a meta-analysis. J Natl Cancer Inst 2007;99(20):1544–50.
17. Preusser M, Lim M, Hafler DA, et al. Prospects of immune checkpoint modulators in the treatment of glioblastoma. Nat Rev Neurol 2015; 11(9):504–14.
18. Dunn GP, Old LJ, Schreiber RD. The three Es of cancer immunoediting. Annu Rev Immunol 2004;22(1): 329–60.
19. Reardon DA, Desjardins A, Schuster J, et al. IMCT-08ReACT: long-term survival from a randomized phase II study of rindopepimut (CDX-110) plus bevacizumab in relapsed glioblastoma. Neuro Oncol 2015;17(Suppl 5):v109.
20. Swartz AM, Li Q-J, Sampson JH. Rindopepimut: a promising immunotherapeutic for the treatment of glioblastoma multiforme. Immunotherapy 2014; 6(6):679–90.
21. Data Safety and Monitoring Board Recommends Celldex's phase 3 study of RINTEGA® (rindopepimut) in newly diagnosed glioblastoma be discontinued as it is unlikely to meet primary overall survival endpoint in patients with minimal residual disease (NASDAQ: CLDX). Available at: http://ir.celldex.com/releasedetail.cfm?ReleaseID=959021. Accessed March 16, 2016.
22. Gan HK, Kaye AH, Luwor RB. The EGFRvIII variant in glioblastoma multiforme. J Clin Neurosci 2009; 16(6):748–54.
23. Tykocinski ES, Grant RA, Kapoor GS, et al. Use of magnetic perfusion-weighted imaging to determine epidermal growth factor receptor variant III expression in glioblastoma. Neuro Oncol 2012; 14(5):613–23.
24. Furnari FB, Fenton T, Bachoo RM, et al. Malignant astrocytic glioma: genetics, biology, and paths to treatment. Genes Dev 2007;21(21):2683–710.
25. Zhao J, Sukhadia S, Fox A, et al. Abstract 4916: development of a NGS-based method for EGFRvIII detection: sequence analysis of the junction. Cancer Res 2015;75(Suppl 15):4916.

26. Lal A, Glazer CA, Martinson HM, et al. Mutant epidermal growth factor receptor up-regulates molecular effectors of tumor invasion. Cancer Res 2002; 62(12):3335–9.

27. Boockvar JA, Kapitonov D, Kapoor G, et al. Constitutive EGFR signaling confers a motile phenotype to neural stem cells. Mol Cell Neurosci 2003;24(4): 1116–30.

28. Montgomery RB, Guzman J, O'Rourke DM, et al. Expression of oncogenic epidermal growth factor receptor family kinases induces paclitaxel resistance and alters beta-tubulin isotype expression. J Biol Chem 2000;275(23):17358–63.

29. Lammering G, Valerie K, Lin P-S, et al. Radiation-induced activation of a common variant of EGFR confers enhanced radioresistance. Radiother Oncol 2004;72(3):267–73.

30. Diedrich U, Lucius J, Baron E, et al. Distribution of epidermal growth factor receptor gene amplification in brain tumours and correlation to prognosis. J Neurol 1995;242(10):683–8.

31. Wikstrand CJ, Hale LP, Batra SK, et al. Monoclonal antibodies against EGFRvIII are tumor specific and react with breast and lung carcinomas and malignant gliomas. Cancer Res 1995;55(14):3140–8.

32. Morgan RA, Johnson LA, Davis JL, et al. Recognition of glioma stem cells by genetically modified T cells targeting EGFRvIII and development of adoptive cell therapy for glioma. Hum Gene Ther 2012;23(10):1043–53.

33. Udono H, Srivastava PK. Comparison of tumor-specific immunogenicities of stress-induced proteins gp96, hsp90, and hsp70. J Immunol 1994; 152(11):5398–403.

34. Bloch O, Crane CA, Fuks Y, et al. Heat-shock protein peptide complex–96 vaccination for recurrent glioblastoma: a phase II, single-arm trial. Neuro Oncol 2014;16(2):274–9.

35. Bloch O, Raizer JJ, Lim M, et al. Newly diagnosed glioblastoma patients treated with an autologous heat shock protein peptide vaccine: PD-L1 expression and response to therapy. ASCO Meet Abstr 2015;33(Suppl 15):2011.

36. Chiocca EA, Aguilar LK, Bell SD, et al. Phase IB study of gene-mediated cytotoxic immunotherapy adjuvant to up-front surgery and intensive timing radiation for malignant glioma. J Clin Oncol 2011; 29(27):3611–9.

37. Oldfield EH, Ram Z, Culver KW, et al. Gene therapy for the treatment of brain tumors using intratumoral transduction with the thymidine kinase gene and intravenous ganciclovir. Hum Gene Ther 1993;4(1):39–69.

38. Sandmair A-M, Loimas S, Puranen P, et al. Thymidine kinase gene therapy for human malignant glioma, using replication-deficient retroviruses or adenoviruses. Hum Gene Ther 2000;11(16):2197–205.

39. Mineta T, Rabkin SD, Yazaki T, et al. Attenuated multi-mutated herpes simplex virus-1 for the treatment of malignant gliomas. Nat Med 1995;1(9):938–43.

40. Puduvalli VK, Kyritsis AP, Hess KR, et al. Patterns of expression of Rb and p16 in astrocytic gliomas, and correlation with survival. Int J Oncol 2000;17(5):963–9.

41. Chiocca EA, Abbed KM, Tatter S, et al. A phase I open-label, dose-escalation, multi-institutional trial of injection with an E1B-Attenuated adenovirus, ONYX-015, into the peritumoral region of recurrent malignant gliomas, in the adjuvant setting. Mol Ther J Am Soc Gene Ther 2004;10(5):958–66.

42. Fueyo J, Gomez-Manzano C, Alemany R, et al. A mutant oncolytic adenovirus targeting the Rb pathway produces anti-glioma effect in vivo. Oncogene 2000;19(1):2–12.

43. Fueyo J, Alemany R, Gomez-Manzano C, et al. Preclinical characterization of the antiglioma activity of a tropism-enhanced adenovirus targeted to the retinoblastoma pathway. J Natl Cancer Inst 2003; 95(9):652–60.

44. Lang FF, Conrad C, Gomez-Manzano C, et al. First-in-human phase I clinical trial of oncolytic delta-24-RGD (DNX-2401) with biological endpoints: implications for viro- immunotherapy. Neuro Oncol 2014;16 (Suppl 3):iii39.

45. Merrill MK, Bernhardt G, Sampson JH, et al. Poliovirus receptor CD155-targeted oncolysis of glioma. Neuro Oncol 2004;6(3):208–17.

46. Gromeier M, Lachmann S, Rosenfeld MR, et al. Intergeneric poliovirus recombinants for the treatment of malignant glioma. Proc Natl Acad Sci U S A 2000;97(12):6803–8.

47. Goetz C, Gromeier M. Preparing an oncolytic poliovirus recombinant for clinical application against glioblastoma multiforme. Cytokine Growth Factor Rev 2010;21(2–3):197–203.

48. Kirn DH, Thorne SH. Targeted and armed oncolytic poxviruses: a novel multi-mechanistic therapeutic class for cancer. Nat Rev Cancer 2009;9(1):64–71.

49. Dix AR, Brooks WH, Roszman TL, et al. Immune defects observed in patients with primary malignant brain tumors. J Neuroimmunol 1999;100(1–2):216–32.

50. Sampson JH, Archer GE, Mitchell DA, et al. An epidermal growth factor receptor variant III-targeted vaccine is safe and immunogenic in patients with glioblastoma multiforme. Mol Cancer Ther 2009;8(10): 2773–9.

51. Phuphanich S, Wheeler CJ, Rudnick JD, et al. Phase I trial of a multi-epitope-pulsed dendritic cell vaccine for patients with newly diagnosed glioblastoma. Cancer Immunol Immunother 2013;62(1):125–35.

52. Wen P, Reardon D, Phuphanich S, et al. At-60a randomized double blind placebo-controlled phase 2 trial of dendritic cell (DC) vaccine ICT-107 following standard treatment in newly diagnosed patients with GBM. Neuro Oncol 2014;16(Suppl 5):v22.

53. Prins RM, Soto H, Konkankit V, et al. Gene expression profile correlates with T-cell infiltration and relative survival in glioblastoma patients vaccinated with dendritic cell immunotherapy. Clin Cancer Res 2011;17(6):1603–15.

54. Polyzoidis S, Ashkan K. DCVax®-L—developed by Northwest Biotherapeutics. Hum Vaccines Immunother 2014;10(11):3139–45.

55. Rosenberg SA, Yang JC, Sherry RM, et al. Durable complete responses in heavily pretreated patients with metastatic melanoma using T-cell transfer immunotherapy. Clin Cancer Res 2011;17(13):4550–7.

56. Hong JJ, Rosenberg SA, Dudley ME, et al. Successful treatment of melanoma brain metastases with adoptive cell therapy. Clin Cancer Res 2010;16(19):4892–8.

57. Parkhurst MR, Joo J, Riley JP, et al. Characterization of genetically modified T-cell receptors that recognize the CEA:691-699 peptide in the context of HLA-A2.1 on human colorectal cancer cells. Clin Cancer Res 2009;15(1):169–80.

58. Li Y, Moysey R, Molloy PE, et al. Directed evolution of human T-cell receptors with picomolar affinities by phage display. Nat Biotechnol 2005;23(3):349–54.

59. Facoetti A. Human leukocyte antigen and antigen processing machinery component defects in astrocytic tumors. Clin Cancer Res 2005;11(23):8304–11.

60. Maude SL, Frey N, Shaw PA, et al. Chimeric antigen receptor T cells for sustained remissions in leukemia. N Engl J Med 2014;371(16):1507–17.

61. Linette GP, Stadtmauer EA, Maus MV, et al. Cardiovascular toxicity and titin cross-reactivity of affinity-enhanced T cells in myeloma and melanoma. Blood 2013;122(6):863–71.

62. Johnson LA, Scholler J, Ohkuri T, et al. Rational development and characterization of humanized anti-EGFR variant III chimeric antigen receptor T cells for glioblastoma. Sci Transl Med 2015;7(275):275ra22.

63. O'Rourke D, Desai A, Morrissette J, et al. IMCT-15PI-LOT study of T cells redirected to EGFRvIII with a chimeric antigen receptor in patients with EGFRvIII+ glioblastoma. Neuro Oncol 2015;17(Suppl 5):v110–1.

64. Cobbs CS, Harkins L, Samanta M, et al. Human cytomegalovirus infection and expression in human malignant glioma. Cancer Res 2002;62(12):3347–50.

65. Dziurzynski K, Wei J, Qiao W, et al. Glioma-associated cytomegalovirus mediates subversion of the monocyte lineage to a tumor propagating phenotype. Clin Cancer Res 2011;17(14):4642–9.

66. Charles NA, Holland EC, Gilbertson R, et al. The brain tumor microenvironment. Glia 2011;59(8):1169–80.

67. Waziri A. Glioblastoma-derived mechanisms of systemic immunosuppression. Neurosurg Clin N Am 2010;21(1):31–42.

68. Khong HT, Restifo NP. Natural selection of tumor variants in the generation of "tumor escape" phenotypes. Nat Immunol 2002;3(11):999–1005.

69. Sampson JH, Heimberger AB, Archer GE, et al. Immunologic escape after prolonged progression-free survival with epidermal growth factor receptor variant III peptide vaccination in patients with newly diagnosed glioblastoma. J Clin Oncol 2010;28(31):4722–9.

70. Hegde M, Corder A, Chow KKH, et al. Combinational targeting offsets antigen escape and enhances effector functions of adoptively transferred T cells in glioblastoma. Mol Ther J Am Soc Gene Ther 2013;21(11):2087–101.

71. Grada Z, Hegde M, Byrd T, et al. TanCAR: a novel bispecific chimeric antigen receptor for cancer immunotherapy. Mol Ther Nucleic Acids 2013;2:e105.

72. Peng W, Liu C, Xu C, et al. PD-1 blockade enhances T-cell migration to tumors by elevating IFN-γ inducible chemokines. Cancer Res 2012;72(20):5209–18.

73. Lugade AA, Sorensen EW, Gerber SA, et al. Radiation-induced IFN-gamma production within the tumor microenvironment influences antitumor immunity. J Immunol 2008;180(5):3132–9.

74. Gupta A, Young RJ, Shah AD, et al. Pretreatment dynamic susceptibility contrast MRI perfusion in glioblastoma: prediction of EGFR gene amplification. Clin Neuroradiol 2015;25(2):143–50.

75. Anguille S, Smits EL, Lion E, et al. Clinical use of dendritic cells for cancer therapy. Lancet Oncol 2014;15(7):e257–67.

76. Wolchok JD, Hoos A, O'Day S, et al. Guidelines for the evaluation of immune therapy activity in solid tumors: immune-related response criteria. Clin Cancer Res 2009;15(23):7412–20.

77. Okada H, Weller M, Huang R, et al. Immunotherapy response assessment in neuro-oncology: a report of the RANO working group. Lancet Oncol 2015;16(15):e534–42.

CHAPTER 20

Early Detection of Glioblastoma

Javier M. Figueroa, MD, PhD, Bob S. Carter, MD, PhD*

HISTORICAL CONTEXT AND BIOLOGICAL BASIS

Early detection of solid tumors is vital for extending survival and possibly curing patients with cancer. This idea is especially relevant to patients with the most common and most lethal malignant brain tumor, glioblastoma (GBM), because earlier detection would likely increase not only survival but also quality of life. Historically, the more common malignancies, such as breast and colon cancer, paved the way for early discovery of these solid tumors, with mammogram and colonoscopy screenings saving countless lives. However, detecting solid tumors of the brain is a far more difficult task given that it is enclosed in the calvarium and imaging studies are not yet at the technical level to be considered fully diagnostic. In this regard, population-based screening with neurologic examinations and imaging is neither beneficial nor cost-effective.[1] As with other cancers, screening for GBM would require a diagnostic test that has low false-positive rates in order to prevent unnecessary and costly imaging studies and further clinical work-up. Thus, clinicians and researchers have been pursuing biomarkers in the serum and cerebrospinal fluid (CSF) in order to detect GBM early enough for meaningful treatment.

Analyzing biofluids for markers of malignancy was initially pioneered in colorectal cancer with the detection of increased carcinoembryonic antigen (CEA) levels in the serum.[2] However, levels of this normal physiologic protein were not always increased and were associated with numerous other cancer types, limiting its use as a diagnostic biomarker. Other biomarkers soon came to the forefront, such as prostate-specific antigen for prostate cancer and cancer antigen 125 (CA-125) for ovarian cancer; however, the specificities of these tests again failed to meet

requirements for a diagnostic test.[3,4] At present there are more than 20 US Food and Drug Administration–approved tumor biomarker proteins, most of which are used to monitor disease progression and response to therapy.[5] However, GBM does not have a reliable serum biomarker, and initial detection currently relies solely on the presentation of symptoms related to the tumor size and/or location. For this reason, early detection is essential in order to initiate treatment before the patient is symptomatic, which is likely to affect quality of life and progression-free survival.

The ability to detect GBM early, ideally before clinical symptoms arise, is beneficial in 2 distinct ways in the current paradigm of therapeutic management. First, early discovery results in surgical resection of a smaller tumor volume, with likely less impact on surrounding structures compared with that of a larger tumor that is detected only after clinical symptoms are presented (eg, symptoms of speech difficulty, seizures, paralysis). Given that GBM invades into the surrounding tissue, the primary resection of a smaller tumor may necessitate less removal of normal brain parenchyma to prevent recurrence. Secondly, on a molecular genetic level, the total cell count of smaller tumors indicates less genetic variation between the tumor stem cells and their progeny, which can affect their ability to escape both chemotherapy and radiation treatment. Larger tumors have more genetic diversity in their cells, some of which aids in resistance to therapy, evasion of immunosurveillance, and initiation of recurrence.

Specific surface markers and mutations present in GBM may allow early detection in the serum and/or CSF. CSF is especially interesting given that the brain is bathed in this fluid, and there is a greater chance of finding relevant biomarkers because there is no blood-brain barrier

Department of Neurosurgery, UC San Diego, 3855 Health Sciences Drive, La Jolla, CA 92093, USA
* Corresponding author.
E-mail address: BobCarter@ucsd.edu

to cross. However, collecting CSF is a more invasive process than collecting blood, hence discovery of a serum biomarker would be ideal. In addition, not all GBMs are alike and some respond better to different chemotherapeutic/radiation therapeutic regimens, so an ideal biomarker would be able to distinguish between the various molecular subtypes. Certain aberrations found in many GBMs, such as in the epithelial growth factor receptor (EGFR) and RNA profiling, as well as circulating tumor cells (CTCs) and extracellular vesicles (EVs), have the potential to diagnose GBM and also discriminate between classic, mesenchymal, and proneural subtypes. Thus, a reliable liquid biopsy from the serum or CSF would serve not only to improve GBM diagnosis but also would also affect treatment and surveillance for recurrence.

DEVELOPMENT AND EVIDENCE FOR BIOMARKERS

Early detection of GBM has focused on the search for tumor-specific biomarkers in the blood and CSF. In this regard, current research concentrates on identifying 3 distinct tumor-related elements; extracellular macromolecules, EVs, and CTCs. Investigations into these 3 categories span the range of biological locales for tumor-specific biomarker discovery, and combined have the potential to affect GBM screening and diagnosis.

Detection of Extracellular Macromolecules

Detection of free nucleic acid species in the serum and CSF is of particular interest in GBM because tumor-specific aberrations in DNA, messenger RNA (mRNA), or microRNA (miRNA) may be used to distinguish malignancy from normal tissue. Furthermore, nucleic acid signatures may be able to speciate between the various subtypes of GBM, provide prognostic information, and direct tumor-specific therapies.

Recently, the presence of circulating tumor DNA (ctDNA) in the serum of patients with brain tumors was reported by several groups.[6,7] As cells within the tumor begin to die and release intracellular content, ctDNA can be isolated from the serum and can give tumor-specific information about the molecular genetics of the malignancy. Specifically, methylation status of tumor suppressor genes and loss of heterozygosity (LOH) can be determined by analyzing ctDNA from patients with high-grade gliomas (HGGs).[6] Serum ctDNA analysis can determine the methylation status of O^6-methylguanine methyltransferase (MGMT) and phosphatase and tensin homolog (PTEN), as well as LOH in chromosomes 1p, 19q, and 10q,

with a sensitivity of 50% to 55% and a specificity of 100%.[6] Similarly, serum ctDNA can detect the presence of methylation in MGMT, RASSF1A, p15INK4B, and p14ARF in patients with malignant gliomas,[7] with a sensitivity of 50% and a specificity of 100%.[7] The poor sensitivity for these biomarkers in detecting intracranial tumors is likely related to the low concentration of tumor-specific ctDNA in serum, and suggests that CSF analysis could improve false-negative rates. Analysis of CSF has shown significantly higher concentrations of tumor-specific ctDNA compared with serum.[8,9] Isolated circulating tumor DNA (ctDNA) has been shown to detect tissue-concordant mutations in the following genes: NF2, AKT1, BRAF, NRAS, KRAS and EGFR.[8] Although the concentration of total ctDNA is less in CSF than in serum, the concentration of mutation-specific ctDNA and the mutant allelic frequency are higher in the CSF.[8,9] Furthermore, mutations in EGFR, PTEN, ESR1, IDH1, ERBB2, and FGFR2 are readily detectable in CSF ctDNA, with a sensitivity of 58%, compared with 0% for serum.[9] Together, the results of these studies indicate that analysis of free ctDNA in biofluids may be useful for early detection of mutation-specific intracranial brain tumors.

Because of the heterogeneity of tumors, not all malignant cells express the same genetic mutations, and investigating the RNA expression profile from biofluids may provide a more accurate real-time representation of the malignant process. Investigations into serum miRNA profiles show that patients with GBM have greater than 100 miRNAs that are significantly upregulated (highest: miR-340, miR-576-5p, and miR-626), as well as greater than 20 that are significantly downregulated (lowest: let-7g-5p, miR-7-5p, and miR-320), compared with normal healthy controls.[10] Others have shown that the serum levels of miR-185 are significantly increased in patients with GBM, and that these levels returned to normal after surgery and subsequent chemotherapy and radiation.[11] In addition, serum levels of miR-210 in patients with GBM correlate with both tumor grade and patient outcomes, compared with healthy controls.[12] In contrast, serum levels of miR-205 are significantly decreased in patients with gliomas, and correlate with tumor grade, Karnofsky Performance Scale, and overall survival.[13] Analysis of miRNA in the CSF of patients with GBM has also yielded some interesting results. CSF levels of miR-10b and miR-21 are significantly increased in patients with GBM, and miR-200 levels are only increased in patients with metastatic tumors of the central nervous system (CNS), enabling clinicians to distinguish metastases from primary malignancies with an accuracy of 91% to 99%.[14]

Similarly, levels of miR-223, miR-451, and miR-711 are also significantly increased in the CSF of patients with gliomas.[15] The results of these studies indicate that the panels of miRNAs in the CSF may be used to not only diagnose GBM but also distinguish it from other CNS tumors in the future.

The search for protein biomarkers in GBM has focused on aberrations in levels of normal physiologic secreted proteins, given that no tumor-specific proteins have been identified. This approach relies on the detection of proteins secreted into the serum or CSF from cells within the malignancy, in hopes of identifying levels at which clinicians can diagnose lesions as GBMs.

By far the most studied serum protein in patients with GBM is glial fibrillary acidic protein (GFAP), an intermediate filament highly expressed in glial cells. Several reports have found that increased GFAP levels in the serum can accurately diagnose GBM.[16-18] Overall, a GFAP level of greater than 0.05 ng/mL yields a sensitivity of 75% to 85% and a specificity of 70% to 100% for diagnosing patients with malignant gliomas.[16-18] Furthermore, increased GFAP levels correlate with a lack of IDH1 mutation,[18] and patients with non-GBM tumors did not have any detectable GFAP in their serum.[16] Several other studies have focused on proteins other than GFAP. Increased serum levels of both YKL-40 and matrix metalloproteinase 9 correlated with active intracranial tumors and decreased overall survival.[19] In addition, detecting increased serum levels of BMP2, HSP70, and CXCL10 results in a sensitivity of 96% and a specificity of 89% for diagnosing patients with HGGs.[20] The analysis of serum EGFR levels appeals to GBM researchers given that most of these tumors have increased DNA amplifications and RNA expression of wild-type EGFR (wtEGFR).[21] Patients with GBM with increased serum EGFR levels have poorer outcomes and decreased overall survival.[22] As with the other extracellular macromolecules, the search for protein biomarkers in the CSF may yield more GBM-specific proteins than in the serum. GFAP levels of greater than 0.04 μg/mL in the CSF correlate with the diagnosis of GBM, distinguishing this from other CNS malignancies and healthy controls.[23] Similarly, myelin basic protein (MBP), a protein unique to the CNS, is of interest as a biomarker in the CSF of patients with GBM. MBP levels greater than 4.0 ng/mL in the CSF correlate with active tumors, and these levels decreased after surgery and chemotherapy.[24] Other growth factors and cytokines have also been identified as possible CSF biomarkers of GBM. Most patients with malignant gliomas have increased levels of vascular endothelial growth factor (VEGF) and interleukin-6 (IL-6) in the CSF,

distinguishing them from patients with low-grade gliomas and normal healthy controls.[25,26] Thus, these proteins may serve as a basis for improving CSF biomarkers of GBM.

Recently, investigators have also started studying tumor metabolomics in serum and CSF. Increased serum levels of the cysteine metabolite correlate with GBM diagnosis, enabling distinction from oligodendrogliomas, which have increased levels of lysine and 2-oxoisocaproic acid metabolites.[27] In addition, increased serum levels of myoinositol and hexadecenoic acid metabolites at the time of GBM diagnosis were of prognostic value in terms of long-term survival.[27] In the CSF, metabolites from the amino acid, lipid, pyrimidine, and central carbon metabolism pathways are significantly different compared with those of healthy controls.[28] Note that CSF levels of 2-hydroxyglutarate are increased in patients with GBM, indicating the presence of the IDH1 mutation in the tumor. Clinically, increased CSF levels of metabolites involved in tryptophan and histidine metabolism can be used to distinguish primary GBM from recurrent disease.[28] Although metabolomic biomarkers are fairly new, they have the ability to study the inner workings of the malignant process, and have potential as a biomarker for GBM.

Detection of Extracellular Vesicles

Detection of EVs as a biomarker of GBM in both the serum and CSF is not as well investigated as that of extracellular macromolecules. However, given the harsh environment of the serum, and CSF to some extent, free circulating nucleic acids, and even proteins, are more prone to degradation than are EVs. The secretion of EVs is a normal physiologic process described in nearly every cell type, and is a broad term that includes microvesicles and exosomes.[29] Microvesicles, typically 200 to 500 nm in diameter, are released via blebbing of the cell membrane and can contain elements in the cytoplasm at that time, such as mRNA and miRNA. Exosomes, typically 40 to 100 nm in diameter, are packaged and secreted via the endosomal system within the cell, and the mRNA and miRNA content is more regulated compared with microvesicles.[29] However, both subgroups can contain elements of the cell membrane that are tumor specific and that, in addition to nucleic acid species, can be used as diagnostic biomarkers for GBM in the serum and CSF.

Given that EVs contain a measurable amount of nucleic acids, researchers have analyzed these profiles for GBM-specific biomarkers. The mRNA expression pattern of serum-derived EVs in patients with GBM contains significantly lower levels of genes associated with ribosome functions: RPL11, RPS12, TMSL3, and B2M.[30] Similarly, mRNA expression of the EGFR variant III (EGFRvIII) mutation can be detected in serum-derived microvesicles, which can direct receptor-specific therapy in addition to surgery.[31] Given that noncoding RNA can regulate mRNA expression, it is also prudent to investigate their utility as a GBM biomarker. Increased levels of RNU6-1, miR-320, and miR-574-3p in serum-derived EVs correlate with the diagnosis of GBM with a sensitivity of 87% and a specificity of 86%.[32] Similar to free circulating macromolecules, GBM-specific EVs are more likely to be found in the CSF compared with the serum. CSF-derived EVs from patients with GBM express an average of 10-fold more miR-21 compared with those of nononcologic controls, and are able to diagnose this malignancy with a sensitivity of 87% and a specificity of 93%.[33] Although microvesicles contain more total RNA, most of the miRNA in CSF-derived EVs is enriched in exosomes; greater than 40 miRNA compared with ~10 miRNA in microvesicles.[34] These intriguing results indicated that the miRNA profile of CSF-derived EVs may be used to diagnose GBM in the future.

Proteins within serum-derived EVs can also potentially be used as a biomarker for GBM. Serum-derived EVs of patients with GBM express significant levels of angiogenin, FGF-alpha, IL-6, VEGF, TIMP-1, and TIMP-2.[31] In addition, using micro nuclear magnetic resonance (μNMR) technology on a quad panel of proteins (EGFR, EGFRvIII, PDPN, and IDH1) in serum-derived EVs has a sensitivity of 85% and a specificity of 80% for diagnosing GBM, and is able to predict response to temozolomide chemotherapy.[35] More recently, researchers have also investigated CSF-derived EVs for the expression of GBM-specific genetic aberrations. Our group has recently found that the EGFRvIII mutation can be detected in CSF-derived EVs from patients with GBM, with a sensitivity of 60% and a specificity of 98% for diagnosing EGFRvIII-positive GBMs (Figueroa and colleagues, unpublished data, 2016). In addition, EGFRvIII-positive CSF-derived EVs have significantly increased expression of wtEGFR, which is known to be overexpressed in the classic subtype of GBM.[36] These novel diagnostic tests have potential for not only diagnosing GBM but also determining EGFRvIII status and distinguishing between GBM subtypes.

Detection of Circulating Tumor Cells

The least studied strategy for the early diagnosis of GBM is the detection of CTCs. Typically, researchers investigate methods to isolate rogue malignant cells that have separated from the primary tumor mass and entered either the circulatory system or the CSF. However, the term CTC does not only apply to malignant cells but also includes subverted cells within the tumor stroma, such as endothelial cells and immune cells. At present, there are reports of serum CTCs identified in patients with GBM, but there are no studies investigating CTCs in the CSF.

The search for CTCs in GBM is difficult because there is no established tumor-defining cell surface marker. Instead, researchers have relied on various antibody cocktails that may target GBM-specific CTCs. A panel of antibodies, anti-CD14, anti-CD16, and anti-CD45, validated by analysis of known genetic aberrations in GBM, is able to detect CTCs in the serum that correlate with specific GBM subtypes.[36] Similarly, using an adenoviral probe for human telomerase reverse transcriptase, which is known to be at increased levels in GBM, serum CTCs were isolated and validated by analysis for the overexpression of nestin, GFAP, and EGFR, as well as the absence of epithelial cell adhesion molecule, in patients with malignant gliomas.[37] These promising results indicate that CTC detection is possible in GBM, and may be improved in the future to become a useful diagnostic protocol.

SUMMARY

The ability to diagnose GBM early in the malignant process by analyzing the serum and CSF is still evolving. Researchers have investigated numerous free nucleic acid and protein signatures in biofluids with fairly good results. The expanding field of EV isolation, and their relative RNA and protein contents, provides another intriguing diagnostic method for clinicians. In addition, more work is needed in the area of CTC detection, which has proved to be a promising modality for tumor diagnosis. In the future, these approaches may not only be used as screening tools for the early diagnosis of GBM but may also provide tumor-specific information that can direct appropriate therapeutic strategies.

REFERENCES

1. Raizer JJ, Fitzner KA, Jacobs DI, et al. Economics of malignant gliomas: a critical review. J Oncol Pract 2015;11(1):e59–65.
2. Gold P, Freedman SO. Specific carcinoembryonic antigens of the human digestive system. J Exp Med 1965;122(3):467–81.
3. Vihko P, Sajanti E, Jänne O, et al. Serum prostate-specific acid phosphatase: development and validation of a specific radioimmunoassay. Clin Chem 1978;24(11):1915–9.

4. Bast RC Jr, Klug TL, St John E, et al. A radioimmuno-assay using a monoclonal antibody to monitor the course of epithelial ovarian cancer. N Engl J Med 1983;309(15):883–7.

5. Füzéry AK, Levin J, Chan MM, et al. Translation of proteomic biomarkers into FDA approved cancer diagnostics. Clin Proteomics 2013;10(1):13.

6. Lavon I, Refael M, Zelikovitch B, et al. Serum DNA can define tumor-specific genetic and epigenetic markers in gliomas of various grades. Neuro Oncol 2010;12(2):173–80.

7. Majchrzak-Celińska A, Paluszczak J, Kleszcz R, et al. Detection of MGMT, RASSF1A, p15INK4B, and p14ARF promoter methylation in circulating tumor-derived DNA of central nervous system cancer patients. J Appl Genet 2013;54(3):335–44.

8. Pan W, Gu W, Nagpal S, et al. Brain tumor mutations detected in cerebral spinal fluid. Clin Chem 2015;61(3):514–22.

9. De Mattos-Arruda L, Mayor R, Ng CK, et al. Cerebrospinal fluid-derived circulating tumour DNA better represents the genomic alterations of brain tumours than plasma. Nat Commun 2015;10(6):8839.

10. Dong L, Li Y, Han C, et al. MicroRNA microarray reveals specific expression in the peripheral blood of glioblastoma patients. Int J Oncol 2014;45(2):746–56.

11. Tang H, Liu Q, Liu X, et al. Plasma miR-185 as a predictive biomarker for prognosis of malignant glioma. J Cancer Res Ther 2015;11(3):630–4.

12. Lai NS, Wu DG, Fang XG, et al. Serum microRNA-210 as a potential noninvasive biomarker for the diagnosis and prognosis of glioma. Br J Cancer 2015;112(7):1241–6.

13. Yue X, Lan F, Hu M, et al. Downregulation of serum microRNA-205 as a potential diagnostic and prognostic biomarker for human glioma. J Neurosurg 2016;124(1):122–8.

14. Teplyuk NM, Mollenhauer B, Gabriely G, et al. MicroRNAs in cerebrospinal fluid identify glioblastoma and metastatic brain cancers and reflect disease activity. Neuro Oncol 2012;14(6):689–700.

15. Drusco A, Bottoni A, Laganà A, et al. A differentially expressed set of microRNAs in cerebro-spinal fluid (CSF) can diagnose CNS malignancies. Oncotarget 2015;6(25):20829–39.

16. Jung CS, Foerch C, Schänzer A, et al. Serum GFAP is a diagnostic marker for glioblastoma multiforme. Brain 2007;130(12):3336–41.

17. Tichy J, Spechtmeyer S, Mittelbronn M, et al. Prospective evaluation of serum glial fibrillary acidic protein (GFAP) as a diagnostic marker for glioblastoma. Neurooncol 2016;126(2):361–9.

18. Kiviniemi A, Gardberg M, Frantzén J, et al. Serum levels of GFAP and EGFR in primary and recurrent high-grade gliomas: correlation to tumor volume, molecular markers, and progression-free survival. Neuro Oncol 2015;124(2):237–45.

19. Hormigo A, Gu B, Karimi S, et al. YKL-40 and matrix metalloproteinase-9 as potential serum biomarkers for patients with high-grade gliomas. Clin Cancer Res 2006;12(19):5698–704.

20. Elstner A, Stockhammer F, Nguyen-Dobinsky TN, et al. Identification of diagnostic serum protein profiles of glioblastoma patients. Neuro Oncol 2011;102(1):71–80.

21. Benito R, Gil-Benso R, Quilis V, et al. Primary glioblastomas with and without EGFR amplification: relationship to genetic alterations and clinical-pathological features. Neuropathology 2010;30(4):392–400.

22. Quaranta M, Divella R, Daniele A, et al. Epidermal growth factor receptor serum levels and prognostic value in malignant gliomas. Tumori 2007;93(3):275–80.

23. Szymaś J, Morkowski S, Tokarz F. Determination of the glial fibrillary acidic protein in human cerebrospinal fluid and in cyst fluid of brain tumors. Acta Neurochir 1986;83(3–4):144–50.

24. Nakagawa H, Yamada M, Kanayama T, et al. Myelin basic protein in the cerebrospinal fluid of patients with brain tumors. Neurosurgery 1994;34(5):825–33.

25. Sampath P, Weaver CE, Sungarian A, et al. Cerebrospinal fluid (vascular endothelial growth factor) and serologic (recoverin) tumor markers for malignant glioma. Cancer Control 2004;11(3):174–80.

26. Shen F, Zhang Y, Yao Y, et al. Proteomic analysis of cerebrospinal fluid: toward the identification of biomarkers for gliomas. Neurosurg Rev 2014;37(3):367–80.

27. Mörén L, Bergenheim AT, Ghasimi S, et al. Metabolomic screening of tumor tissue and serum in glioma patients reveals diagnostic and prognostic information. Metabolite 2015;5(3):502–20.

28. Locasale JW, Melman T, Song S, et al. Metabolomics of human cerebrospinal fluid identifies signatures of malignant glioma. Mol Cell Proteomics 2012;11(6). M111.014688.

29. Kalra H, Simpson RJ, Ji H, et al. Vesiclepedia: a compendium for extracellular vesicles with continuous community annotation. PLoS Biol 2012;10(12):e1001450.

30. Noerholm M, Balaj L, Limperg T, et al. RNA expression patterns in serum microvesicles from patients with glioblastoma multiforme and controls. BMC Cancer 2012;12:22.

31. Skog J, Würdinger T, van Rijn S, et al. Glioblastoma microvesicles transport RNA and proteins that promote tumour growth and provide diagnostic biomarkers. Nat Cell Biol 2008;10(12):1470–6.

32. Manterola L, Guruceaga E, Gállego Pérez-Larraya J, et al. A small noncoding RNA signature found in

exosomes of GBM patient serum as a diagnostic tool. Neuro Oncol 2014;16(4):520–7.

33. Akers JC, Ramakrishnan V, Kim R, et al. MiR-21 in the extracellular vesicles (EVs) of cerebrospinal fluid (CSF): a platform for glioblastoma biomarker development. PLoS One 2013;8(10):e78115.

34. Akers JC, Ramakrishnan V, Kim R, et al. MicroRNA contents of cerebrospinal fluid extracellular vesicles in glioblastoma patients. Neuro Oncol 2015;123(2): 205–16.

35. Shao H, Chung J, Balaj L, et al. Protein typing of circulating microvesicles allows real-time monitoring of glioblastoma therapy. Nat Med 2012;18(12):1835–40.

36. Sullivan JP, Nahed BV, Madden MW, et al. Brain tumor cells in circulation are enriched for mesenchymal gene expression. Cancer Discov 2014;4(11):1299–309.

37. Macarthur KM, Kao GD, Chandrasekaran S, et al. Detection of brain tumor cells in the peripheral blood by a telomerase promoter-based assay. Cancer Res 2014;74(8):2152–9.

CHAPTER 21

Health-related Quality of Life and Neurocognitive Functioning After Glioblastoma Treatment

Florien W. Boele, PhD[a], Linda Dirven, PhD[b],
Johan A.F. Koekkoek, MD, PhD[b,c],
Martin J.B. Taphoorn, MD, PhD[b,c,*]

INTRODUCTION

With a median survival of 12 to 14 months, the prognosis of patients with glioblastoma multiforme (GBM) remains poor.[1] Treatment is therefore not only designed to prolong survival but also to maintain an optimal level of health-related quality of life (HRQOL). HRQOL is determined by self-report, and is a multidimensional concept. It includes people's perception of their physical, cognitive, and affective state, as well as their perception of their interpersonal relationships and social roles,[2] specifically related to the impact of health or illness. Cognitive functioning is, as such, part of the concept of HRQOL. Although HRQOL is assessed through self-report, cognitive complaints as reported by patients do not accurately reflect the results of formal neuropsychological testing.[3] Therefore, formal neuropsychological assessment is required to obtain a clear idea of the patient's cognitive deficits, which may include problems with attention, memory storage and retrieval, working memory, information processing, psychomotor speed, and executive functioning.

This chapter first describes the impact of the diagnosis and treatment of GBM on patients' HRQOL and cognitive functioning. It then provides an overview of cognitive tests that may be used to assess cognitive dysfunction in patients

with GBM, and describes how cognitive functioning might be improved, so that perhaps HRQOL might be improved as well.

Impact of Disease and Treatment on Health-related Quality of Life

Both the disease and its treatment can affect HRQOL. Common disease-specific symptoms that may negatively influence HRQOL include paresis, sensory loss, visual-perceptual deficits, cognitive deficits, and symptoms associated with increased intracranial pressure, such as nausea and headache.[4–6] Moreover, fatigue and mood issues can contribute to poorer HRQOL.[7,8] Patients with newly diagnosed GBM experience significantly lower levels of HRQOL than healthy controls, shortly after surgery.[9,10] Compared with other neurologic patient groups, HRQOL among patients with stable high-grade glioma is similar,[11] but patients with GBM report less positive affect, more depression, and more illness intrusiveness than other patients with cancer.[12]

The impact of antitumor treatment (surgery followed by radiotherapy and/or chemotherapy) on HRQOL can be both negative and positive.[13] Surgery can either improve HRQOL by reducing tumor mass and the disease-specific symptoms associated with increased intracranial pressure,[14] or it can decrease HRQOL by damaging functional

Disclosure: The authors report no conflict of interest.
[a] Edinburgh Centre for Neuro-Oncology, Western General Hospital, Crewe Road, Edinburgh EH4 2XU, UK;
[b] Department of Neurology, Leiden University Medical Center, PO Box 9600, Leiden 2300 RC, The Netherlands;
[c] Department of Neurology, Medical Center Haaglanden, PO Box 432, The Hague 2501 CK, The Netherlands
* Corresponding author. Department of Neurology, Leiden University Medical Center, PO Box 9600 (Postal Zone K5-Q), Leiden 2300 RC, The Netherlands.
E-mail address: M.J.B.Taphoorn@lumc.nl

tissue.[15] In patients with low-grade glioma, treatment with radiotherapy has generally been associated with a negative impact on HRQOL, because increased fatigue and cognitive deficits can hinder everyday functioning.[16–19] These late toxic effects of treatment play a less prominent role in patients with high-grade glioma, who have a poorer prognosis. On the group level, the HRQOL of patients with high-grade glioma does not seem to be negatively influenced by a treatment regimen consisting of radiotherapy and chemotherapy.[10,20–23] However, specific aspects of HRQOL, such as social and cognitive functioning, may be affected temporarily.[23,24] In long-term survivors (>2.5 years) of anaplastic glioma treated with radiotherapy and chemotherapy, lower levels of motor functioning and social, cognitive, and emotional aspects of HRQOL have been reported.[25] The side effects that occur with chemotherapy, such as nausea or vomiting, appetite loss, and drowsiness, can also negatively influence patients' functioning and HRQOL.[23]

Adding bevacizumab, an antiangiogenic agent that may benefit progression-free survival in a subgroup of patients with recurrent GBM,[26] does not seem to affect HRQOL,[27–30] although one study reports a decrease in HRQOL.[31] Other medications commonly administered to manage symptoms, such as antiepileptic drugs (AEDs) and corticosteroids, can influence HRQOL. Decreasing seizure frequency may improve HRQOL, but side effects or drug-drug interactions may decrease HRQOL.[32] However, second-generation AEDs such as levetiracetam and oxcarbazepine cause fewer side effects and do not seem to significantly influence HRQOL in the longer term.[33,34] Similarly, corticosteroids may improve HRQOL by relieving symptoms of increased intracranial pressure but can also cause adverse effects that may harm HRQOL. Therefore, it is advised to administer corticosteroids in the lowest effective dose to minimize side effects.[35]

Of note, the HRQOL results of studies including patients with GBM are often biased, because those patients participating in trials are often young and have a good performance status. In addition, patients who show clinical deterioration are more frequently lost to follow-up.[36] Thus, HRQOL could be overestimated, especially in studies with long follow-up.[36] As GBM recurs or the disease progresses, HRQOL seems to become worse.[30,37,38] However, in long-term survivors of GBM (ie, survival ≥16 months) HRQOL can return to a level comparable with normal controls.[37] Despite the poor prognosis, patients often long to return to a normal everyday life, including return to work and social activities after primary

treatment. It is especially during this phase of life that HRQOL may be correlated with cognitive functioning, because even subtle cognitive deficits might hamper patients' autonomy and professional life (Fig. 21.1).[39,40]

The Association Between Health-related Quality of Life and Neurocognitive Functioning

Almost all patients with GBM experience cognitive deficits,[9] which can include dysfunction in the domains of information processing, attention, psychomotor speed, executive functioning, and verbal and working memory. Shortly after diagnosis, memory storage and retrieval, categorical word fluency and also information processing capacity and more complex executive functioning tasks seem to be most commonly affected.[9] In general, cognitive functioning declines as the disease progresses,[41] although long-term survivors (>3 years) may only show mild cognitive impairment.[42]

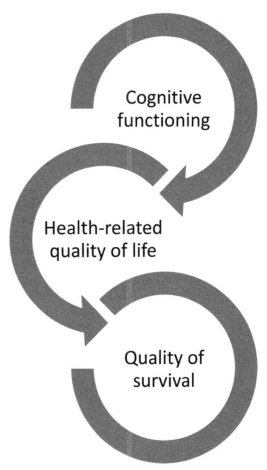

Fig. 21.1 The relationships between cognition, health-related quality of life, and quality of survival in patients with GBM.

Cognitive functioning is part of the concept of HRQOL, because even mild deficits may affect patients' ability to function independently, affecting their social and emotional functioning to a great extent. When severe, cognitive deficits can also affect patients' ability to accurately report on their HRQOL, complicating the association between cognition and HRQOL. Studies on the relationships between HRQOL measures and objective cognitive functioning throughout the GBM disease trajectory are rare, although some evidence exists. A recent longitudinal study showed preoperative cognitive symptoms to be predictive of HRQOL during the first year of GBM.[43] In patients with newly diagnosed GBM, information processing speed was associated with mental health.[9] Moreover, in patients with temporal lobe glioma, verbal learning, processing speed, and executive functioning were shown to be related to general, social, and functional well-being, respectively.[44] Furthermore, self-reported cognitive complaints are related to HRQOL in patients with GBM,[9] although self-reported measures of cognition are only moderately correlated with the performance on formal neuropsychological assessments.[3] It is important to keep track of cognitive functioning throughout the disease trajectory, not only because of the link between HRQOL and cognitive functioning but also because it is known to predict functional decline and even survival.[45–49]

Neurocognitive Issues Associated with Glioblastoma Treatment

Cognitive functioning is influenced by the patient's premorbid level of cognitive functioning and psychological distress, but cognitive deficits can also be the result of the brain tumor, its symptoms, and its treatment (eg, surgery, radiotherapy, chemotherapy, epilepsy, use of AEDs and corticosteroids).[50] The invasive nature of GBM can cause damage to functional brain tissue, disrupting neural networks and causing cognitive problems.[51] Depending on the size and location of the tumor, this may lead to specific (eg, language deficits) or more global cognitive dysfunction (eg, attentional deficits).[52] Before resection, larger tumors have been shown to result in more cognitive deficits, especially in the areas of verbal and visual memory, verbal fluency, shifting between different tasks, and visuospatial abilities.[53] Cognitive deficits caused by increased intracranial pressure or disruption of functional brain networks may be alleviated after surgical resection of the tumor,[51,54–56] although worsening of symptoms may also be observed shortly after surgery.[55,57] Removal of functional tissue in an attempt to dissect the tumor may cause specific cognitive deficits depending on the location in the brain.[52] For example, lesions of the supplementary motor area can lead to agraphia.[58]

Radiotherapy has long been associated with cognitive effects, which may be transient (acute or early-delayed toxicity), or lasting and progressive (late-delayed toxicity).[59] Vascular abnormalities, demyelination, radionecrosis, and cerebral atrophy are recognized as a late-delayed effects (>6 months after irradiation).[52,59] However, cognitive deficits may occur independently from radiographic or clinical evidence of injury to the brain.[59] It is estimated that 50% to 90% of patients with brain tumors treated with fractionated whole-brain radiotherapy experience cognitive impairment 6 months later.[59] Verbal and spatial memory, attention, and problem-solving seem to be particularly affected.[59] Cognitive deficits may remain present even many years after low-dose radiotherapy, because patients with irradiated low-grade gliomas experienced a decline in attentional functioning compared with nonirradiated patients as much as 12 years after treatment.[17] In long-term survivors (>2.5 years) of anaplastic glioma treated with radiotherapy and chemotherapy, scores on tests of working memory, attention, psychomotor speed, information processing, and executive functioning were significantly worse than in healthy controls matched for age, sex, and educational level.[25] Although most studies investigating radiation effects have been performed in patients with low-grade glioma, note that many patients with glioblastoma also survive long enough (>6 months) to be affected by cognitive sequelae.

Chemotherapy is also known to affect cognitive functioning.[60] Risk factors for developing neurotoxicity after chemotherapy include higher doses, treatment with multiple chemotherapeutic agents, treatment with both chemotherapy and radiotherapy either concurrently or subsequently, intra-arterial administration with disruption of the blood-brain barrier, and intrathecal administration.[60] Across different cancer groups, attention, concentration, memory, and visual functioning are vulnerable after chemotherapy.[61] In patients with high-grade glioma specifically, diminished learning ability, information processing, and attentional functioning and concentration seem to be linked to chemotherapy treatment.[62] However, other studies show mild cognitive effects, or even no cognitive effects of chemotherapy. For example, in elderly patients with GBM with poor performance status, treatment with chemotherapy alone did not seem to influence HRQOL or cognitive functioning before disease progression occurred.[63] Moreover, a small study assessing progression-free patients with GBM during their treatment with radiotherapy plus concomitant and adjuvant chemotherapy did not show a decline in cognitive functioning.[64] Similarly, the cognitive effects of the antiangiogenic agent bevacizumab in patients with GBM remain ambiguous.[65] Some studies find no clear negative cognitive effects of bevacizumab treatment,[66,67] whereas a large randomized controlled trial shows a decline in both HRQOL and cognitive functioning in patients with GBM, especially after longer treatment with bevacizumab.[31]

Apart from antitumor treatment, medications for symptom management can lead to cognitive dysfunction. Both epileptic seizures and AEDs have been associated with cognitive deterioration.[68] First-generation AEDs (eg, carbamazepine, phenytoin, and valproic acid) are known to affect cognitive functioning.[69] Cognitive slowing and attention deficits can result in subsequent poor performance on other cognitive tests. Fatigue associated with AED use can also hamper neuropsychological test performance. In patients with glioma specifically, seizures and AEDs seem to be related to deficits in processing speed, attention, and executive functioning.[18,52] Corticosteroids can lead to cognitive improvement with decreased intracranial pressure, but long-term use may cause behavioral problems as well as attention and memory disturbances.[52,70] These issues largely depend on the steroid dose and treatment duration, and may be reversible after treatment cessation.[70] Of note, the treatment regimen in GBM almost invariably includes multimodal treatments, making it difficult to decipher to what degree cognitive deficits are the result of any specific treatment.

EVALUATION AND TREATMENT OF NEUROCOGNITIVE ISSUES

When cognitive problems are suspected, a neuropsychologist performs a formal cognitive evaluation to determine the extent to which cognitive dysfunction occurs in the patient. Ideally, neuropsychologists should be part of the multidisciplinary treatment team, but this may not be feasible in all hospitals. Brief cognitive screening can be done by physicians during a neurologic examination or by the nurse specialists during their consultation. Because screening instruments do not require thorough understanding of the psychometric properties of the tests, and are quick and easy to administer, this may be a viable alternative. If cognitive difficulties are suspected, referral to a neuropsychologist is warranted so that an assessment of the need for cognitive rehabilitation and supportive care can be made.

Instruments to Evaluate and Monitor Cognitive Deficits

To screen for cognitive deficits in clinical practice, the Mini-Mental State Examination (MMSE) is often used.[71] This instrument is scored on a 0 to 30 scale, with higher scores indicating better functioning. A score less than 25 is considered cognitively impaired, but this may be too insensitive to detect more subtle cognitive problems, so a score less than 26 or 27 has also been used as a cutoff point in clinical trials (eg, Refs.[72,73]). It touches on 7 cognitive areas: orientation in time, orientation in place, working memory, verbal memory, concentration and calculation, language, and visuoperceptual functioning. Other screening measures are the Montreal Cognitive Assessment (MoCA)[74] and the Addenbrooke Cognitive Examination–Revised (ACE-R).[75] ACE-R incorporates the MMSE and has additional questions, making it a more comprehensive screening instrument. MoCA consists of 30 items and can be administered in about 10 minutes. MoCA taps into the domains of orientation in time and place, attention, working memory and verbal memory, visuospatial functioning, executive functioning, language, and fluency. All 3 screening instruments have been translated into various languages and are widely used. However, the usefulness of cognitive screening measures per se can be debated, because these are crude measures and subtle cognitive dysfunction may go unnoticed. However, major cognitive problems are likely to be detected.

After cognitive screening, a comprehensive neuropsychological assessment by a trained neuropsychologist may be warranted. Because of their background and training, neuropsychologists are especially suitable to provide insight and interpret neuropsychological test results.[76] For example, a poor performance on a test of visual memory can be the result of a deficit in 1 or more components of memory (eg, capacity to learn new material, encoding, retrieval, consolidation) but also may be influenced by problems in attention, visual-perceptual deficits, or executive functioning (eg, planning a learning strategy). Motivation, fatigue, and mood play crucial roles as well. Neuropsychologists make an estimation of the contribution of each of these factors in their reports.

A full neuropsychological assessment can be burdensome for patients with GBM. Depending on the degree of cognitive dysfunction and the patient's insight into problems, it can be uncomfortable for patients to be confronted with their cognitive issues in such a straightforward way. Therefore, neuropsychologists generally aim to limit the number of tests performed in areas in which, based on the patient's history and test performance, there does not seem to be a problem. In cognitive domains in which a patient's test scores lag behind, more than 1 neuropsychological test may be necessary to determine the exact nature of the problem. In clinical practice, differences between institutes exist, but in general about 1 to 1.5 hours is considered sufficient to obtain a cognitive profile.

However, in a research setting, a test battery covering a wide range of cognitive domains, but not in depth, is more appropriate. The test battery should be short and not take more than approximately 30 minutes to administer, it should be suitable for repeated assessments over time (ie, alternate versions should be available to limit practice effects), and it should have good psychometric properties.[76,77] Naturally, it must also be possible to detect change in functioning over time.[76,77] Using often-used tests makes it easier to compare across different studies and populations. **Table 21.1** presents an overview of neuropsychological tests that are often used or are suggested by leading investigators, including the International Cancer and Cognition Task Force.[76,78–82] Of note, for the working memory domain no specific tests were suggested because none of the tests met all requirements in terms of psychometric properties.[82] Moreover, neuropsychological tests often tap into multiple cognitive domains. For example, fluency is sometimes considered executive functioning because it requires the patient to use strategies to retrieve words from memory, or language functioning, because of the heavy verbal component, but can also be scored as a separate domain. Domains and tests displayed in the table are merely examples. Deciding on any particular set of tests remains dependent on the goal of the research study.

When interpreting published results on cognition in patients with GBM, note that estimates of

TABLE 21.1			
Suggestions for cognitive assessment in research studies in patients with GBM			
Cognitive Domain	**Cognitive Test**	**Description**	**Time to Administer (min)**[a]
Processing speed	Trail Making Test Part A[105]	Circles labeled 1–25 to be connected as quickly as possible	2–3
Working memory	Digit span[106]	A sequence of digits is read aloud and the patient is to repeat (trial: forward) or repeat in reverse order (trial: backward). Spans range 2–8 digits	4
Verbal memory	Hopkins Verbal Learning Test–Revised[107]	12 words are read aloud to the patient with 2-s intervals. Direct recall is scored for trials 1–3. After an interval of 20–25 min, delayed recall (trial 4) and recognition are scored	15, plus 5
Executive functioning	Trail Making Test Part B[105]	Circles labeled 1–13 and A–L to be connected in alternating successive order (ie, 1-A, 2-B, and so forth) as quickly as possible	4–5
Fluency	Controlled Oral Word Association[108]	Naming as many words as possible belonging to a category or beginning with a certain letter within 1 min	2–3
Psychomotor speed Visuospatial functioning	Grooved pegboard test[109]	Placing pins in holes as quickly as possible in the right orientation, using the dominant, nondominant, and both hands	10
Visuoconstruction	Rey-Osterrieth Complex Figure (copy)[110]	The patient is asked to copy a figure as precisely as possible	5

[a] This is an estimation and depends heavily on the individual patient.

the prevalence of cognitive deficits may vary because of differences in the patient populations studied, the neuropsychological tests administered, or the normative data and cutoff scores used.[83] Similar to the overestimation bias reported in HRQOL,[36] results on cognitive functioning as an outcome measure in clinical trials should be interpreted with caution because patients who deteriorate (and are thus likely to have cognitive decline) may drop out of the study, whereas patients who perform well remain. Moreover, the nuanced report of a neuropsychologist is lost in clinical trials, in which factors such as fatigue, motivation, and mood may be disregarded and only pure test performance is taken into consideration.

Treatment of Cognitive Deficits in Patients with Glioblastoma Multiforme

After neuropsychological assessment, an estimation of the need for treatment or support in coping with cognitive deficits can be made. Here, it is important to keep in mind that cognitive performance can be influenced by the antitumor treatment and symptom management, as described earlier. These effects can be reversible (eg, in the case of corticosteroid use or AEDs) or irreversible, as is the case in surgery. However, the brain's plasticity should not be underestimated because, even in adults, spontaneous recovery of cognitive functions can occur after acquired brain damage.[84,85] This regenerative process mostly occurs within 6 months after brain injury, but may continue for a longer period.[84] Although starting treatment of cognitive deficits early in the disease process can make it difficult to determine whether recovery occurred as a result of the therapy or because of spontaneous neuronal regeneration, it may help speed up the recovery process and could have a positive influence on HRQOL. It is especially relevant to achieve recovery early in patients with GBM, who are faced with a prognosis that is usually measured in months, rather than years.

In determining the need for treatment or supportive care, not only the patient's cognitive profile plays a role but also their motivation to improve cognitive functioning, and the burden of cognitive dysfunction experienced by the patient and their family members, are equally important to consider. Therefore, a participatory approach should be used, taking into account the opinions of the patients and their families. Discussion in multidisciplinary meetings in which physicians, (neuro)psychologists, nurse specialists, and social workers are present may further assist in determining what kind of support is most suitable for individual patients with GBM.

Nonpharmacologic treatment strategies for cognitive deficits include cognitive rehabilitation and psychoeducation or coaching. Programs available for cognitive rehabilitation vary and can be intense, with patients undergoing therapy for several hours a day, over the course of multiple weeks. This schedule may be too demanding for a subset of patients with GBM, especially those on active treatment. Moreover, as described earlier, cognitive deficits generally improve gradually over the course of weeks to months following surgery.[84,85] Perhaps because of this, those patients referred to cognitive rehabilitation have generally finished their primary treatment and are in a period of stable disease. However, there is increasing attention on the early treatment of cognitive deficits. As early inpatient rehabilitation focused on physical functioning proved feasible and effective in patients with newly diagnosed GBM,[86] cognition may also be improved early in the disease trajectory. It would be interesting to perform a study comparing early cognitive rehabilitation with cognitive rehabilitation provided during stable disease, but, to our knowledge, no such trial has been initiated so far.

Several studies have been performed that show some beneficial effects of cognitive rehabilitation in patients with glioma.[87–91] Furthermore, a multidisciplinary rehabilitation intervention found subjective improvement in cognitive functioning, although formal neuropsychological assessments were not performed.[92] Of note, study populations are often small, and study designs generally lack a control condition. One randomized controlled trial has been performed in patients with glioma with favorable prognosis.[87] After 6 months, attention, verbal memory, and mental fatigue improved compared with a care-as-usual control group. However, this was a very intensive rehabilitation program and patients with GBM were not included, thereby limiting the ability to generalize to this patient group. In a meta-analysis, Langenbahn and colleagues[93] conclude that there is still too little evidence for the effectiveness of cognitive rehabilitation studies in adult patients with brain tumors.

As an example of less intensive treatment, psychoeducation in the form of feedback from neuropsychological assessment early in the disease trajectory can help patients and their families understand the cognitive difficulties that patients experience, which may substantially improve the home and family situation. Patients and family caregivers indicate that this kind of support is currently often lacking in health care.[94] The feedback could help health care professionals and families in assessing what kind of formal or informal support the patients need at home, and it might be helpful in determining whether and when return to work may be feasible. Other interventions include restructuring of the home environment to aid patients to rely less on their impaired functions, providing advice on using external aids and technology, teaching strategies to cope with their cognitive problems, and retraining specific cognitive skills.[83] This support may also lead to better mental adjustment as well as functional improvement and can help patients maintain independence.

Other nonpharmacologic alternatives are also being investigated in research studies. An online application of the rehabilitation program investigated in a randomized controlled setting[87] is now under development, allowing patients to access training at a time of their choosing.[95] Interventions based on physical exercise also show promising results in improving cognitive functioning.[96,97] Although potentially useful for some patients, here, too, subsets of patients with GBM are excluded: those with difficulty using computers and those whose physical status prevents them from exercising.

Pharmacologic treatment of cognitive deficits is also possible. Sometimes, psychostimulants are prescribed to try to improve cognitive functioning. Studies evaluating the use of methylphenidate,[98,99] modafinil,[99,100] armodafinil,[101] memantine,[102] and donepezil[103] have been performed and show modest effects on cognitive functioning at best. Most studies have included patients with GBM, although these made up most of the sample in only 1 report.[101] Several studies included patients who were undergoing radiotherapy[98,101,102] or chemotherapy,[99] although some focused on patients in a stable disease phase.[100,103] After psychostimulant use, performance on cognitive screening measures[98] or tests of working memory,[100] attention,[103] processing speed,[99] information processing,[100] executive functioning,[99] and sometimes even verbal[102,103] and visual memory[103] may improve. However, these may be attributable to a placebo effect because there are often no reported differences in cognitive performance when comparing 2 psychostimulants,[99] or when comparing the psychostimulant with placebo.[98,100,101] In a recent systematic review, Day and colleagues[104] discussed treatment interventions for fatigued patients during cranial irradiation, and similarly concluded that, although pharmacologic interventions such as memantine or donepezil may have beneficial effects, studies were limited by small sample sizes and high risk of bias.

SUMMARY

Patients with GBM frequently experience diminished HRQOL and cognitive deficits, which can result from the tumor and its symptoms, antitumor treatment, or symptom management. Although HRQOL and cognitive functioning may return to an almost normal level in survivors, both decline as the disease progresses. Because HRQOL and cognitive functioning are interlinked, treatment of cognitive deficits may improve patients' HRQOL. Perhaps because of the unfavorable prognosis of GBM, early treatment of cognitive deficits rarely occurs, whereas (low-intensity) treatment and support may be feasible and effective shortly after surgery. In referring patients with GBM to cognitive treatment or support, the multidisciplinary treatment team plays a key role. Cognitive screening may be performed by physicians or nurses, after which full neuropsychological assessment may be performed if necessary. Nurses or psychologists may provide guidance in dealing with everyday consequences of cognitive deficits, whereas a more intensive cognitive rehabilitation program generally requires a multidisciplinary treatment team, including, for example, psychologists, physiotherapists, occupational therapists, and speech therapists. To determine which form of treatment, be it nonpharmacologic or pharmacologic, is most effective, further research studies with strong methodological design are required.

REFERENCES

1. Stupp R, Mason WP, van den Bent MJ, et al. Radiotherapy plus concomitant and adjuvant temozolomide for glioblastoma. N Engl J Med 2005;352(10): 987–96.

2. WHOQOL Group. The World Health Organization quality of life assessment (WHOQOL): position paper from the World Health Organization. Soc Sci Med 1995;41(10):1403–9.

3. Gehring K, Taphoorn M, Sitskoorn M, et al. Predictors of subjective versus objective cognitive functioning in patients with stable grade II and III glioma. Neurooncol Pract 2015;2(1):20–31.

4. Bergo E, Lombardi G, Guglieri I, et al. Neurocognitive functions and health-related quality of life in glioblastoma patients: a concise review of the literature. Eur J Cancer Care 2015. [Epub ahead of print].

5. Mukand JA, Blackinton DD, Crincoli MG, et al. Incidence of neurologic deficits and rehabilitation of patients with brain tumors. Am J Phys Med Rehabil 2001;80(5):346.

6. Young R, Jamshidi A, Davis G, et al. Current trends in the surgical management and treatment of adult glioblastoma. Ann Transl Med 2015;3(9):121–36.

7. Aprile I, Chiesa S, Padua L, et al. Occurrence and predictors of the fatigue in high-grade glioma patients. Neurol Sci 2015;36(8):1363–9.

8. Rooney AG, Carson A, Grant R. Depression in cerebral glioma patients: a systematic review of observational studies. J Natl Cancer Inst 2011; 103(1):61–76.

9. Klein M, Taphoorn MJ, Heimans JJ, et al. Neurobehavioral status and health-related quality of life in newly diagnosed high-grade glioma patients. J Clin Oncol 2001;19(20):4037–47.

10. Taphoorn M, Stupp R, Coens C, et al. Health-related quality of life in patients with glioblastoma: a randomised controlled trial. Lancet Oncol 2005; 6(12):937–44.

11. Giovagnoli AR. Quality of life in patients with stable disease after surgery, radiotherapy, and chemotherapy for malignant brain tumour. J Neurol Neurosurg Psychiatry 1999;67:358–63.

12. Edelstein K, Coate L, Massey C, et al. Illness intrusiveness and subjective well-being in patients with glioblastoma. J Neurooncol 2016;126(1):127–35.

13. Dirven L, Aaronson N, Heimans J, et al. Health-related quality of life in high-grade glioma patients. Chin J Cancer 2014;33(1):40–5.

14. Brown P, Maurer M, Rummans T, et al. A prospective study of quality of life in adults with newly diagnosed high-grade gliomas: the impact of the extent of resection on quality of life and survival. Neurosurgery 2005;57(3):495–504.

15. Taphoorn MJB, Klein M. Cognitive deficits in adult patients with brain tumors. Lancet Neurol 2004; 3(3):159–68.

16. Aaronson NK, Taphoorn MJ, Heimans JJ, et al. Compromised health-related quality of life in patients with low-grade glioma. J Clin Oncol 2011; 29(33):4430–5.

17. Douw L, Klein M, Fagel SS, et al. Cognitive and radiological effects of radiotherapy in patients with low-grade glioma: long-term follow-up. Lancet Neurol 2009;8(9):810–8.

18. Klein M, Heimans JJ, Aaronson NK, et al. Effect of radiotherapy and other treatment-related factors on mid-term to long-term cognitive sequelae in low-grade gliomas: a comparative study. Lancet 2002;360(9343):1361–8.

19. Postma T, Klein M, Verstappen C, et al. Radiotherapy-induced cerebral abnormalities in patients with low-grade glioma. Neurology 2002; 59(1):121–3.

20. Ernst-Stecken A, Ganslandt O, Lambrecht U, et al. Survival and quality of life after hypofractionated stereotactic radiotherapy for recurrent malignant glioma. J Neurooncol 2007;81(3):287–94.

21. Keime-Guibert F, Chinot O, Taillandier L, et al. Radiotherapy for glioblastoma in the elderly. N Engl J Med 2007;356(15):1527–35.

22. Minniti G, Scaringi C, Baldoni A, et al. Health-related quality of life in elderly patients with newly diagnosed glioblastoma treated with short-course radiation therapy plus concomitant and adjuvant temozolomide. Int J Radiat Oncol Biol Phys 2013; 86(2):285–91.

23. Taphoorn MJ, van den Bent MJ, Mauer ME, et al. Health-related quality of life in patients treated for anaplastic oligodendroglioma with adjuvant chemotherapy: results of a European Organisation for Research and Treatment of Cancer randomized clinical trial. J Clin Oncol 2007;25(36):5723–30.

24. Reddy K, Gaspar L, Kavanagh B, et al. Prospective evaluation of health-related quality of life in patients with glioblastoma multiforme treated on a phase II trial of hypofractionated IMRT with temozolomide. J Neurooncol 2013;114(1):111–6.

25. Habets EJ, Taphoorn MJ, Nederend S, et al. Health-related quality of life and cognitive functioning in long-term anaplastic oligodendroglioma and oligoastrocytoma survivors. J Neurooncol 2014;116:161–8.

26. Erdem-Eraslan L, van den Bent M, Hoogstrate Y, et al. Identification of patients with recurrent glioblastoma who may benefit from combined bevacizumab and CCNU therapy: a report from the BELOB trial. Cancer Res 2016;76(3):525–34.

27. Chinot O, Wick W, Mason W, et al. Bevacizumab plus radiotherapy-temozolomide for newly diagnosed glioblastoma. N Engl J Med 2014;370(8): 709–22.

28. Dirven L, van den Bent M, Bottomley A, et al. The impact of bevacizumab on health-related quality of life in patients treated for recurrent glioblastoma: results of the randomised controlled phase 2 BELOB trial. Eur J Cancer 2015;51(10):1321–30.

29. Poulsen H, Urup T, Michaelsen S, et al. The impact of bevacizumab treatment on survival and quality of life in newly diagnosed glioblastoma patients. Cancer Manag Res 2014;6:373–87.

30. Taphoorn M, Henriksson R, Bottomley A, et al. Health-related quality of life in a randomized phase III study of bevacizumab, temozolomide, and radiotherapy in newly diagnosed glioblastoma. J Clin Oncol 2015;33(19):2166–75.

31. Gilbert M, Dignam J, Armstrong T, et al. A randomized trial of bevacizumab for newly diagnosed glioblastoma. N Engl J Med 2014;370(8): 699–708.

32. Klein M, Engelberts NH, van der Ploeg HM, et al. Epilepsy in low-grade gliomas: the impact on cognitive function and quality of life. Ann Neurol 2003;54(4):514–20.

33. Maschio M, Dinapoli L, Sperati F, et al. Levetiracetam monotherapy in patients with brain tumor-related epilepsy: seizure control, safety, and quality of life. J Neurooncol 2011;104(1):205–14.

34. Maschio M, Dinapoli L, Sperati F, et al. Oxcarbazepine monotherapy in patients with brain tumor-related epilepsy: open-label pilot study for assessing the efficacy, tolerability and impact on quality of life. J Neurooncol 2012;106(3):651–6.

35. Kaal E, Vecht C. The management of brain edema in brain tumors. Curr Opin Oncol 2004;16(6):593–600.

36. Dirven L, Reijneveld JC, Aaronson NK, et al. Health-related quality of life in patients with brain tumors: limitations and additional outcome measures. Curr Neurol Neurosci Rep 2013;13(7):1–9.

37. Bosma I, Reijneveld J, Douw L, et al. Health-related quality of life of long-term high-grade glioma survivors. Neuro Oncol 2009;11(1):51–8.

38. Yavas C, Zorlu F, Ozyigit G, et al. Health-related quality of life in high-grade glioma patients: a prospective single-center study. Support Care Cancer 2012;20(10):2315–25.

39. Giovagnoli AR, Boiardi A. Cognitive impairment and quality of life in long-term survivors of malignant brain tumors. Ital J Neurol Sci 1994;15(9):481–8.

40. Mitchell A, Kemp S, Benito-Leon J, et al. The influence of cognitive impairment on health-related quality of life in neurological disease. Acta Neuropsychiatr 2010;22(1):2–13.

41. Bosma I, Vos M, Heimans J, et al. The course of neurocognitive functioning in high-grade glioma patients. Neuro Oncol 2007;9(1):53–62.

42. Flechl B, Ackerl M, Sax C, et al. Neurocognitive and sociodemographic functioning of glioblastoma long-term survivors. J Neurooncol 2012;109(2):331–9.

43. Sagberg L, Solheim O, Jakola A. Quality of survival the 1st year with glioblastoma: a longitudinal study of patient-reported quality of life. J Neurosurg 2015;124(4):989–97.

44. Noll K, Bradshaw M, Weinberg J, et al. Relationships between neurocognitive functioning, mood, and quality of life in patients with temporal lobe glioma. Psychooncology 2015. [Epub ahead of print].

45. Brown PD, Buckner JC, O'Fallon JR, et al. Importance of baseline mini-mental state examination as a prognostic factor for patients with low-grade glioma. Int J Radiat Oncol Biol Phys 2004;59(1):117–25.

46. Johnson DR, Sawyer AM, Meyers CA, et al. Early measures of cognitive function predict survival in patients with newly diagnosed glioblastoma. Neuro Oncol 2012;14(6):808–16.

47. Klein M, Postma TJ, Taphoorn MJB, et al. The prognostic value of cognitive functioning in the survival of patients with high-grade glioma. Neurology 2003;61(12):1796–8.

48. Meyers CA, Hess KR, Yung WA, et al. Cognitive function as a predictor of survival in patients with recurrent malignant glioma. J Clin Oncol 2000;18(3):646.

49. Meyers CA, Hess KR. Multifaceted end points in brain tumor clinical trials: cognitive deterioration precedes MRI progression. Neuro Oncol 2003;5(2):89–95.

50. Klein M. Neurocognitive functioning in adult WHO grade II gliomas: impact of old and new treatment modalities. Neuro Oncol 2012;14(Suppl 4):iv17–24.

51. Derks J, Reijneveld J, Douw L. Neural network alterations underlie cognitive deficits in brain tumor patients. Curr Opin Oncol 2014;26(6):627–33.

52. Klein M, Duffau H, de Witt Hamer P. Cognition and resective surgery for diffuse infiltrative glioma: an overview. J Neurooncol 2012;108:309–18.

53. Tucha O, Smely C, Preier M, et al. Cognitive deficits before treatment among patients with brain tumors. Neurosurgery 2000;47(2):324–34.

54. Agner C, Dujovny M, Gaviria M. Neurocognitive assessment before and after cranioplasty. Acta Neurochir (Wien) 2002;144(10):1033–40.

55. Talacchi A, Santini B, Savazzi S, et al. Cognitive effects of tumour and surgical treatment in glioma patients. J Neurooncol 2011;103(3):541–9.

56. Tucha O, Smely C, Preier M, et al. Preoperative and postoperative cognitive functioning in patients with frontal meningiomas. J Neurosurg 2003;98(1):21–31.

57. Yoshii Y, Tominaga D, Sugimoto K, et al. Cognitive function of patients with brain tumor in pre- and postoperative stage. Surg Neurol 2008;69(1):51–61.

58. Scarone P, Gatignol P, Guillaume S, et al. Agraphia after awake surgery for brain tumor: new insights into the anatomo-functional network of writing. Surg Neurol 2009;72(3):223–41.

59. Greene-Schloesser D, Robbins M. Radiation-induced cognitive impairment - from bench to bedside. Neuro Oncol 2012;14:iv37–44.

60. Wefel J, Schagen S. Chemotherapy-related cognitive dysfunction. Curr Neurol Neurosci Rep 2012;12(3):267–75.

61. Abrey L. The impact of chemotherapy on cognitive outcomes in adults with primary brain tumors. J Neurooncol 2012;108:285–90.

62. Lucas M. The impact of chemo brain on the patient with a high-grade glioma. Adv Exp Med Biol 2010;678:21–5.

63. Perez-Larraya G, Ducray F, Chinot O, et al. Temozolomide in elderly patients with newly diagnosed glioblastoma and poor performance status: an ANOCEF phase II trial. J Clin Oncol 2011;29(22):3050–5.

64. Hilverda K, Bosma I, Heimans J, et al. Cognitive functioning in glioblastoma patients during radiotherapy and temozolomide treatment: initial findings. J Neurooncol 2010;97(1):89–94.

65. Fathpour P, Obad N, Espedal H, et al. Bevacizumab treatment for human glioblastoma. Can it induce cognitive impairment? Neuro Oncol 2014; 16(5):754–6.

66. Henriksson R, Asklund T, Poulsen H. Impact of therapy on quality of life, neurocognitive function and their correlates in glioblastoma multiforme: a review. J Neurooncol 2011;104(3):639–46.

67. Wefel J, Cloughesy T, Zazzali J, et al. Neurocognitive function in patients with recurrent glioblastoma treated with bevacizumab. Neuro Oncol 2011;13(6):660–8.

68. van Breemen M, Wilms E, Vecht C. Epilepsy in patients with brain tumours: epidemiology, mechanisms, and management. Lancet Neurol 2007; 6(5):421–30.

69. Carreno M, Donaire A, Sanchez-Carpintero R. Cognitive disorders associated with epilepsy: diagnosis and treatment. Neurologist 2008;14(6): S26–34.

70. Fietta P, Fietta P, Delsante G. Central nervous system effects of natural and synthetic glucocorticoids. Psychiatry Clin Neurosci 2009;63(5):613–22.

71. Folstein M, Folstein S, McHugh P. 'Mini-mental state': a practical method for grading the cognitive state of patients for the clinician. J Psychiatr Res 1975;12(3):189–98.

72. Gorlia T, Van den Bent MJ, Hegi M, et al. Nomograms for predicting survival of patients with newly diagnosed glioblastoma: prognostic factor analysis of EORTC and NCIC trial 26981-22981/CE.3. Lancet Oncol 2008;9(1):29–38.

73. Larner A. Screening utility of the Montreal Cognitive Assessment (MoCA): in place of - or as well as - the MMSE? Int Psychogeriatr 2012;24(3):391–6.

74. Nasreddine Z, Phillips N, Bedirian V, et al. The Montreal Cognitive Assessment, MoCA: A brief screening tool for mild cognitive impairment. J Am Geriatr Soc 2005;53(4):695–9.

75. Mioshi E, Dawson K, Mitchell J, et al. The Addenbrooke's Cognitive Examination Revised (ACE-R): a brief cognitive test battery for dementia screening. Int J Geriatr Psychiatry 2006;21(11):1078–85.

76. Meyers C, Brown P. Role and relevance of neurocognitive assessment in clinical trials of patients with CNS tumors. J Clin Oncol 2006;24(8):1305–9.

77. Schagen S, Klein M, Reijneveld J, et al. Monitoring and optimising cognitive function in cancer patients: present knowledge and future directions. EJC Suppl 2014;12(1):29–40.

78. Correa DD, DeAngelis LM, Shi W, et al. Cognitive functions in low-grade gliomas: disease and treatment effects. J Neurooncol 2007;81(2):175–84.

79. Lageman S, Cerhan J, Locke D, et al. Comparing neuropsychological tasks to optimize brief cognitive batteries for brain tumor clinical trials. J Neurooncol 2010;96(2):271–6.

80. Lin N, Wefel J, Lee E, et al. Challenges relating to solid tumour brain metastases in clinical trials, part 2: neurocognitive, neurological, and quality-of-life outcomes. A report from the RANO group. Lancet Oncol 2013;14(10):e407–16.

81. Van den Bent MJ, Wefel JS, Schiff D, et al. Response assessment in neuro-oncology (a report of the RANO group): assessment of outcome in trials of diffuse low-grade gliomas. Lancet Oncol 2011;12(6):583–93.

82. Wefel J, Vardy J, Ahles T, et al. International Cognition and Cancer Task Force recommendations to harmonise studies of cognitive function in patients with cancer. Lancet Oncol 2011;12(7): 703–8.

83. Gehring K, Aaronson NK, Taphoorn MJ, et al. Interventions for cognitive deficits in patients with a brain tumor: an update. Expert Rev Anticancer Ther 2010;10(11):1779–95.

84. Munoz-Cespedes J, Rios-Lago M, Paul N, et al. Functional neuroimaging studies of cognitive recovery after acquired brain damage in adults. Neuropsychol Rev 2005;15(4):169–83.

85. Stein D, Hoffman S. Concepts of CNS plasticity in the context of brain damage and repair. J head Trauma Rehabil 2003;18(4):317–41.

86. Roberts PS, Nuño M, Sherman D, et al. The impact of inpatient rehabilitation on function and survival of newly diagnosed patients with glioblastoma. Phys Med Rehabil 2014;6:514–21.

87. Gehring K, Sitskoorn MM, Gundy CM, et al. Cognitive rehabilitation in patients with gliomas: a randomized, controlled trial. J Clin Oncol 2009; 27(22):3712–22.

88. Hassler MR, Elandt K, Preusser M, et al. Neurocognitive training in patients with high-grade glioma: a pilot study. J Neurooncol 2010;97(1):109–15.

89. Locke DE, Cerhan JH, Wu W, et al. Cognitive rehabilitation and problem-solving to improve quality of life of patients with primary brain tumors: a pilot study. J Support Oncol 2008;6(8):383–91.

90. Sacks-Zimmerman A, Duggal D, Liberta T. Cognitive remediation therapy for brain tumor survivors with cognitive deficits. Cureus 2015;7(10):e350.

91. Sherer M, Meyers CA, Bergloff P. Efficacy of post-acute brain injury rehabilitation for patients with primary malignant brain tumors. Cancer 1997; 80(2):250–7.

92. Khan F, Amatya B, Physio B, et al. Effectiveness of integrated multidisciplinary rehabilitation in primary brain cancer survivors in an Australian community cohort: a controlled clinical trial. J Rehabil Med 2014;46(8):754–60.

93. Langenbahn DM, Ashman T, Cantor J, et al. An evidence-based review of cognitive rehabilitation in medical conditions affecting cognitive function. Arch Phys Med Rehabil 2013;94(2):271–86.

94. Piil K, Juhler M, Jakobsen J, et al. Daily life experiences of patients with a high-grade glioma and their caregivers: a longitudinal exploration of rehabilitation and supportive care needs. J Neurosci Nurs 2015;47(5):271–84.

95. Gehring K, Hoogendoorn P, Sitskoorn M. The development of a web-based application of an evidence-based cognitive rehabilitation program for patients with primary brain tumors. Neuro Oncol 2013;15(Suppl 3):iii92–7.

96. Gomez-Pinilla F, Hillman C. The influence of exercise on cognitive abilities. Compr Physiol 2013;3:403–28.

97. Hötting K, Röder B. Beneficial effects of physical exercise on neuroplasticity and cognition. Neurosci Biobehav Rev 2013;37(9):2243–57.

98. Butler JM Jr, Case LD, Atkins J, et al. A phase III, double-blind, placebo-controlled prospective randomized clinical trial of d-threo-methylphenidate HCl in brain tumor patients receiving radiation therapy. Int J Radiat Oncol Biol Phys 2007;69(5):1496–501.

99. Gehring K, Patwardhan SY, Collins R, et al. A randomized trial on the efficacy of methylphenidate and modafinil for improving cognitive functioning and symptoms in patients with a primary brain tumor. J Neurooncol 2012;107(1):165–74.

100. Boele FW, Douw L, de Groot M, et al. The effect of modafinil on fatigue, cognitive functioning, and mood in primary brain tumor patients: a multicenter randomized controlled trial. Neuro Oncol 2013;15(10):1420–8.

101. Page B, Shaw E, Lu L, et al. Phase II double-blind placebo-controlled randomized study of armodafinil for brain radiation-induced fatigue. Neuro Oncol 2015;17(10):1393–401.

102. Brown PD, Pugh S, Laack NN, et al. Memantine for the prevention of cognitive dysfunction in patients receiving whole-brain radiotherapy: a randomized, double-blind, placebo-controlled trial. Neuro Oncol 2013;15(10):1429–37.

103. Shaw EG, Rosdhal R, D'Agostino RB, et al. Phase II study of donepezil in irradiated brain tumor patients: effect on cognitive function, mood, and quality of life. J Clin Oncol 2006;24(9):1415–20.

104. Day J, Zienius K, Gehring K, et al. Interventions for preventing and ameliorating cognitive deficits in adults treated with cranial irradiation. Cochrane Database Syst Rev 2014;(12):CD011335.

105. Reitan R. Validity of the trail making test as an indicator of organic brain damage. Percept Mot Skills 1958;8(3):271–6.

106. Wechsler D. Wechsler adult intelligence scale–fourth edition. San Antonio (TX): Pearson; 2008.

107. Benedict R, Schretlen D, Groninger L, et al. Hopkins Verbal Learning Test–Revised: normative data and analysis of inter-form and test-retest reliability. Clin Neuropsychol 1998;12(1):43–55.

108. Ruff R, Light R, Parker S, et al. Benton Controlled Oral Word Association Test: reliability and updated norms. Arch Clin Neuropsychol 1996;11(4):329–38.

109. Ruff R, Parker S. Gender- and age-specific changes in motor speed and eye-hand coordination in adults: normative values for the finger tapping and grooved pegboard tests. Perceptual Mot skills 1993;76(3c):1219–30.

110. Strauss E, Sherman E, Spreen O. A compendium of neuropsychological tests: administration, norms, and commentary. New York: Oxford University Press; 2006.

CHAPTER 22

Socioeconomics and Survival

Maya A. Babu, MD, MBA

INTRODUCTION

Accounting for 52% of all primary brain tumors, glioblastoma is the most common and most aggressive.[1] Glioblastomas account for 20% of all intracranial tumors.[1] Disparities in risk factors,[2,3] incidence,[4,5] treatment,[6,7] and follow-up[8,9] have been shown in the literature for several types of cancer. For patients with glioblastoma, the influence of socioeconomic factors, including gender, race, ethnicity, income level, marital status, and occupation, have been explored in several articles. This issue reviews the literature on socioeconomic status (SES) and glioblastoma.

PROPOSED RISK FACTORS FOR GLIOBLASTOMA

Although there are no definable risk factors for glioblastoma, several studies have explored putative risk factors. In one article, 80% of patients with newly diagnosed glioblastoma had detectable cytomegalovirus (CMV) DNA in their peripheral blood, whereas seropositive normal donors and other surgical patients did not show detectable virus.[1] Challenging this finding, another study reported that a series of 5 patients with glioblastoma showed no circulating CMV detected either with reverse transcription polymerase chain reaction or blood culture.[1] Several investigators hypothesized that CMV could be a factor in the genesis of glioblastoma if age at infection is taken into account, because the incidence of both glioblastoma and CMV infection are inversely related to SES. CMV infection in early childhood, which is most common in lower socioeconomic groups, may be protective against glioblastoma, whereas CMV infection in later childhood or adulthood may be a risk factor for glioblastoma. If so, glioblastoma occurrence would resemble paralytic polio, in which low SES, poor hygiene, and early infection are protective.[1] This hypothesis has not been supported in the literature.

Some investigators suggest a relationship between glioblastoma and neurocysticercosis. In a case-control study, 6 of 8 patients with neurocysticercosis and a cerebral glioma had calcified parasitic lesions within and around the tumor. The investigators hypothesized that the intense astrocytic gliosis that surrounds calcified cysticerci, together with the suppression of the cellular immune response induced by cysticerci, may contribute to the development of malignant glial cells in patients with neurocysticercosis.[10] However, the relationship between glioblastoma and neurocysticercosis was not statistically significant.

In terms of behavioral risk factors, a study of cigarette smoking, alcohol intake, and risk of glioma in the National Institutes of Health–AARP (American Association for Retired Persons) Diet and Health Study of 477,095 American men and women found that smoking and alcohol consumption did not increase the risk of glioma.[11]

SOCIOECONOMIC STATUS AND THE DIAGNOSIS OF GLIOBLASTOMA

The negative impact of SES on many medical conditions is widely understood; patients without financial resources, who lack transportation, and who do not have the means to access timely primary care services often experience delays in diagnosis. Early diagnosis in patients with glioblastoma of differing SES has not explicitly been explored in the literature. However, several articles have examined the incidence of glioblastoma and its relation to SES. For instance, one study found associations between age, sex, Medicaid enrollment, and the incidence of primary malignant brain tumors in Michigan from 1996 to 1997 examining the Michigan Cancer Surveillance Program (1006 cases). Persons enrolled in Medicaid were more likely than nonenrolled persons to develop a malignant brain tumor of any type, including glioblastoma or astrocytoma. Incidence

Department of Neurological Surgery, Mayo Clinic, 200 First Street SW, Rochester, MN 55905, USA
E-mail address: Babu.Maya@mayo.edu

rates for malignant brain tumors in persons enrolled in Medicaid peaked at a younger age.[12]

Another study examined the incidence and epidemiology of glioblastoma in Los Angeles County, California, from 1974 to 1999. Men had a higher overall incidence of glioblastoma compared with women. In this study, non–Latin American white people had the highest incidence rates (2.5 per 100,000) followed by Latin American white people (1.8 per 100,000), and African Americans (1.5 per 100,000). Glioblastoma incidence increased in Los Angeles County after 1989, suggesting that the introduction of MRI may have contributed to an increase in diagnosis. Older age, male gender, higher SES, and non–Latin American white race increased the risk of glioblastoma in this article.[13] Similarly, another study examined 880 patients with a diagnosis of glioblastoma who had surgery between 2006 and 2012; increasing glioblastoma incidence was associated with increasing wages, employment status, lower population density, and greater ownership of cars.[14]

Several other studies have found an association between higher SES and a higher risk of glioblastoma. For instance, one study showed that, relative to persons living in census areas with the lowest SES quintile, the highest SES quintile had a higher rate of glioblastoma.[15] Similar associations were seen in population subgroups defined by age, sex, and race. A study of men aged 20 years and older who died of brain tumors in Washington State between 1969 and 1978 found that increasing SES was associated with a higher risk for all brain tumors, including gliomas and astrocytomas. After adjustment for SES, stationary engineers were found to be at excess risk across all tumor types. Increased numbers of astrocytic tumors were observed for petroleum refinery workers, forestry workers, and cleaning service workers.[16] The strong association between higher SES and glioblastoma risk is unlikely to represent an ascertainment effect because glioblastoma is rapidly progressive and ultimately fatal. An ascertainment effect represents a systematic failure to represent equally all classes of cases or people supposed to be represented in a sample (ie, a sampling bias). In this context, an ascertainment effect would suggest that lower SES patients have not been appropriately included within the sampling, such that it seems that higher SES is correlative as a risk factor for glioblastoma. The investigators of this study do not believe that ascertainment effect explains these findings, and suggest instead that several previously proposed glioma risk factors may be correlated with SES, including atopy and allergy rates.[15]

In terms of brain tumors among children, several investigators reviewed the California Cancer Registry to examine primary central nervous system tumors (PCNST) from 2001 to 2005. Children younger than 5 years old had the highest incidence of malignant PCNST (2.6 per 100,000). Teens aged 15 to 19 years had the highest incidence of benign PCNST (1.8 per 100,000). There was no statistically significant difference in the incidence of malignant PCNST by race/ethnicity in any age group assessed by this study.[17]

SOCIOECONOMIC STATUS AND THE TREATMENT AND FOLLOW-UP OF GLIOBLASTOMA

Studies have revealed that glioblastoma long-term survival was most related to prognostically favorable clinical factors, in particular young age and good initial functional performance score, as well as O(6)-methylguanine-DNA methyltransferase promoter hypermethylation.[18] Socioeconomic, environmental, and occupational factors did not correlate with survival. The influence of site of treatment has been explored in the literature. In one study, survival of patients treated in private hospitals was statistically superior to that of patients treated in public hospitals.[19]

A retrospective study of Michigan Medicaid and Medicare patients with a first primary astrocytoma diagnosis between 1996 and 2000 revealed that controlling for age, income, surgical intervention, comorbidities, gender, and stage, African Americans were less likely to report having received radiation treatment than white people.[20] Patients with dual eligibility in Medicare and Medicaid were less likely to report having received radiation treatment than those with Medicare only. These differences were not seen with chemotherapy. When only those with a glioblastoma were examined, dual eligible patients and African Americans were much less likely to report radiation treatment. These data suggest that disparities in race and insurance status may exist in receiving standard-of-care treatment of astrocytomas.[20] Another study examined 22,777 patients diagnosed with glioblastoma between 1988 and 2007. Overall, 74% received radiation, whereas 26% did not. Factors associated with omission of radiation included older age, lower annual income, African American race, Hispanic race, Asian American race, unmarried status, and subtotal resection/biopsy. The use of radiation was significantly associated with improved overall survival (2-year survival, 14.6% vs 4.2%).[21] Several investigators evaluated surgical intervention and postoperative radiation therapy receipt, and patient data for patients diagnosed with glioblastoma were obtained from the years 2004 to 2008 from a National Cancer Institute database. Younger, married patients in hospital services areas with higher median incomes were significantly more likely to receive both gross total resection and postoperative radiation therapy. The density of radiation oncology–equipped hospitals was also a significant predictor of postoperative radiation therapy receipt. These findings suggest regional variations in of neuro-oncology services and income.[22]

A study of the Surveillance, Epidemiology, and End Results program from 2000 to 2010 of 26,481 patients found that, from lowest to highest SES quintile, median survival ranged from 5 months to 9 months, respectively.[23] The association between SES and survival was not driven solely by poor outcomes in the lowest SES group; the difference in survival between the middle and highest quintiles was also statistically significant. SES remained highly associated with survival in a multivariable model including patient age, sex, race/ethnicity, radiation therapy usage, and surgery type (gross total resection vs other surgery vs no surgery). This study suggests a strong association between higher SES and increased survival after diagnosis of glioblastoma in the United States.

Another retrospective cohort study compared early versus late hospice enrollment of patients with primary malignant brain tumors admitted to the home hospice program of a large urban, not-for-profit home health care agency between 2009 and 2013. Of 160 patients with primary malignant brain tumors followed to death in hospice care, 22.5% were enrolled within 7 days of death. Compared with patients referred to hospice more than 7 days before death, a greater proportion of those with late referral were bed bound at admission, aphasic, unresponsive, or dyspneic. In multivariable analysis, male patients who were receiving Medicaid or charitable care and were without a health care proxy were more likely to enroll in hospice within 1 week of death. Patients with primary malignant brain tumors enrolled late in hospice are severely neurologically debilitated at the time hospice is initiated may not derive optimal benefit from multidisciplinary hospice care.[24] Similarly, a study examining 197 patients with brain tumors found that 53% of patients died at home, 34% at hospice, and 12.5% at the hospital. A positive impact on caregivers for home assistance was recorded in 97% of cases, and 72% of patients had an improvement in their quality of life scores caused by rehabilitation. The decision-making process at the end of life stage is time consuming, but the degree of distress of the family is inversely proportional to the extent of the preparatory period.[25]

INTERNATIONAL EXPERIENCES

The United Kingdom's National Health Service holds that the concomitant administration of temozolomide with radiotherapy in the treatment of patients with newly diagnosed glioblastoma improves survival. The West of Scotland, a semiautonomous region within the United Kingdom, has a population with poor SES and has had a poor record of implementing this treatment paradigm. Prospectively collected clinical data were analyzed in 105 consecutive patients receiving concurrent chemoradiotherapy following surgical treatment of glioblastoma. These data were compared with data from 106 patients with glioblastoma who had radical radiotherapy after surgery. The median overall survival for the treatment cohort was 15.3 months, with 1-year and 2-year overall survival rates of 65.7% and 19%, respectively. Multivariate Cox regression analysis showed that independent prognostic factors for better survival were younger age, greater extent of surgical resection, and a postoperative chemoradiotherapy regimen.[26] In another United Kingdom study, of 553 patients diagnosed with glioblastoma between 2001 and 2011, 81% had 1 operation and 19% had more than 2 operations. Patients who had more than 2 operations were significantly younger (median age, 55 years vs 64 years), less likely to have multifocal or bilateral disease, and more likely to have initial macroscopic resection than those who had only 1 operation.[27]

Data from 529 Australian patients with glioblastoma diagnosed from 1998 to 2010 were divided into poor (<6 months), average (6–24 months), and long-term (>24 months) survivors. Those surviving longer than 24 months were younger and significantly more likely to be in a higher SES, be of a better performance status, have a frontal lobe tumor, have a craniotomy (rather than a biopsy), have a macroscopic resection, have 2 or more operations, and participate in a clinical trial. No statistically significant sociodemographic differences were found when comparing long-term and poor survivors with glioblastoma.[28] A study of 156,242 male Alberta, Saskatchewan, and Manitoba Canadian farmers found a statistically significant association between risk of dying from glioblastoma and increasing fuel/oil expenditures. Low income was associated with a significantly reduced risk of brain cancer mortality.[29] A prospective study of 56 Greek patients with gliomas found that 46.5% of the patients were of low SES, 25% of middle SES, and 28.5% of high SES.[30]

A retrospective study of 171 patients with glioblastoma between 2003 and 2011 in Brazil in public and private institutions found that the median survival for patients treated in private institutions was 17.4 months compared with 7.1 months for patients treated in public institutions.[31] The time from the first symptom to surgery was longer in the public setting (median of 64 days for the public hospital and 31 days for the private institution). Patients at the private hospital received radiotherapy concurrent with chemotherapy in 59.3% of cases; at the public hospital, only 21.4% received this concurrent regimen. Despite these differences, the institution of treatment was not an independent predictor of outcome. Karnofsky Performance Status and any additional treatment after surgery were predictors of survival. Survival was directly influenced by additional treatment after surgery. The investigators concluded that increasing access to treatment resources in developing countries like Brazil is necessary to benefit patients.

POTENTIAL REMEDIES FOR THE ISSUE OF ACCESS TO CARE

With literature finding disparities in treatment received by patients with differing SES and race, there is meaningful concern about how standard-of-care radiation and chemotherapeutic regimens can be administered to patients. First, making oncologists and neurosurgeons aware of treatment disparities and providing education as to how these disparities can be addressed must occur at all levels of training. Medical schools are beginning to include cultural competency as part of the standard curriculum, but this must be reinforced for residents, fellows, and practicing physicians.[32] Continuing Medical Education provides one vehicle to help educate and increase practitioner awareness regarding disparities in treatment. Second, systemic barriers to accessing care must be addressed. It had been hoped that, by mandating insurance in the United States, more individuals who were impoverished would be able to access health care. However, programs such as Medicaid, which in many states provides marginal insurance for patients, coupled with shortages in primary care physicians and long wait times for appointments in many parts of the country, have led to delays in accessing care.[33,34] For patients with an aggressive malignancy such as a glioblastoma with favorable genetic characteristics, timely initiation of treatment can help alleviate symptoms and delay morbidity. Third,

ensuring that there are enough specialists to treat underserved populations remains a challenge. Accessing tertiary care centers, which often means traveling several hundred kilometers, can be difficult for patients without sufficient financial reserves.[35] Fourth, continuing to study how patients of all SESs, races, religions, geographies, and genders access care for the treatment of glioblastoma helps inform public policy. Without continued attention to understanding diagnosis and treatment disparities, these inequities cannot be appropriately addressed.

REFERENCES

1. Lehrer S. Cytomegalovirus infection in early childhood may be protective against glioblastoma multiforme, while later infection is a risk factor. Med Hypotheses 2012;78(5):657–8.
2. Golden SH, Brown A, Cauley JA, et al. Health disparities in endocrine disorders: biological, clinical, and nonclinical factors–an Endocrine Society scientific statement. J Clin Endocrinol Metab 2012;97(9): E1579–639.
3. Doubeni CA, Major JM, Laiyemo AO, et al. Contribution of behavioral risk factors and obesity to socioeconomic differences in colorectal cancer incidence. J Natl Cancer Inst 2012;104(18):1353–62.
4. Hebert JR, Daguise VG, Hurley DM, et al. Mapping cancer mortality-to-incidence ratios to illustrate racial and sex disparities in a high-risk population. Cancer 2009;115(11):2539–52.
5. O'Keefe EB, Meltzer JP, Bethea TN. Health disparities and cancer: racial disparities in cancer mortality in the United States, 2000-2010. Front Public Health 2015;3:51.
6. Golden SH, Purnell T, Halbert JP, et al. A community-engaged cardiovascular health disparities research training curriculum: implementation and preliminary outcomes. Acad Med 2014;89(10):1348–56.
7. Chin MH, Clarke AR, Nocon RS, et al. A roadmap and best practices for organizations to reduce racial and ethnic disparities in health care. J Gen Intern Med 2012;27(8):992–1000.
8. Chu KC, Chen MS Jr, Dignan MB, et al. Parallels between the development of therapeutic drugs and cancer health disparity programs: implications for disparities reduction. Cancer 2008;113(10): 2790–6.
9. Palmer NR, Kent EE, Forsythe LP, et al. Racial and ethnic disparities in patient-provider communication, quality-of-care ratings, and patient activation among long-term cancer survivors. J Clin Oncol 2014;32(36): 4087–94.
10. Del Brutto OH, Castillo PR, Mena IX, et al. Neurocysticercosis among patients with cerebral gliomas. Arch Neurol 1997;54(9):1125–8.

11. Braganza MZ, Rajaraman P, Park Y, et al. Cigarette smoking, alcohol intake, and risk of glioma in the NIH-AARP Diet and Health Study. Br J Cancer 2014;110(1):242–8.

12. Sherwood PR, Stommel M, Murman DL, et al. Primary malignant brain tumor incidence and Medicaid enrollment. Neurology 2004;62(10):1788–93.

13. Chakrabarti I, Cockburn M, Cozen W, et al. A population-based description of glioblastoma multiforme in Los Angeles County, 1974-1999. Cancer 2005;104(12):2798–806.

14. Muquit S, Parks R, Basu S. Socio-economic characteristics of patients with glioblastoma multiforme. J Neurooncol 2015;125(2):325–9.

15. Porter AB, Lachance DH, Johnson DR. Socioeconomic status and glioblastoma risk: a population-based analysis. Cancer Causes Control 2015;26(2):179–85.

16. Demers PA, Vaughan TL, Schommer RR. Occupation, socioeconomic status, and brain tumor mortality: a death certificate-based case-control study. J Occup Med 1991;33(9):1001–6.

17. Brown M, Schrot R, Bauer K, et al. Incidence of first primary central nervous system tumors in California, 2001-2005: children, adolescents and teens. J Neurooncol 2009;94(2):263–73.

18. Krex D, Klink B, Hartmann C, et al. Long-term survival with glioblastoma multiforme. Brain 2007; 130(Pt 10):2596–606.

19. Lynch JC, Welling L, Escosteguy C, et al. Socioeconomic and educational factors interference in the prognosis for glioblastoma multiform. Br J Neurosurg 2013;27(1):80–3.

20. Sherwood PR, Dahman BA, Donovan HS, et al. Treatment disparities following the diagnosis of an astrocytoma. J Neurooncol 2011;101(1):67–74.

21. Aizer AA, Ancukiewicz M, Nguyen PL, et al. Underutilization of radiation therapy in patients with glioblastoma: predictive factors and outcomes. Cancer 2014;120(2):238–43.

22. Aneja S, Khullar D, Yu JB. The influence of regional health system characteristics on the surgical management and receipt of post operative radiation therapy for glioblastoma multiforme. J Neurooncol 2013; 112(3):393–401.

23. Leeper HE, D.R.J. Socioeconomic status predicts survival in patients with newly diagnosed glioblastoma. Neuro Oncol 2014;16(Suppl 2):ii97.

24. Diamond EL, Russell D, Kryza-Lacombe M, et al. Rates and risks for late referral to hospice in patients with primary malignant brain tumors. Neuro Oncol 2016;18(1):78–86.

25. Pompili A, Telera S, Villani V, et al. Home palliative care and end of life issues in glioblastoma multiforme: results and comments from a homogeneous cohort of patients. Neurosurg Focus 2014; 37(6):E5.

26. Teo M, Martin S, Owusu-Agyemang K, et al. A survival analysis of glioblastoma patients in the West of Scotland pre- and post-introduction of the Stupp regime. Br J Neurosurg 2014;28(3): 351–5.

27. Sia Y, Field K, Rosenthal M, et al. Socio-demographic factors and their impact on the number of resections for patients with recurrent glioblastoma. J Clin Neurosci 2013;20(10):1362–5.

28. Field KM, Rosenthal MA, Yilmaz M, et al. Comparison between poor and long-term survivors with glioblastoma: review of an Australian dataset. Asia Pac J Clin Oncol 2014;10(2):153–61.

29. Morrison HI, Semenciw RM, Morison D, et al. Brain cancer and farming in western Canada. Neuroepidemiology 1992;11(4–6):267–76.

30. Gousias K, Markou M, Voulgaris S, et al. Descriptive epidemiology of cerebral gliomas in northwest Greece and study of potential predisposing factors, 2005-2007. Neuroepidemiology 2009;33(2):89–95.

31. Loureiro LV, Pontes Lde B, Callegaro-Filho D, et al. Initial care and outcome of glioblastoma multiforme patients in 2 diverse health care scenarios in Brazil: does public versus private health care matter? Neuro Oncol 2014;16(7):999–1005.

32. American Medical Association. Med school curriculum changes aim to eliminate health care disparities. Chicago: AMA Wire; 2014.

33. Felland LE, Lechner AE, Sommers A. Improving access to specialty care for Medicaid patients: policy issues and options. New York: The Commonwealth Fund; 2013.

34. Rosenthal E. The health care waiting game. New York: New York Times; 2014.

35. Rabalais GP. Telemedicine and the pediatric tertiary care center: presented as the 2002 Melinda J. Pouncey Memorial Lecture. Ochsner J 2003;5(2): 11–4.

CHAPTER 23

National and Global Economic Impact of Glioblastoma

YouRong Sophie Su, MD*, Kalil G. Abdullah, MD

INTRODUCTION

The cost of cancer treatment has progressively increased over the past decade as newer chemotherapy and immunotherapy agents have been established. Glioblastoma, in particular, has a significant cost in the health care system because of both the severity of neurologic dysfunction that is associated with the disease and the wide range of treatment options offered in order to prolong survival. The costs of glioblastoma can be divided into medical, emotional, and financial burdens. Although often overlooked, the economic costs and burden associated with glioblastoma can affect the short-term and long-term outcomes of patients with glioblastoma.

ECONOMIC BACKGROUND AND TREATMENT COSTS

The diagnosis of glioblastoma has become streamlined in many centers as imaging modalities have become more ubiquitous. The National Brain Tumor Society estimates that 700,000 people currently live with a primary brain tumor in the United States and that 78,000 people will be diagnosed in 2016. As rates of diagnosis have increased, so has the general scale of treatment modalities, ranging from the standard of care to more personalized treatment regimens. In describing the utility of the various treatments, economic studies use the term cost-effectiveness as the additional cost per life-year gained and compares the cost-effectiveness of different treatments to determine the least costly approach that yields the greatest outcome. Economic terms often used in cost-analysis studies are listed in **Table 23.1**, as defined by the National

Institute for Health and Clinical Excellence (NICE). Many clinical studies cite incremental cost-effectiveness ratios (ICERs) with respect to quality-adjusted life-years (QALYs) to measure the cost-effectiveness of a health care intervention.

Costs for cancer therapy can be divided into direct medical, direct nonmedical, and indirect costs. Direct medical costs include imaging, surgery, medications, radiotherapy, and chemotherapy, whereas direct nonmedical costs include transportation to treatments, parking, food, telephone bills, housing, cost of any required medical and physical therapy equipment, and payment for home nurse or therapist. Before the use of chemotherapeutic agents, 71% of the direct medical costs could be accounted for by the initial hospitalization with surgery and inpatient care.[1] Indirect costs refer to the financial losses from the patient's sick leave and/or early retirement and the time invested by the patient's caregiver.

In general, brain tumors have the highest initial cost for any cancer type, with a mean net cost greater than $100,000 per patient in 2010 US dollars.[2] Comparing ICER data from Greenberg and colleagues and Uyl-de Groot and colleagues,[3] treatment of glioblastoma with temozolomide has the highest ICER compared with treatment of other cancer types (**Fig. 23.1**).

Chang and colleagues[4] in 2004 also ranked brain cancer fourth out of 7 cancers in terms of direct medical costs for treatment at an average monthly cost of $8478 (annual $101,736), even when the study focused on treatment costs before the integration of temozolomide. Despite overall high direct medical costs, 75% of the total costs of brain tumors is attributed to indirect costs.[1] This finding reflects prior studies that

Department of Neurosurgery, University of Pennsylvania, 3 Silverstein Pavilion, 3400 Spruce Street, Philadelphia, PA 19104, USA
* Corresponding author.
E-mail address: Sophie.Su@uphs.upenn.edu

TABLE 23.1
Common terminology in economic studies

Term	Definition
Cost-effectiveness analysis	Economic study comparing the costs and health outcomes of different health interventions to determine the benefit of the intervention; the benefits are often measured in units of health
Direct cost	Costs of inpatient and outpatient care, including medical and nonmedical costs
Indirect cost	Costs to patients from loss of productivity caused by missed time at work or inability to work
Cost-effectiveness ratio	Cost of an intervention per unit of health effects produced
Unit of health	Ways to assess the value that an individual places on a health state, as measure by QALYs, DALYs, or HYEs; the most commonly used unit of health is QALY
ICER	(Difference between the cost of 2 interventions)/(difference in health effects produced by the 2 interventions); a higher number means more cost to generate each additional unit of health effect
QALY	Measures of the health of an individual in terms of the length of life are adjusted based on the quality of living as determined by the person's ability to perform activities of daily living, freedom from pain, and mental burden; 1 QALY = 1 y of life in perfect health
Willingness-to-pay threshold	Monetary threshold for what society deems is acceptable for costs of health intervention

Abbreviations: DALYs, disability-adjusted life years; HYE, healthy year equivalents; ICER, incremental cost-effectiveness ratio; QALY, quality-adjusted life-year.

show, not only for brain cancer but even for other cancer types, that the burden of costs is greatest for initial care and end-of-life care.[5]

The recommended treatment of glioblastoma is maximal surgical resection, adjuvant radiation, and chemotherapy. Various studies have found that the economic costs of these 3 different modalities of treatment of glioblastoma are significantly higher compared with other types of cancer

treatments. Although outdated, Silverstein and colleagues[6] reported mean and median total costs of direct medical services in 1996 as $99,253 and $91,368, with radiotherapy and imaging as the top two contributors to costs. In their review of costs for malignant gliomas, Raizer and colleagues[7] cite a similar range, from $50,600 to $92,700, for the cost of surgery and radiation prior to any treatment with chemotherapy. The average

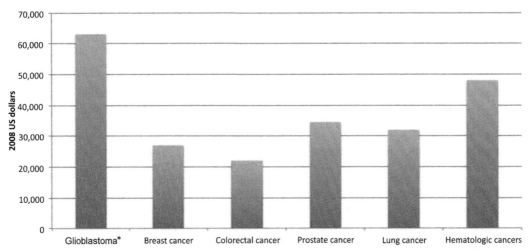

Fig. 23.1 Median reported ICER. * Although the cost listed directly refer to the median reported ICER for Glioblastoma, which is one of the most aggressive brain tumors, overall, brain tumors inclusively have the highest cost of all cancer types.

cost of craniotomy has been estimated between $12,178 and $16,292,[8,9] with modern-day costs ostensibly even higher given inflation and advances in technology. Meanwhile, mean and median monthly out-of-pocket direct expenses range from $1341 to $2450 (yearly cost, $16,092–$29,400) in order to cover the costs of medical copayments, transportation, and hospital bills. Using data from the National Institute for Clinical Excellence in the United Kingdom, Raizer and colleagues[7] estimated the cost per progression-free week to be $1955 for glioblastoma and the cost per life-year gained to be $78,185.

Temozolomide (Temodar), an alkylating agent, is dosed per body weight at 75 mg/m^2 for 42 days concomitant with focal radiotherapy followed by a maintenance dose of 150 mg/m^2 for 5 days out of a 28-day cycle for 6 cycles. If patients can tolerate higher dosing and have no significant side effects on their hematologic studies, then 200 mg/m^2/d is given for maintenance cycles 2 to 6. The estimated retail price for 5 capsules of temozolomide is $1584.57 (First Databank). The base case prices listed from the Veterans Affairs Federal Supply Schedule price a 100-mg and 20-mg capsule of temozolomide at $110 and $22, respectively.[10] The average cost per life-year gained from temozolomide ranges from $39,012 to $42,054 with the 2011 inflation-adjusted cost being $45,822.55 to $61,140.20.[7] The cost per QALY ranged from $55,731 to $72,251. The US counterpart to Raizer and colleagues'[7] study was conducted by Lamers and colleagues[11] in 2008, and examined the direct cost-effectiveness of concomitant and adjuvant temozolomide with radiotherapy in patients with newly diagnosed glioblastoma. Their study listed the cost per life-year gained for patients treated with temozolomide at $57,858 and the cost per progression-free life-year at $53,572. Although another study found the average cost of temozolomide to be lower at $31,274 compared with other studies, the main finding from this study was that the use of temozolomide as a concomitant and adjuvant treatment increased medical costs 8-fold.[12] Most of the cost of temozolomide is related to upfront acquisition costs.

Temozolomide has widely replaced other chemotherapeutic agents because of its favorable toxicity profile and ease of administration, which are considerations factored in economic studies of the cost-effectiveness for QALY in addition to cost per life-month gained or progression-free life-month.[13] Gliadel, a carmustine wafer implanted in the resection cavity of tumors, is both US Food and Drug Administration (FDA) approved in de novo and recurrent glioblastoma and has been shown to increase overall survival for several months. Westphal and colleagues[14] found that carmustine wafers increased 1-year survival by roughly 2.5 months without increasing complication rates, although more recent meta-analyses have shown that long-term complication rates may be substantial.[15] Furthermore, when carmustine wafers were used in combination with temozolomide, median survival increased by 4 months for both young and old patients with glioblastoma.[16,17] Cost associated with implantation of carmustine wafers followed by radiotherapy was £54,5000 ($101,000) per additional QALY compared with surgery with radiotherapy only.[18] This cost was similarly reflected in another study, which found that carmustine wafers required an additional £54,501 (average 2004 $99,900) per QALY.[19] Using the cost-effective standards of United Kingdom, carmustine wafers were deemed to have less than 10% probability of being cost-effective with a willingness-to-pay threshold of £30,0000 ($55,635) per QALY.[18]

For eligible patients, bevacizumab, an antibody against the vascular endothelial growth factor, is given if patients have recurrence or progression of disease after initial treatments. Bevacizumab was first approved as monotherapy for recurrent glioblastoma in found that bevacizumab reduced tumor size, increased progression-free survival, and reduced tumor-associated edema which subsequently reduced the need for steroids.[20] However, a study in 2014, found that the benefit of bevacizumab was limited to progression-free survival, including patients with and without MGMT (O_6-methylguanine-DNA-methyltransferase) status, whereas bevacizumab provided no benefit in median overall survival.[21] Dosed at 10 mg/kg every 2 weeks, Raizer and colleagues[7] estimated the monthly cost of bevacizumab to be $10,000 to $20,000. A Canadian study focusing on the cost-utility found that bevacizumab required $97,000 over a 2-year period but only increased QALY by 0.13 in newly diagnosed glioblastoma.[22] In the United Kingdom, bevacizumab is estimated to cost £21,000 (average $28,400). Most of the costs associated with bevacizumab were related to outpatient administration of the intravenous medication, management and treatment of side effects, additional physician visits and hospitalizations.[22] Despite the differences in cost, the overall consensus is that bevacizumab has a low probability of being cost-effective regardless of the willingness-to-pay threshold.

Temozolomide, carmustine wafers, and bevacizumab are the only chemotherapy agents directly approved for glioblastoma, but patients are often prescribed additional medications secondary to significant chemotherapeutic side effects. Furthermore, patients with malignant gliomas often have higher costs because of a greater need for specialty equipment (ie, wheelchair, commode) or physical, occupational, cognitive, and/or speech therapy depending on the neurologic deficits from the location and size of the mass.[23] Comparing out-of-pocket medical costs for a variety of cancer types, the American Cancer Society reports that 66% of the total costs associated with cancer treatments are typically nonmedical, and thus not covered by insurance companies. These nonmedical costs consist of transportation to clinic appointments, imaging, or physical therapy, childcare, bills for telephone, food, and housing expenses. These costs are often overlooked in terms of the burden they place on patients and their families, not only in terms of the monetary aspect of bills and loans but also in terms of the emotional stress of planning and strategizing for the costs.[24]

The most significant portion of indirect costs is related to productivity loss experienced by patients and families as patients are no longer able to functionally maintain their jobs and families must balance careers with caregiving. The National Brain Tumor Foundation cites that, of the patients who were diagnosed with brain tumors, only 33% of them remained employed after diagnosis compared with the 91% employed before diagnosis. Disability from brain tumors makes job security and financial stability difficult to maintain, and many families and caregivers of patients have to change their work practices, taking leave of absences, switching to part-time employment, and/or leaving their careers to become full-time care providers. Even for direct medication costs, patients must often bear the burden of covering for novel chemotherapeutic medications, unless they are eligible and selected for a clinical trial, because insurance companies may refuse to cover medications not approved by the FDA or still undergoing investigation.

EFFECTS OF INCOME DISPARITY ON STANDARD-OF-CARE TREATMENT AND FOLLOW-UP

The socioeconomics behind diagnosing and managing glioblastoma are difficult because patients with high-grade tumors present to the clinical setting with acute and/or rapid deterioration that requires urgent interventions and more than half of the patients develop long-lasting cognitive deficits that require therapy and support. As a result, for many patients diagnosed with cancer, the predominant viewpoint is to utilize any therapy that can provide incremental improvement in the outcome, regardless of how small or how costly that increment is. However, with costs as high as those described for the treatment of glioblastoma, it is possible that many patients cannot afford their treatment and can easily become bankrupt. It is also logical to surmise that income disparity plays a large role in the options available to patients. Higher incomes allow patients to afford better quality insurance to cover standard-of-care treatment, any out-of-pocket costs for investigational medications not covered by insurance, subsequent surgical procedures should there be recurrence, and/or ancillary equipment to facilitate a better quality of life. Twenty-five percent of families in the United States use up most or all of their savings for cancer treatment.

Although few studies address the income disparities on brain tumor treatment, Lawrence and colleagues[25] (2012) analyzed the median household income for patients with glioblastoma treated with temozolomide as part of a larger study on factors that improved prognosis. Among those who showed a survival benefit with the use of temozolomide, patients living in high-income districts had an overall survival 2 months longer than patients living in low-income districts. Although patients with higher incomes were also more likely to receive gross total resection and radiation therapy, which can confound the survival benefit, Lawrence and colleagues'[25] work reinforces that income can lead to disparities in treatment regimens and, subsequently, outcomes. Analyzing prognosis over time between high-income and low-income patients, the disparity in survival seems to be increasing over time, suggesting that income can be a separate prognostic factor for glioblastoma.

Supporting Lawrence and colleagues'[25] work, Aneja and colleagues[26] (2013) similarly found that income plays a role in the management of glioblastoma. Younger patients and patients with higher median incomes were more likely to receive gross total resection and postoperative radiation therapy. Specifically, Aneja and colleagues[26] found that every $10,000 increase in the median income correlated with a 7% increase in the rate of gross total resection for patients with glioblastoma, separate from factors including the patient's ethnicity and the density of neurosurgeons in the same geographic region.

Admission to, and care in, private versus public hospital settings also affects survival outcomes because different hospitals have access to different levels of resources.[27] Loureiro and colleagues[27] found that private and public hospitals had different access to adjuvant therapy, including type and frequency, which led to longer median overall survival times for patients treated at a private hospital (17.4 months) compared with public hospital (7.1 months).

Few patients are aware of the high costs until treatments have already been initiated. When patients are initially hospitalized for changes in their mental status or decreased arousal and are found to have a concerning intracranial lesion, there is often no hesitancy among patients to proceed with further imaging and surgical intervention. In the outpatient setting, few oncologists broach the subject of the costs of chemotherapy when they meet and discuss plans, even though they report that patients should have access to cancer treatment only if the treatments are cost-effective.[28] Although the volume of studies of the economics of glioblastoma treatment is low, it is expected that the prognosis and outcomes for glioblastoma are affected not only by tumor characteristics, patient's age, and comorbid medical conditions, but also by socioeconomic factors such as income and education.

Studies have found that patients with lower socioeconomic status often have more advanced disease at the time of diagnosis, delayed or infrequent health care, and higher recurrence rates.[29,30] The most common explanation for this negative association is that patients with lower socioeconomic status may be limited financially in their ability to acquire continuity or standard of care. They may live in regions that lack health care staff, equipment, or the resources to provide timely and easily accessible care. Furthermore, patients of lower socioeconomic status may not be able or willing to see physicians regarding mild symptoms or may even attribute their neurologic symptoms of headaches, fatigue, or blurry vision to financial insecurities, working multiple jobs, or stress. Patients with lower socioeconomic status are often associated with other chronic comorbidities (ie, obesity, diabetes, hypertension, cardiac disease) that can affect the overall health state of patients. In addition, low socioeconomic status is associated with a lower education status, which can make it more difficult to process complex treatment plans without proper instruction from the providing care team.

The quality of a patient's insurance can strongly influence diagnosis and treatment decisions for patients. In the United States health system, insurance status often acts as a proxy for socioeconomic status. High-income patients often have third-party private insurance. Lower-income patients may have limited or no health insurance, which decreases the chances of early work-up and diagnosis of a brain mass. Although the Affordable Care Act in the United States will decrease the uninsured status, the underinsured status may continue to be a concern, especially with the duration and high costs of cancer therapy. In addition, deductibles, coinsurance, and copayments can even force patients with private, high-quality insurance to experience financial strain. Studies of patients with glioblastoma, who were covered under private insurance, Medicare, or Medicaid, revealed different outcomes in terms of mortality and adverse discharges. Patients covered by Medicaid had increased mortality compared with patients on Medicare, whereas patients with private insurance had the lowest mortality.[31] Depending on insurance, patients were also evaluated at different types of hospitals, with Medicare patients more commonly treated at community hospitals with lower neurosurgical oncology volumes. For outcomes after neurosurgical procedures, El-Sayed[32] (2011) found that disparities existed between government-issued versus private insurance for critical care needs, length of hospitalization, and number of complications. Underinsured or uninsured patients were thought to have worse outcomes because of their inability to afford the ancillary facilities or staff not covered by insurance (ie, visiting home nurse for wound checks, physical therapy for rehabilitation).

NATIONAL AND INTERNATIONAL PERSPECTIVES ON THE ECONOMICS OF GLIOBLASTOMA

The United States has generally taken a more aggressive stance toward expensive treatment agents compared with other industrialized countries. Part of this stance stems from a nonsocialized, individualistic approach to patient care that does not favor cost-sparing approaches. Economic evaluations for health care are often used in countries with socialized health care, such as Australia, Canada, the United Kingdom, to evaluate cost-effectiveness of treatments and subsequently determine how best to allocate limited funds. The NICE of the United Kingdom's National Health Service is perhaps the most notable and cited database for cost-effectiveness studies on whether new treatments or therapies provide better value than treatments currently in use. Since 1999, NICE has set the willingness-to-pay threshold at £20,000 to £30,000 per QALY gained (equivalent to 2016 US\$28,445.70 to US\$42,668.55). In contrast, many cost-effectiveness studies from the United States perspective assume a willingness-to-pay threshold of \$150,000 per QALY, although few practices limit treatments based on ICER or cost-effectiveness. Regardless, many novel cancer drugs are associated with a steep increase in cost, but not an equivalent increase in benefit compared with existing cancer treatments, leading to a higher ICER. Fortunately for specific populations of patients at the end of their life, NICE has recently adopted a new approach for determining ICER per QALY for end-of-life drugs that allows the ICER to remain outside the current threshold,[33–35] creating opportunities for patients to receive previously denied treatment and medications.

As historically noted with carmustine and lomustine, nitrosourea agents gained usage in the United States in the 1980s and 1990s after clinical trials reported benefit. However, it was not until 2007 that NICE issued guidance on carmustine wafers, limiting their use for only a specific population of patients with newly diagnosed high-grade gliomas who could undergo surgery with at least 90% resection.[36] Retrospective studies after this implementation have found that carmustine wafers in combination with temozolomide improved median survival longer than previously reported.[37] However, given the lack of randomized controlled trials and concern regarding potential toxicities, many European countries continue to have conservative stances regarding the use of carmustine wafers.[38,39]

Similarly, although bevacizumab has been efficacious in some cancer types by prolonging overall survival,[40] clinical improvements have not been as dramatic in glioblastoma. Two more recent phase 3 trials found that benefits of bevacizumab were restricted only to progression-free survival and not overall survival; however, the rate of adverse events with bevacizumab was also significantly higher. One of the first studies of bevacizumab looked at its use in recurrent glioblastoma with irinotecan, an agent with topoisomerase inhibitor activity, with findings that 46% of patients had 6-month progression-free survival and 77% of patients had 6-month overall survival with only moderate toxicities.[41] The FDA accelerated approval for bevacizumab in 2009 for recurrent glioblastoma after radiation and temozolomide based on phase II studies that reported median progression-free survival of 3.7 to 4.2 months and median overall survival of 7.2 to 9.2 months.[42] However, the rate of adverse events and the high cost associated with bevacizumab can significantly influence the quality of life for patients with glioblastoma and, as a result, may explain why some countries, including the European Union, have not approved the use of bevacizumab because of their concerns of limited efficacy, cost-effectiveness, and survival benefits.[43] Note that the Committee to Evaluate Drugs recommended against the use of bevacizumab even for recurrent

glioblastoma in 2014 after a study found that patients with recurrent glioblastoma treated with bevacizumab alone not only had lower 9-month overall survival rates compared with lomustine only and combination therapies but also more toxicity.[44]

The willingness-to-pay threshold varies widely between patients based on socioeconomic status and between different countries based on medical health system. In the US third party payer system, patients bear the burden of more out-of-pocket expenses compared to patients who have subsidized costs in a nationalized medical health system. The World Health Organization endorses a willingness-to-pay threshold of 3 times the price of the gross domestic product of the country where the intervention is to be used. For example, in the United States, the willingness-to-pay threshold for temozolomide is $150,000 per QALY. In the United Kingdom, the threshold changes to €30,000 (~$34,200) per QALY.

In another example of differential thresholds for willingness to pay, Wu and colleagues[45] examined China as a nation with limited health resources and examined the Chinese approach to the treatment of patients with glioblastoma. The payment capacity of China is insufficient to cover the high costs of temozolomide. As a result, to treat their patients with glioma, many hospitals in China continue to use nitrosourea agents that have a lower cost at the expense of being less effective for patients. In China, the payment threshold is $11,034; note that the incremental costs per QALY to produce benefits for radiation and nitrosourea therapy are $87,940.60 and $94,968.30, respectively.

SUMMARY

Despite the high costs associated with glioblastoma, several studies have found that median costs of care for glioblastoma are lower compared with costs for lower-grade gliomas, in part because of how aggressive glioblastomas are and because many patients, despite optimal therapy, have significantly shorter survival periods. Patients with glioblastomas also tend to be on the older spectrum with more comorbid medical problems that may be prohibitive to certain treatments. Nonetheless, the evidence on the economics of glioblastoma can be expanded even to the broader population of patients with glioma; the costs of care can place a great financial burden on patients and create disparities in treatment. More transparency and focus need to be placed on the economics of glioblastoma for these disparities to resolve. Part of this improvement needs to begin with cost-effectiveness studies, which have only recently become integrated into glioblastoma scientific literature, despite being highly prevalent in other surgical fields. With more options available for chemotherapy and increasing medical costs, attention to cost-effectiveness and cost-utility is increasingly important. At the same time, it is important that socioeconomic disparities between patient populations, and even developed and developing countries, do not hinder patients from accessing the appropriate standard of care. A better understanding of the economic burden of glioblastoma treatment is needed to provide the most appropriate care to individual patients and local, national, and international communities.

REFERENCES

1. Blomqvist P, Lycke J, Strang P, et al. Brain tumors in Sweden 1996: care and costs. J Neurol Neurosurg Psychiatr 2000;69(6):792–8.

2. Mariotto AB, Yabroff KR, Shao Y, et al. Projections of the cost of cancer care in the United States: 2010-2020. J Natl Cancer Inst 2011;103(2):117–28.

3. Uyl-de Groot CA, Stupp R, van der Bent M. Cost-effectiveness of temozolomide for the treatment of newly diagnosed glioblastoma multiforme. Expert Rev Pharmacoecon Outcomes Res 2009;9(3):235–41 [Erratum appears in J Clin Oncology 2007;25(30):4722–9].

4. Chang S, Long SR, Kutikova L, et al. Estimating the cost of cancer: results on the basis of claims data analyses for cancer patients diagnosed with seven types of cancer during 1999 to 2000. J Clin Oncol 2004;22:3524–30.

5. Yabroff KR, Lund J, Kepka D, et al. Economic burden of cancer in the US: estimates, projections, and future research. Cancer Epidemiol Biomarkers Prev 2011;20(10):2006–14.

6. Silverstein MD, Cascino TL, Harmsen WS. High-grade astrocytomas: resource use, clinical outcomes, and cost of care. Mayo Clin Proc 1996;71:936–44.

7. Raizer JJ, Fitzner KA, Jacobs DI, et al. Economics of malignant gliomas: a critical review. J Oncol Pract 2015;11(1):e59–65.

8. Long D, Gordon T, Boman H, et al. Outcome and cost of craniotomy performed to treat tumors in regional academic referral centers. Neurosurgery 2003;62(5):1056–65.

9. Polinsky MN, Greer CP, Ross DA. Stereotaxy reduces cost of brain tumor resection. Surg Neurol 1997;48:542–50.

10. Messali A, Villacorta R, Hay JW. A review of the economic burden of glioblastoma and the cost effectiveness of pharmacologic treatments. Pharmacoeconomics 2014;32:1201–12.

11. Lamers LM, Stupp R, van den Bent M, et al. Cost-effectiveness of temozolomide for the treatment of newly diagnosed glioblastoma multiforme. Cancer 2008;112(6):1337–44.

12. Wasserfallen JB, Ostermann S, Pica A, et al. Can we afford to add chemotherapy to radiotherapy for glioblastoma multiforme? Cost-identification analysis of concomitant and adjuvant treatment with temozolomide until patient death. Cancer 2004;101(9):2098–105.

13. Martikainen JA, Kivioja A, Hallinen T, et al. Economic evaluation of temozolomide in the treatment of recurrent glioblastoma multiforme. Pharmacoeconomics 2005;23(8):803–15.

14. Westphal M, Ram Z, Riddle V, et al. Gliadel wafer in initial surgery for malignant glioma: long-term follow-up of a multicenter controlled trial. Acta Neurochir (Wien) 2006;148(3):269–75.

15. Bregy A, Shah A, Diaz M, et al. The role of Gliadel wafers in the treatment of high-grade gliomas. Expert Rev Anticancer Ther 2013;13(12):1453–61.

16. Affronti ML, Heery CR II, Herndon JE 2nd, et al. Overall survival of newly diagnosed glioblastoma patients receiving carmustine wafers followed by radiation and concurrent temozolomide plus rotational multi-agent chemotherapy. Cancer 2009;115(15):3501–11.

17. Chaichana KL, Zaidi H, Pendleton C, et al. The efficacy of carmustine wafers for older patients with glioblastoma multiforme: prolonging survival. Neurol Res 2011;33(7):759–64.

18. Rogers G, Garside R, Mealing S, et al. Carmustine implants for the treatment of newly diagnosed high-grade gliomas: a cost-utility analysis. Pharmacoeconomics 2008;26(1):33–44.

19. Garside R, Pitt M, Anderson R, et al. The effectiveness and cost-effectiveness of carmustine implants and temozolomide for the treatment of newly diagnosed high-grade glioma: a systematic review and economic evaluation. Health Technol Assess 2007;11(45):1–258.

20. Gilbert MR, Dignam JJ, Armstrong TS, et al. A randomized trial of bevacizumab for newly diagnosed glioblastoma. N Engl J Med 2014;370:699–708.

21. Chinot OL, Wick W, Mason W, et al. Bevacizumab plus radiotherapy-temozolomide for newly diagnosed glioblastoma. N Engl J Med 2014;370:709–22.

22. Kovic B, Xie F. Economic evaluation of bevacizumab for the first-line treatment of newly diagnosed glioblastoma multiforme. J Clin Oncol 2015;33(20):2296–302.

23. Kumthekar P, Stell BV, Jacobs DI, et al. Financial burden experienced by patients undergoing treatment for malignant gliomas. Neurooncol Pract 2014;1(2):71–6.

24. Bradley S, Sherwood PR, Donovan HS, et al. I could lose everything: Understanding the cost of a brain tumor. J Neurooncol 2007;85:329–38.

25. Lawrence YR, Mishra MV, Werner-Wasik M, et al. Improving prognosis of glioblastoma in the 21st century: who has benefited most? Cancer 2012; 118:4228–34.

26. Aneja S, Khuller D, Yu JB. The influence of regional health system characteristics on the surgical management and receipt of post operative radiation therapy for glioblastoma multiforme. J Neurooncol 2013; 112(3):393–401.

27. Loureiro L, de Barros Pontes L, Callegaro-Filho D, et al. Initial care and outcome of glioblastoma multiforme patients in 2 diverse health care scenarios in Brazil: does public versus private health care matter? Neuro Oncol 2014; 16(7):999–1005.

28. Neumann PJ, Palmer JA, Nadler E, et al. Cancer therapy costs influence treatment: a national survey of oncologists. Health Aff (Milwood) 2010;29(1): 196–202.

29. Curry WT, Carter BS, Barker FG. Racial, ethnic, and socioeconomic disparities in patient outcomes after craniotomy for tumor in adult patients in the US. 1988-2004. Neurosurgery 2010;66(3):427–37.

30. Dropcho EJ. Should the cost of care for patients with glioblastoma influence treatment decision. Continuum (Minneap Minn) 2012;18(2):416–20.

31. Curry WT, Barker FG II. Racial, ethnic, and socioeconomic disparities in the treatment of brain tumors. J Neurooncol 2009;93:25–39.

32. El-Sayed AM. Insurance status and inequalities in outcomes after neurosurgery. World Neurosurg 2011;76(5):459–66.

33. Collins M, Latimer N. NICE's end of life decision making scheme: impact on population health. BMJ 2013;346:f1363.

34. Greenberg D, Earle C, Fang CH, et al. When is cancer care cost-effective? A systematic overview of cost-utility analysis in oncology. J Natl Cancer Inst 2010;102:82–8.

35. Lai A, Tran A, Nghiemphu PL, et al. Phase II study of bevacizumab plus temozolomide during and after radiation therapy for patients with newly diagnosed glioblastoma multiforme. J Clin Oncol 2011;29(2): 142–8.

36. National Institute of Health and Clinical Excellence. TA121 glioma (newly diagnosed and high grade) - carmustine implants and temozolomide. Available at: http://www.niceorg/uk/nicemedia/live/11620/34049/34049.peft.2007.London:NICE. Accessed February 4, 2016.

37. Barr JG, Grundy PL. The effects of the NICE Technology Appraisal 121 (Gliadel and Temozolomide) on survival in high-grade glioma. Br J Neurosurg 2012;26(6):818–22.

38. Messali A, Hay JW, Villacorta R. The cost-effectiveness of temozolomide in the adjuvant treatment of newly diagnosed glioblastoma in the United States. Neuro Oncol 2013;15(11):1532–42.

39. Price SJ, Whittle IR, Ashkan K, et al. NICE guidance on the use of carmustine wafers in high grade gliomas: a national study on variation in practice. Br J Neurosurg 2012;26(3):331–5.

40. Tewari KS, Sill MW, Long HJ, et al. Improved survival with bevacizumab in advanced cervical cancer. N Engl J Med 2014;370:734–43.

41. Vredenburgh JJ, Desjardins A, Herndon JE, et al. Bevacizumab plus irinotecan in recurrent glioblastoma multiforme. J Clin Oncol 2007;25(30):4722–9.

42. Kreisl TN, Kim L, Moore K, et al. Phase II trial of single-agent bevacizumab followed by bevacizumab plus irinotecan at tumor progression in recurrent glioblastoma. J Clin Oncol 2009;27:740–5.

43. Wick W, Weller M, van den Bent M, et al. Bevacizumab and recurrent malignant gliomas: a European perspective. J Clin Oncol 2010;28(12):e188–9.

44. Taal W, Oosterkamp HM, Walenkamp AME, et al. Single-agent bevacizumab or lomustine versus a combination of bevacizumab plus lomustine in patients with recurrent glioblastoma (BELOB trial): a randomised controlled phase 2 trial. Lancet Oncol 2014;15(9):943–53.

45. Wu B, Miao Y, Bai Y, et al. Subgroup economic analysis for glioblastoma in a health resource-limited setting. PLoS One 2012;7(4):e34588.

CHAPTER 24

Lessons Learned
Clinical Trials and Other Interventions for Glioblastoma

Rodica Bernatowicz, MD, David Peereboom, MD*

Glioblastoma (GBM) remains the most common primary malignant brain tumor in adults and accounts for 16% of all primary brain tumors and for 45% of malignant primary brain tumors.[1] Despite ample research to find better treatments the prognosis of GBM remains grim, with a less than 10% 5-year survival with maximal medical treatment.[2]

In 2004, the European Organization for Research and Treatment of Cancer and National Cancer Institute of Canada Trails Group conducted a randomized phase III trial that led to the establishment of the current standard treatment consisting of surgical resection, radiotherapy with concomitant temozolomide, followed by temozolomide alone.[2–4] Since then, multiple single and multicenter trials have sought to advance treatment of GBM further but without great success. This chapter examines lessons learned from clinical research in GBM with the hope that future patients will benefit from more effective trials and practice.

SURGERY

Several retrospective[5–11] as well as prospective[12,13] studies have shown that extent of resection plays a key role in the overall survival and performance status of patients with GBM. Surgery is an instant way to reduce tumor burden (debulking) and, by removing mass effect, often leads to improvement and even resolution of symptoms. However, not all tumors are resectable and, especially in GBM, the tumor border is rarely clearly defined. Removing too little tumor may lead to earlier progression, whereas resecting too much brain tissue may cause unnecessary neurologic deficits. In addition, variable resectability implies a treatment bias: easily resectable tumors may have a better prognosis simply because they are less invasive, not necessarily because they were removed completely, and vice versa.

INTRAOPERATIVE TECHNIQUES

The recognition that maximal resection is an independent predictor of survival in patients with GBM led to the search for techniques to identify tumor tissue intraoperatively. Intraoperative visualization of the tumor enables the surgeon to gauge the extent of resection in real time and perform further resection if needed. Several methods for intraoperative visualization of tumor tissue have been studied, including intraoperative ultrasonography, MRI, and various tumor cell markers.

Intraoperative MRI

Intraoperative MRI (iMRI) has been studied extensively in the past decade. Although several groups have reported increased extent of resection with iMRI,[14–20] few data exist regarding the clinical benefit of iMRI as measured by overall and progression-free survival as well as performance status.[21] Thus far only 1 randomized controlled study confirmed that the use of iMRI led to higher rates of complete tumor resection compared with conventional surgery. This study also showed that postoperative complications and new neurologic deficits were comparable in both groups and therefore that the use of iMRI was safe. However, no improvement of progression-free survival was observed.[22] The use of iMRI has implications in terms of cost and operative time. iMRI prolongs the surgical procedure and overall time spent in the operating room.[22,23] In an era of medical care cost escalation, clinicians must decide

Cleveland Clinic, 9500 Euclid Avenue, R35, Cleveland, OH 44195, USA
* Corresponding author.
E-mail address: peerebd@ccf.org

whether the benefits outweigh the costs of acquisition and maintenance associated with MRI equipment located in the operating room. The authors have learned that difficult decisions such as these will become part of the success or failure of medical innovation in the future.

5-Aminolevulinic Acid as a Tumor Marker

In 2006, the ALA-Glioma Study Group conducted the only prospective randomized study that assessed the efficacy and safety of using 5-aminolevulinic acid (5-ALA) for the resection of malignant gliomas. 5-ALA is a hemoglobin precursor that leads to accumulation of fluorescent porphyrins in malignant glioma cells but not in healthy brain tissue. The use of 5-ALA and fluorescence-guided surgery was compared with traditional microsurgery using white light. Although the use of 5-ALA led to increased rates of complete resection and to longer progression-free survival, which were the 2 primary end points of the study, no benefit was found in overall survival, postoperative neurologic status, or Karnofsky Performance Score.[24]

Barone and colleagues[25] performed a systematic review of the role of imaging guidance in brain tumor surgery, including iMRI, fluorescence-guided surgery using 5-ALA, neuronavigation, and ultrasonography. Three large databases and an extensive literature review, including 4 randomized controlled trials, were performed up to 2013. Their goal was to answer 2 essential questions: (1) is image-guided surgery more effective at removing brain tumors than surgery without image guidance? (2) Is one image guidance technology or tool better than another? Based on their review, there is low to very low evidence (according to GRADE [Grading of Recommendations Assessment, Development and Evaluation] criteria) that image-guided surgery using iMRI, 5-ALA, or diffusion-tensor imaging neuronavigation increases the proportion of patients with high-grade glioma who have a complete tumour resection on postoperative MRI.[25] Similarly, there was poor evidence that image-guided surgery increases overall or progression-free survival or quality of life.[25] Thus, although the 5-ALA randomized trial did meet its primary end points, it did not extend survival or quality of life, showing that a well-executed trial that does not show improvement in these metrics may fail to attain regulatory approval (at least in the United States) and acceptance as a standard of care.

Carmustine Wafers

Biodegradable polymers (wafers) containing carmustine have proved safe when implanted in the glioma tumor cavity after resection.[26–28] The US Food and Drug Administration (FDA) approved this agent for the treatment of recurrent GBM based on the results of a multicenter, randomized controlled study.[28] Carmustine wafers were inserted into the tumor bed following gross total resection of recurrent high-grade gliomas. A clear survival benefit was found in patients with GBM treated with carmustine wafers compared with placebo wafers.

The benefit of carmustine wafers in patients with newly diagnosed GBM is less clear. The first prospective, randomized, double-blinded study using carmustine wafers in newly diagnosed high-grade gliomas was performed in Finland.[29] The subgroup analysis of patients diagnosed with GBM showed a significant survival benefit in the carmustine wafer group compared with the placebo group.[29] Four years later, a phase III trial in 240 patients with newly diagnosed high-grade gliomas was performed.[30] Although patients treated with carmustine wafers had a long-term overall survival benefit compared with the placebo group,[31] no significant survival benefit was found in the GBM subgroup.[30] None of the aforementioned studies used treatment with temozolomide in the postoperative phase because the studies were performed before temozolomide was established as standard of care for GBM.

Several retrospective studies assessed the safety and efficacy of combining carmustine wafers with radiation therapy and temozolomide (Stupp regimen[3]) in patients with GBM and concluded that the triple regimen was safe.[32–35] Few prospective data are available comparing treatment with carmustine wafers and Stupp regimen with Stupp regimen alone in patients with newly diagnosed GBM. Only 1 prospective, but nonrandomized, study in 787 patients in France compared the survival rates and postoperative complications in both treatment groups. The carmustine plus Stupp regimen arm showed significantly longer progression-free survival, but no statistically significant benefit was observed for overall survival.[36] In contrast with previous studies, patients receiving carmustine wafers and Stupp regimen had significantly more postoperative complications such as postoperative infections and increased intracranial pressure caused by edema compared with patients treated with the Stupp regimen only.

The advantages of carmustine wafers seem obvious: they provide localized treatment without significant systemic side effects and they are complementary to systemic therapy. However, the complications mentioned earlier associated with the wafers can also be significant. Note that most data on carmustine wafers do not differentiate between GBM and non-GBM gliomas and caution should be used when extrapolating the results to the subgroup of patients with GBM. In addition, carmustine wafers can interfere with the interpretation of MRIs because of local increase in enhancement caused by the wafers. For this reason, many GBM clinical trials exclude patients who have received carmustine wafers. Overall, despite being FDA approved, the enthusiasm for general use of the wafers seems modest based on modest efficacy and the clinical trial exclusion described earlier.

However, a phase 1 trial that increased the percentage of carmustine in wafers reached a maximum tolerated dose of 20% carmustine by weight, representing a 5-fold increase compared with the standard 3.8% wafer.[37] However, a phase II trial at this dose was never conducted, representing a missed opportunity in drug development.[38] Such a trial may have improved the efficacy of the wafer, showing that the phase II trials are critical to the further development of promising therapies. Further development of this technology should be explored using other agents.

RADIATION THERAPY

Stereotactic radiosurgery (SRS) focuses a radiation plan on a small tumor (usually ≤2–3 cm) using several techniques whereby multiple beams converge on a target to create a highly conformal delivery of a single or several high-dose fractions. SRS offers the hope that large-fraction doses, when added to radiation therapy, could overcome the radioresistance of GBM. Several trials have shown the benefit of SRS when added to whole-brain radiation therapy for patients with brain metastases.[39,40] The same paradigm has been attempted in high-grade glioma trials of standard radiation therapy with or without SRS.[41] In contrast with the benefits shown in brain metastases, the trials in high-grade gliomas have been uniformly negative and SRS has not developed a role in the management of GBM. These trials have taught clinicians that, despite the ability to target enhancing disease with SRS, the biology and infiltrative pattern of GBM, and all gliomas, is such that SRS fails to address a sufficient volume of nonenhancing tumor. As a result, newer local therapies, such as convection-enhanced delivery of chemotherapy, treat the infiltrative nonenhancing tumor that surrounds the enhancing disease. Future efforts to improve outcomes for patients with GBM will need to incorporate effective therapy for the nonenhancing tumor.

Various radiation therapy techniques have become standard management for several malignancies.[42] These methods include brachytherapy, intraoperative radiation therapy, and targeted radionuclide therapy. These methods have largely failed in GBM trials. Two randomized trials of brachytherapy[43,44] failed to produce a survival advantage, as did a trial using I-125 in a liquid solution placed in a balloon catheter inside the surgical cavity.[45] Similarly, several radiosensitizers (eg, bromodeoxyuridine, misonidazole, motexafin gadolinium) have failed to improve local control more than radiation therapy alone.[46–48] These various attempts to intensify local radiation therapy show that, most likely, the maximum safe dose of radiation therapy has not been enough to overcome radioresistance in GBM. Furthermore, it is likely that improvements in the initial therapy for GBM will require improvements in systemic agents that have activity as adjuvant agents after the completion of concurrent radiation with chemotherapy.

CHEMOTHERAPY

Angiogenesis Inhibitors

Like many malignancies, GBM requires an ample supply of blood vessels to support its high oxygen demand and metabolic activity.[49,50] Angiogenesis, the formation of new blood vessels, is a hallmark of malignant tumors and is crucial for tumor growth.[51] New blood vessels formed within tumors are abnormal, hindering delivery of oxygen and chemotherapeutic agents to the tumor.[52] One of the main tumor-associated regulators is vascular endothelial growth factor (VEGF) A.[53,54] Preclinical studies suggest that VEGF inhibitors lead to decreased formation and even regression of blood vessels in tumors and subsequently to tumor cell apoptosis.[55,56] Inhibition of angiogenesis normalizes blood vessels and improves delivery of oxygen and chemotherapeutic agents, which may enhance the effects of chemotherapy and radiotherapy.[57,58]

VEGF inhibitors prolong overall survival in metastatic colorectal and non–small-cell lung cancer[59] as well as progression-free survival in metastatic renal cell[60] and breast cancer.[61] The VEGF inhibitor used predominantly in cancer research is bevacizumab (Avastin), a recombinant humanized monoclonal immunoglobulin G1 antibody that binds and neutralizes VEGF.

Based on the standard combination consisting of bevacizumab and irinotecan used in colorectal cancer, oncologist Stark Vance[62] reported a series using the same regimen in patients with recurrent GBM. These striking results ultimately led to 3 trials that resulted in FDA approval of bevacizumab in recurrent GBM. Despite the benefits of bevacizumab in recurrent disease, the initial expectation of bevacizumab as a new standard of care for newly diagnosed GBM did not materialize in 2 major independent, randomized, double-blind, placebo-controlled studies (AVAglio[63,64] and RTOG 0825[65]). The lack of survival benefit showed that encouraging results in recurrent disease (typically a more resistant setting than newly diagnosed disease) do not a priori support the use of such agents; rigorous, adequately powered clinical trials must be done in both settings. This lesson will become more relevant with the advent of newer agents such as vaccines and other immunotherapies.

Dose-dense Temozolomide

Methylation status of O^6-methylguanine DNA methyltransferase (MGMT) is an important prognostic and predictive factor in newly diagnosed GBM. GBMs with MGMT promoter methylation are associated with improved overall and progression-free survival in patients treated with temozolomide.[66–70] Patients with unmethylated and therefore preserved activity of MGMT are relatively resistant to temozolomide and have a significantly weaker response to treatment with the drug. Several trials, the largest of which treated 90 and 120 patients, have been conducted seeking to overcome this resistance by altering the temozolomide regimen.[71,72] The theory behind these trials is that a more sustained exposure to temozolomide would lead to depletion of cellular MGMT and thereby overcome resistance to temozolomide.[73] In addition, some preclinical studies have suggested that metronomic dosing of temozolomide has an antiangiogenic effect on tumor cells.[74,75] However, a phase III randomized trial, RTOG 0525 (Radiation Therapy Oncology Group), compared dose-intensive adjuvant temozolomide with standard adjuvant temozolomide in patients with newly diagnosed GBM and did not show a benefit in overall or progression-free survival in patients treated with the dose-dense temozolomide regimen compared with standard dosing.[76,77]

Contradictory data exist regarding the use of dose-dense temozolomide in recurrent GBM. Although a randomized trial comparing standard-dose with dose-dense temozolomide showed significantly higher rates of progression-free and overall survival in the standard-dose arm,[78] a meta-analysis of 33 phase II and retrospective studies showed a significant progression-free and overall survival benefit with individual dose-dense regimens.[79] No differences were detected in objective response or clinical benefit in either report.

At this time, there is no level 1 evidence favoring the use of dose-dense temozolomide more than the current standard therapy. More is not always better, and parameters like adverse reactions and quality of life must be considered when using higher or prolonged doses of a cytotoxic medication. A prospective randomized controlled study may shed light on the question of which dose regimen is superior for a given agent. Although such a trial using temozolomide is unlikely to be performed, future agents may need to be evaluated in this manner if dose intensity for the given agent is thought to be potentially important. As has been shown in other solid tumors, even in the most chemotherapy-sensitive tumors,[80] dose intensity most often does not translate into improved outcomes.

Epidermal Growth Factor Receptor Inhibitors

Epidermal growth factor receptor (EGFR) is commonly mutated or amplified in GBM cells, which leads to increased tumor growth and aggressiveness.[81–84] EGFR expression is an independent negative prognostic indicator in patients with GBM,[85] a potential treatment target, and a subject of extensive research. Preclinical studies reported promising results on the effect of EGFR inhibitors on GBM cells[86–88] but thus far no large randomized controlled study has been attempted to translate those results into clinical practice. Conflicting data exist regarding the benefit of adding the EGFR inhibitor erlotinib to standard therapy for newly diagnosed GBM. One single-institution prospective phase II study reported significantly longer progression-free survival as well as overall survival in patients who received erlotinib in addition to standard therapy.[89] A multicenter prospective phase I/II trial did not find any survival benefit from adding erlotinib to standard treatment.[90] Yet another trial had to be stopped early because of unacceptable toxicity.[91]

EGFR variant III (EGFRvIII) is the most commonly found EGFR mutation, seen in approximately one-third of GBM.[85,92,93] Sampson and colleagues[94] took a novel treatment approach in a phase II multicenter study of the immune response and survival in patients by adding an EGFRvIII vaccine to standard adjuvant therapy in patients with GBM. The results were promising: patients who received intradermal injection with an EGFRvIII vaccine had significantly longer progression-free and overall survival without an increase in adverse events compared with the control group that received standard therapy alone. Almost half of the vaccinated patients developed a humoral immune response to the vaccine, which was associated with prolonged overall survival. Another striking finding was that 82% of the patients who had received the EGFRvIII vaccine lost EGFRvIII expression at tumor recurrence.

An open-label, phase II trial performed by Schuster and colleagues[95] confirmed the survival advantage by adding rindopepimut, an EGFRvIII vaccine, to standard adjuvant GBM therapy. The same group evaluated the use of rindopepimut in recurrent GBM by adding it to standard-of-care bevacizumab in the randomized phase II ReACT study.[96] Preliminary results of this study are promising with regard to 6-month progression-free survival, overall survival, and 2-year survival, as well as the use of steroids. All 3 studies are phase II trials and the number of patients who received EGFRvIII vaccination was small: 18, 65, and 36, respectively.[94–96] However, in a pattern similar to that of bevacizumab, a large, phase III trial of rindopepimut in patients with newly diagnosed GBM was terminated after an interim analysis determined that the study would likely fail to meet its primary end point of overall survival.[97] Again, in GBM, excellent results in recurrent disease trials do not always portend similar outcomes for patients with newly diagnosed GBM.

TUMOR TREATING FIELDS

Tumor treating fields (TTF) are low-intensity intermediate-frequency alternating electric fields delivered transcutaneously via arrays placed on the scalp. These fields[98] inhibit tumor growth by an antimicrotubule mechanism. A randomized trial in 237 patients with recurrent GBM showed equivalent efficacy but was associated with a better quality of life without chemotherapy toxicities.[99] Recently, a large, randomized controlled, international multicenter study was terminated early after an interim analysis showed that adjuvant temozolomide combined with TTF was associated with significantly increased overall and progression-free survival compared with adjuvant temozolomide alone.[100] The incidence and severity of adverse events were comparable in both groups. However, the final analysis of the study population, including subgroup analysis, is pending at this time.

These results are encouraging and have led to regulatory approval for TTF. This method may face a problem with regard to feasibility and compliance. Patients are required to wear the TTF electrodes more or less around the clock and may have difficulties putting the mask back on correctly. However, this device is in clinical trials in a variety of other malignancies, showing that

central nervous system (CNS) tumors can serve as the preliminary site of development of local noninvasive therapies for cancer given the relative (compared with other tumors) proximity of brain tumors to the exterior surface of the body, thus facilitating the application of novel treatment technologies.

SEIZURES AND ANTIEPILEPTIC AGENTS

From 29% to 49% of patients with GBM present with seizures[101–103] or develop them later in the disease course.[104–106] Controlling seizures in patients with brain tumors is of utmost importance because uncontrolled seizures have a detrimental impact on quality of life and can lead to long-term disability.[107–109] When treating brain tumor–related epilepsy (BTRE), providers encounter certain challenges: BTRE is notorious for its refractoriness and multidrug resistance[110,111]; enzyme-inducing AEDs (EIAEDs) increase the metabolism of some chemotherapeutic agents[112–115] as well as steroids,[116–119] necessitating dose escalation of those medications; side effects from AEDs (AEDs) occur more frequently in patients with BTRE than in the overall population[120,121]; many AEDs lead to worsening of cognitive performance in patients with brain tumors.[122–125] The lesson learned from this experience is that non-EIAEDs are a much preferred group of agents for use in patients with GBM or any brain tumors in patients who need them. Another relevant lesson is that most current GBM trials, especially early-stage studies, now exclude the use of EIAEDs as a criterion for trial eligibility in order to obtain more uniform and predictable pharmacokinetic properties an agent. A current randomized trial (NCT01432171) is comparing lacosamide with placebo to evaluate the role for this non-EIAED in the prophylaxis of seizures in patients with newly diagnosed high-grade gliomas.

CHALLENGES IN ASSESSING TREATMENT EFFICACY AND EFFECTIVENESS

Investigators face several challenges when assessing the efficacy and effectiveness of a therapeutic agent. Most of the trials discussed earlier focused on survival rates, with some reports measuring radiologic or clinical criteria to determine disease stability or progression.

Until recently, the MacDonald criteria, established in 1990, served as the standard tool to assess treatment response in high-grade gliomas.[126] They were based on imaging features, like enhancement and new lesions, and on clinical features such as corticosteroid requirement and clinical disease stability. In 2010, Wen and colleagues[127] published the updated Response Assessment in Neuro-oncology (RANO) criteria, which for the most part have replaced the MacDonald criteria. Implementation of the RANO criteria redefined the radiologic appearance of progressive disease. One of the main reasons for the revised criteria is the phenomenon of pseudoprogression, which is a treatment-related imaging finding typically seen within 3 months after radiochemotherapy. Pseudoprogression radiographically appears to be disease progression but resolves spontaneously without treatment within a few months.[128–131] Diagnosis of disease progression often has implications on disease management (eg, premature withdrawal of adjuvant therapy or reoperation), which can be detrimental for some patients, especially when these measures are unnecessary because of being based on a misleading imaging finding. Therefore, distinguishing treatment-induced imaging changes (pseudoprogression) from true progression is extremely important for patient care.

Pseudoprogression is a phenomenon mainly described after standard therapy with radiation and temozolomide.[131] A complicating factor is that chemoradiation with temozolomide is also associated with early necrosis.[129] Pseudoprogression and treatment-related necrosis have similar, often indistinguishable, appearance on MRI,[132] which poses another challenge for monitoring disease and treatment in patients with GBM.

An additional pitfall in assessing success is treatment-induced pseudoresponse, which is another radiographic phenomenon seen after treatment with antiangiogenic therapy, such as the VEGF inhibitor bevacizumab.[133,134] Radiologic response rates with antiangiogenic agents have been attributed to normalization of tumor vessel permeability[135] and do not necessarily indicate a true antitumor effect. The discrepancy between the striking improvement seen on imaging and the minor benefit on survival should again prompt practitioners to approach a radiologic response after VEGF inhibitor treatment with caution. Similar challenges with imaging analysis have occurred with the advent of TTF and immunotherapy, in which in both instances response can be delayed such that MRI early in the treatment course may falsely suggest progressive disease.[136,137]

DOES THE DRUG REACH THE TUMOR?

One fundamental question to ask when treating any disease, and brain tumors in particular, is whether the therapeutic agent gets to the diseased tissue. Answering this question for brain tumors is particularly difficult because the blood-brain barrier (BBB) prevents the entry of exogenous substances into the CNS.[138,139] In addition, drug concentrations measured in serum or cerebrospinal fluid do not reliably reflect drug concentrations at the target site because of a multitude of factors, including the chemical properties of the drug, physical and chemical obstruction by the BBB, active drug transport mechanisms, and drug metabolism at the BBB and within the brain.[140] Insufficient drug levels within the diseased tissue may lead to treatment failure and poor clinical outcome. One lesson is that molecules capable of BBB penetration should ideally be small (<500 kDa) and generally lipid soluble. In contrast, several agents do not need to cross the BBB to give patients benefit. One example of an agent that does not need to cross the BBB is bevacizumab because it works on the vasculature and not directly on the tumor. Similarly, the emerging group of checkpoint inhibitors and other immune therapies work outside the BBB.

An emerging tool to measure concentrations of a drug at a specific site more directly is microdialysis. Microdialysis is a technique that continuously quantifies the concentration of an agent in the extracellular fluid in a body tissue.[141] Microdialysis to assess chemotherapeutic response or toxicity has been studied in non-CNS tumors with promising results.[142,143] Intracerebral microdialysis is fairly safe[144] and has been applied in conditions like epilepsy,[145] traumatic brain injury,[146] and intracerebral hemorrhage.[146] Few studies have been performed to determine the concentration chemotherapeutic agents at the tumor. These studies found considerable regional differences within the brain with higher drug concentrations measured in contrast-enhancing tissue, which usually consists of tumor or tumor-surrounding tissue, whereas healthy brain tissue accumulated less drug.[147,148] Portnow and colleagues[149] measured temozolomide concentrations in nonenhancing tissue surrounding the resection bed in patients with newly diagnosed GBM. Temozolomide was given orally 1 hour before radiation as per the Stupp protocol. The time to peak of temozolomide concentration in the brain (1.2–3.4 hours after ingestion) was longer than the time to peak in serum (approximately 1 hour after ingestion), as described previously.[150] Based on these findings, the authors instruct patients receiving concurrent radiation and temozolomide to take temozolomide approximately 1.5 to 3 hours before radiation treatment to obtain the maximum radiation sensitization effect. Because the kinetics of brain penetration differ from serum pharmacokinetics, the intracerebral kinetics should be determined if possible and should ideally inform the dosing schedules for drugs for which interaction with radiation will be maximized.

SUMMARY

Over the past several decades, clinical trials both positive and negative have moved the treatment of GBM forward. Although some of the lessons learned parallel those of oncology in general, some lessons are unique to neuro-oncology and arguably have benefitted the larger body of oncology. For example, the small size of the head compared with the trunk, as well as the fixed structure of the skull, has made the CNS ideal as an initial site of investigation of TTF and several radiation therapy platforms. Perhaps the CNS will serve as a proving ground for treatment strategies that use these and other innovative forms of therapy.

REFERENCES

1. Thakkar JP, Dolecek TA, Horbinski C, et al. Epidemiologic and molecular prognostic review of glioblastoma. Cancer Epidemiol Biomarkers Prev 2014;23:1985–96.
2. Stupp R, Hegi ME, Mason WP, et al. Effects of radiotherapy with concomitant and adjuvant temozolomide versus radiotherapy alone on survival in glioblastoma in a randomised phase III study: 5-year analysis of the EORTC-NCIC trial. Lancet Oncol 2009;10:459–66.
3. Stupp R, Mason WP, van den Bent MJ, et al. Radiotherapy plus concomitant and adjuvant temozolomide for glioblastoma. N Engl J Med 2005;352:987–96.
4. Brem SS, Bierman PJ, Brem H, et al. Central nervous system cancers. J Natl Compr Canc Netw 2011;9:352–400.
5. Devaux BC, O'Fallon JR, Kelly PJ. Resection, biopsy, and survival in malignant glial neoplasms. A retrospective study of clinical parameters, therapy, and outcome. J Neurosurg 1993;78:767–75.
6. Noorbakhsh A, Tang JA, Marcus LP, et al. Gross-total resection outcomes in an elderly population with glioblastoma: a SEER-based analysis. J Neurosurg 2014;120:31–9.
7. Ammirati M, Vick N, Liao YL, et al. Effect of the extent of surgical resection on survival and quality of life in patients with supratentorial glioblastomas and anaplastic astrocytomas. Neurosurgery 1987;21:201–6.
8. Winger MJ, Macdonald DR, Cairncross JG. Supratentorial anaplastic gliomas in adults. The prognostic importance of extent of resection and prior low-grade glioma. J Neurosurg 1989;71:487–93.
9. Kreth FW, Warnke PC, Scheremet R, et al. Surgical resection and radiation therapy versus biopsy and radiation therapy in the treatment of glioblastoma multiforme. J Neurosurg 1993;78:762–6.
10. Kiwit JC, Floeth FW, Bock WJ. Survival in malignant glioma: analysis of prognostic factors with special regard to cytoreductive surgery. Zentralbl Neurochir 1996;57:76–88.
11. Stummer W, Reulen HJ, Meinel T, et al. Extent of resection and survival in glioblastoma multiforme: identification of and adjustment for bias. Neurosurgery 2008;62:564–76 [discussion: 564–76].
12. Laws ER, Parney IF, Huang W, et al. Survival following surgery and prognostic factors for recently diagnosed malignant glioma: data from the Glioma Outcomes Project. J Neurosurg 2003;99:467–73.
13. Vuorinen V, Hinkka S, Färkkilä M, et al. Debulking or biopsy of malignant glioma in elderly people – a randomised study. Acta Neurochir (Wien) 2003;145:5–10.
14. Schneider JP, Trantakis C, Rubach M, et al. Intraoperative MRI to guide the resection of primary supratentorial glioblastoma multiforme–a quantitative radiological analysis. Neuroradiology 2005;47:489–500.
15. Nimsky C, Ganslandt O, Buchfelder M, et al. Intraoperative visualization for resection of gliomas: the role of functional neuronavigation and intraoperative 1.5 T MRI. Neurol Res 2006;28:482–7.
16. Nimsky C, Ganslandt O, Buchfelder M, et al. Glioma surgery evaluated by intraoperative low-field magnetic resonance imaging. Acta Neurochir Suppl 2003;85:55–63.
17. Senft C, Franz K, Blasel S, et al. Influence of iMRI-guidance on the extent of resection and survival of patients with glioblastoma multiforme. Technol Cancer Res Treat 2010;9:339–46.
18. Wirtz CR, Knauth M, Staubert A, et al. Clinical evaluation and follow-up results for intraoperative magnetic resonance imaging in neurosurgery. Neurosurgery 2000;46:1112–20 [discussion: 1120–2].
19. Hirschberg H, Samset E, Hol PK, et al. Impact of intraoperative MRI on the surgical results for high-grade gliomas. Minim Invasive Neurosurg 2005;48:77–84.
20. Muragaki Y, Iseki H, Maruyama T, et al. Usefulness of intraoperative magnetic resonance imaging for glioma surgery. Acta Neurochir Suppl 2006;98:67–75.
21. Kubben PL, ter Meulen KJ, Schijns OE, et al. Intraoperative MRI-guided resection of glioblastoma multiforme: a systematic review. Lancet Oncol 2011;12:1062–70.

22. Senft C, Bink A, Franz K, et al. Intraoperative MRI guidance and extent of resection in glioma surgery: a randomised, controlled trial. Lancet Oncol 2011;12:997–1003.

23. Bernstein M, Berger MS. Neuro-oncology: The Essentials 3rd Edition. New York: Thieme; 2015. p. 130–4.

24. Stummer W, Pichlmeier U, Meinel T, et al. Fluorescence-guided surgery with 5-aminolevulinic acid for resection of malignant glioma: a randomised controlled multicentre phase III trial. Lancet Oncol 2006;7:392–401.

25. Barone DG, Lawrie TA, Hart MG. Image guided surgery for the resection of brain tumours. Cochrane Database Syst Rev 2014;(1): CD009685.

26. Brem H, Mahaley MS Jr, Vick NA, et al. Interstitial chemotherapy with drug polymer implants for the treatment of recurrent gliomas. J Neurosurg 1991;74:441–6.

27. Brem H, Ewend MG, Piantadosi S, et al. The safety of interstitial chemotherapy with BCNU-loaded polymer followed by radiation therapy in the treatment of newly diagnosed malignant gliomas: phase I trial. J Neurooncol 1995;26:111–23.

28. Brem H, Piantadosi S, Burger PC, et al. Placebo-controlled trial of safety and efficacy of intraoperative controlled delivery by biodegradable polymers of chemotherapy for recurrent gliomas. The Polymer-brain Tumor Treatment Group. Lancet 1995;345:1008–12.

29. Valtonen S, Timonen U, Toivanen P, et al. Interstitial chemotherapy with carmustine-loaded polymers for high-grade gliomas: a randomized double-blind study. Neurosurgery 1997;41:44–8 [discussion: 48–9].

30. Westphal M, Hilt DC, Bortey E, et al. A phase 3 trial of local chemotherapy with biodegradable carmustine (BCNU) wafers (Gliadel wafers) in patients with primary malignant glioma. Neuro Oncol 2003; 5:79–88.

31. Westphal M, Ram Z, Riddle V, et al. Gliadel wafer in initial surgery for malignant glioma: long-term follow-up of a multicenter controlled trial. Acta Neurochir (Wien) 2006;148:269–75 [discussion: 275].

32. Affronti ML, Heery CR, Herndon JE 2nd, et al. Overall survival of newly diagnosed glioblastoma patients receiving carmustine wafers followed by radiation and concurrent temozolomide plus rotational multiagent chemotherapy. Cancer 2009;115: 3501–11.

33. Pan E, Mitchell SB, Tsai JS. A retrospective study of the safety of BCNU wafers with concurrent temozolomide and radiotherapy and adjuvant temozolomide for newly diagnosed glioblastoma patients. J Neurooncol 2008;88:353–7.

34. Pavlov V, Page P, Abi-Lahoud G, et al. Combining intraoperative carmustine wafers and Stupp regimen in multimodal first-line treatment of primary glioblastomas. Br J Neurosurg 2015;29: 524–31.

35. McGirt MJ, Than KD, Weingart JD, et al. Gliadel (BCNU) wafer plus concomitant temozolomide therapy after primary resection of glioblastoma multiforme. J Neurosurg 2009;110:583–8.

36. Pallud J, Audureau E, Noel G, et al. Long-term results of carmustine wafer implantation for newly diagnosed glioblastomas: a controlled propensity-matched analysis of a French multicenter cohort. Neuro Oncol 2015;17:1609–19.

37. Olivi A, Grossman SA, Tatter S, et al. Dose escalation of carmustine in surgically implanted polymers in patients with recurrent malignant glioma: a New Approaches to Brain Tumor Therapy CNS Consortium trial. J Clin Oncol 2003;21: 1845–9.

38. Kleinberg L. Polifeprosan 20, 3.85% carmustine slow-release wafer in malignant glioma: evidence for role in era of standard adjuvant temozolomide. Core Evid 2012;7:115–30.

39. Andrews DW, Scott CB, Sperduto PW, et al. Whole brain radiation therapy with or without stereotactic radiosurgery boost for patients with one to three brain metastases: phase III results of the RTOG 9508 randomised trial. Lancet 2004;363(9422):1665.

40. Kondziolka D, Patel A, Lunsford LD, et al. Stereotactic radiosurgery plus whole brain radiotherapy versus radiotherapy alone for patients with multiple brain metastases. Int J Radiat Oncol Biol Phys 1999;45(2):427.

41. Souhami L, Seiferheld W, Brachman D, et al. Randomized comparison of stereotactic radiosurgery followed by conventional radiotherapy with carmustine to conventional radiotherapy with carmustine for patients with glioblastoma multiforme: report of Radiation Therapy Oncology Group 93-05 protocol. Int J Radiat Oncol Biol Phys 2004; 60:853–60.

42. DeVita Jr VT, Lawrence TS, Rosenberg SA, et al. Cancer: Principles & Practice of Oncology. 10th Edition. Philadelphia: Lippincott Williams & Wilkins; 2014. p. 136–57.

43. Laperriere NJ, Leung PM, McKenzie S, et al. Randomized study of brachytherapy in the initial management of patients with malignant astrocytoma. Int J Radiat Oncol Biol Phys 1998;41:1005–11.

44. Selker RG, Shapiro WR, Burger P, et al. The Brain Tumor Cooperative Group NIH Trial 87-01: a randomized comparison of surgery, external radiotherapy, and carmustine versus surgery, interstitial radiotherapy boost, external radiation therapy, and carmustine. Neurosurgery 2002;51:343–55 [discussion: 355–7].

45. Wernicke AG, Sherr DL, Schwartz TH, et al. Feasibility and safety of GliaSite brachytherapy in treatment of CNS tumors following neurosurgical resection. J Cancer Res Ther 2010;6:65–74.

46. Prados MD, Seiferheld W, Sandler HM, et al. Phase III randomized study of radiotherapy plus procarbazine, lomustine, and vincristine with or without BUdR for treatment of anaplastic astrocytoma: final report of RTOG 9404. Int J Radiat Oncol Biol Phys 2004;58:147–1152.

47. A study of the effect of misonidazole in conjunction with radiotherapy for the treatment of grades 3 and 4 astrocytomas. A report from the MRC Working Party on misonidazole in gliomas. Br J Radiol 1983;56:673–82.

48. Brachman DG, Pugh SL, Ashby LS, et al. Phase 1/2 trials of temozolomide, motexafin gadolinium, and 60-Gy fractionated radiation for newly diagnosed supratentorial glioblastoma multiforme: final results of RTOG 0513. Int J Radiat Oncol Biol Phys 2015;91:961–7.

49. Liotta LA, Kleinerman J, Saidel GM. Quantitative relationships of intravascular tumor cells, tumor vessels, and pulmonary metastases following tumor implantation. Cancer Res 1974;34:997–1004.

50. Folkman J. What is the evidence that tumors are angiogenesis dependent? J Natl Cancer Inst 1990;82:4–6.

51. Hanahan D, Folkman J. Patterns and emerging mechanisms of the angiogenic switch during tumorigenesis. Cell 1996;86:353–64.

52. Niederhuber JE, Armitage JO, Doroshow JH, et al. Abeloff's Clin Oncology. 5th edition. Philadelphia: Elsevier; 2014. p. 108–26.

53. Plate KH, Breier G, Weich HA, et al. Vascular endothelial growth factor is a potential tumour angiogenesis factor in human gliomas in vivo. Nature 1992;359:845–8.

54. Hicklin DJ, Ellis LM. Role of the vascular endothelial growth factor pathway in tumor growth and angiogenesis. J Clin Oncol 2005;23:1011–27.

55. Holmgren L, O'Reilly MS, Folkman J. Dormancy of micrometastases: balanced proliferation and apoptosis in the presence of angiogenesis suppression. Nat Med 1995;1:149–53.

56. Gimbrone MA, Leapman SB, Cotran RS, et al. Tumor dormancy in vivo by prevention of neovascularization. J Exp Med 1972;136:261–76.

57. Jain RK. Antiangiogenic therapy for cancer: current and emerging concepts. Oncology (Williston Park) 2005;19:7–16.

58. Jain RK. Normalization of tumor vasculature: an emerging concept in antiangiogenic therapy. Science 2005;307:58–62.

59. Johnson DH. Randomized phase II trial comparing bevacizumab plus carboplatin and paclitaxel with carboplatin and paclitaxel alone in previously untreated locally advanced or metastatic non-small-cell lung cancer. J Clin Oncol 2004;22:2184–91.

60. Escudier B, Pluzanska A, Koralewski P, et al. Bevacizumab plus interferon alfa-2a for treatment of metastatic renal cell carcinoma: a randomized, double-blind phase III trial. Lancet 2007;370:2103–11.

61. Miller K, Wang M, Gralow J, et al. Paclitaxel plus bevacizumab versus paclitaxel alone for metastatic breast cancer. N Engl J Med 2007;357:2666–76.

62. Stark-Vance V. Bevacizumab and CPT-11 in the treatment of relapsed malignant glioma. Neuro-Oncol 2005;7:369.

63. Chinot OL, Wick W, Mason W, et al. Bevacizumab plus radiotherapy–temozolomide for newly diagnosed glioblastoma. N Engl J Med 2014;370(8):709–22. Available at: http://www.nejm.org/doi/full/10.1056/NEJMoa1308345. Accessed February 28, 2016.

64. Chinot OL, de La Motte Rouge T, Moore N, et al. AVAglio: phase 3 trial of bevacizumab plus temozolomide and radiotherapy in newly diagnosed glioblastoma multiforme. Adv Ther 2011;28:334–40.

65. Gilbert MR, Dignam JJ, Armstrong TS, et al. A randomized trial of bevacizumab for newly diagnosed glioblastoma. N Engl J Med 2014;370:699–708.

66. Hegi ME, Liu L, Herman JG, et al. Correlation of O6-methylguanine methyltransferase (MGMT) promoter methylation with clinical outcomes in glioblastoma and clinical strategies to modulate MGMT activity. J Clin Oncol 2008;26:4189–99.

67. Hegi ME, Diserens AC, Gorlia T, et al. MGMT gene silencing and benefit from temozolomide in glioblastoma. N Engl J Med 2005;352:997–1003.

68. Crinière E, Kaloshi G, Laigle-Donadey F, et al. MGMT prognostic impact on glioblastoma is dependent on therapeutic modalities. J Neurooncol 2007;83:173–9.

69. Eoli M, Menghi F, Bruzzone MG, et al. Methylation of O6-methylguanine DNA methyltransferase and loss of heterozygosity on 19q and/or 17p are overlapping features of secondary glioblastomas with prolonged survival. Clin Cancer Res 2007;13:2606–13.

70. Chinot OL, Barrié M, Fuentes S, et al. Correlation between O6-methylguanine-DNA methyltransferase and survival in inoperable newly diagnosed glioblastoma patients treated with neoadjuvant temozolomide. J Clin Oncol 2007;25:1470–5.

71. Perry JR, Bélanger K, Mason WP, et al. Phase II trial of continuous dose-intense temozolomide in recurrent malignant glioma: RESCUE study. J Clin Oncol 2010;28(12):2051.

72. Wick A, Felsberg J, Steinbach JP, et al. Efficacy and tolerability of temozolomide in an alternating

weekly regimen in patients with recurrent glioma. J Clin Oncol 2007;25(22):3357–61.

73. Tolcher AW, Gerson SL, Denis L, et al. Marked inactivation of O6-alkylguanine-DNA alkyltransferase activity with protracted temozolomide schedules. Br J Cancer 2003;88:1004–11.

74. Kurzen H, Schmitt S, Näher H, et al. Inhibition of angiogenesis by non-toxic doses of temozolomide. Anticancer Drugs 2003;14:515–22.

75. Kim JT, Kim JS, Ko KW, et al. Metronomic treatment of temozolomide inhibits tumor cell growth through reduction of angiogenesis and augmentation of apoptosis in orthotopic models of gliomas. Oncol Rep 2006;16:33–9.

76. Gilbert MR, Wang M, Aldape KD, et al. Dose-dense temozolomide for newly diagnosed glioblastoma: a randomized phase III clinical trial. J Clin Oncol 2013;31:4085–91.

77. Armstrong TS, Wefel JS, Wang M, et al. Net clinical benefit analysis of radiation therapy oncology group 0525: a phase III trial comparing conventional adjuvant temozolomide with dose-intensive temozolomide in patients with newly diagnosed glioblastoma. J Clin Oncol 2013;31:4076–84.

78. Brada M, Stenning S, Gabe R, et al. Temozolomide versus procarbazine, lomustine, and vincristine in recurrent high-grade glioma. J Clin Oncol 2010;28:4601–8.

79. Wei W, Chen X, Ma X, et al. The efficacy and safety of various dose-dense regimens of temozolomide for recurrent high-grade glioma: a systematic review with meta-analysis. J Neurooncol 2015;125:339–49.

80. Nichols CR, Williams SD, Loehrer PJ, et al. Randomized study of cisplatin dose intensity in advanced germ cell tumors. A Southeastern and Southwest Oncology Group Protocol. J Clin Oncol 1991;9:1163–72.

81. Berens ME, Rief MD, Shapiro JR, et al. Proliferation and motility responses of primary and recurrent gliomas related to changes in epidermal growth factor receptor expression. J Neurooncol 1996;27:11–22.

82. Sugawa N, Yamamoto K, Ueda S, et al. Function of aberrant EGFR in malignant gliomas. Brain Tumor Pathol 1998;15:53–7.

83. Schlegel J, Merdes A, Stumm G, et al. Amplification of the epidermal-growth-factor-receptor gene correlates with different growth behaviour in human glioblastoma. Int J Cancer 1994;56:72–7.

84. Nishikawa R, Ji XD, Harmon RC, et al. A mutant epidermal growth factor receptor common in human glioma confers enhanced tumorigenicity. Proc Natl Acad Sci U S A 1994;91:7727–31.

85. Heimberger AB, Hlatky R, Suki D, et al. Prognostic effect of epidermal growth factor receptor and EGFRvIII in glioblastoma multiforme patients. Clin Cancer Res 2005;11:1462–6.

86. Haas-Kogan DA, Prados MD, Tihan T, et al. Epidermal growth factor receptor, protein kinase B/Akt, and glioma response to erlotinib. J Natl Cancer Inst 2005;97:880–7.

87. Uchida H, Marzulli M, Nakano K, et al. Effective treatment of an orthotopic xenograft model of human glioblastoma using an EGFR-retargeted oncolytic herpes simplex virus. Mol Ther 2013;21:561–9.

88. Wykosky J, Fenton T, Furnari F, et al. Therapeutic targeting of epidermal growth factor receptor in human cancer: successes and limitations. Chin J Cancer 2011;30:5–12.

89. Prados MD, Chang SM, Butowski N, et al. Phase II study of erlotinib plus temozolomide during and after radiation therapy in patients with newly diagnosed glioblastoma multiforme or gliosarcoma. J Clin Oncol 2009;27:579–84.

90. Brown PD, Krishnan S, Sarkaria JN, et al. Phase I/II trial of erlotinib and temozolomide with radiation therapy in the treatment of newly diagnosed glioblastoma multiforme: North Central Cancer Treatment Group Study N0177. J Clin Oncol 2008;26:5603–9.

91. Peereboom DM, Shepard DR, Ahluwalia MS, et al. Phase II trial of erlotinib with temozolomide and radiation in patients with newly diagnosed glioblastoma multiforme. J Neurooncol 2010;98:93–9.

92. Wong AJ, Ruppert JM, Bigner SH, et al. Structural alterations of the epidermal growth factor receptor gene in human gliomas. Proc Natl Acad Sci U S A 1992;89:2965–9.

93. Wikstrand CJ, McLendon RE, Friedman AH, et al. Cell surface localization and density of the tumor-associated variant of the epidermal growth factor receptor, EGFRvIII. Cancer Res 1997;57:4130–40.

94. Sampson JH, Heimberger AB, Archer GE, et al. Immunologic escape after prolonged progression-free survival with epidermal growth factor receptor variant III peptide vaccination in patients with newly diagnosed glioblastoma. J Clin Oncol 2010;28:4722–9.

95. Schuster J, Lai RK, Recht LD, et al. A phase II, multi-center trial of rindopepimut (CDX-110) in newly diagnosed glioblastoma: the ACT III study. Neuro Oncol 2015;17:854–61.

96. Reardon DA, Desjardins A, Schuster J, et al. Long-term survival benefit demonstrated in phase 2 ReACT Study of RINTEGA® in recurrent bevacizumab-naive glioblastoma (NASDAQ: CLDX). 2015. Available at: http://ir.celldex.com/releasedetail.cfm?ReleaseID=943877. Accessed March 26, 2016.

97. Available at: http://ir.celldex.com/releasedetail.cfm?ReleaseID=959021. Accessed April 12, 2016.

98. Kirson ED, Dbaly V, Tovarys F, et al. Alternating electric fields arrest cell proliferation in animal tumor models and human brain tumors. Proc Natl Acad Sci U S A 2007;104:10152–7.

99. Stupp R, Wong ET, Kanner AA, et al. NovoTTF-100A versus physician's choice chemotherapy in recurrent glioblastoma: a randomised phase III trial of a novel treatment modality. Eur J Cancer 2012;48:2192–202.

100. Stupp R, Taillibert S, Kanner AA, et al. Maintenance therapy with tumor-treating fields plus temozolomide vs temozolomide alone for glioblastoma. JAMA 2015;314:2535.

101. Lote K, Stenwig AE, Skullerud K, et al. Prevalence and prognostic significance of epilepsy in patients with gliomas. Eur J Cancer 1998;34:98–102.

102. Tandon PN, Mahapatra AK, Khosla A. Epileptic seizures in supratentorial gliomas. Neurol India 2001;49:55–9.

103. Penfield W. Relation of intracranial tumors and symptomatic epilepsy. Arch Neurol Psychiatry 1940;44:300.

104. Glantz MJ, Cole BF, Forsyth PA, et al. Practice parameter: anticonvulsant prophylaxis in patients with newly diagnosed brain tumors. Report of the Quality Standards Subcommittee of the American Academy of Neurology. Neurology 2000;54:1886–93.

105. Pace A, Bove L, Innocenti P, et al. Epilepsy and gliomas: incidence and treatment in 119 patients. J Exp Clin Cancer Res 1998;17:479–82.

106. Telfeian AE, Philips MF, Crino PB, et al. Postoperative epilepsy in patients undergoing craniotomy for glioblastoma multiforme. J Exp Clin Cancer Res 2001;20:5–10.

107. Taylor RS, Sander JW, Taylor RJ, et al. Predictors of health-related quality of life and costs in adults with epilepsy: a systematic review. Epilepsia 2011;52:2168–80.

108. Mendez MF. Depression in epilepsy. Arch Neurol 1986;43:766.

109. Sperling MR. The consequences of uncontrolled epilepsy. CNS Spectr 2004;9:98–109.

110. Löscher W, Potschka H. Role of multidrug transporters in pharmacoresistance to antiepileptic drugs. J Pharmacol Exp Ther 2002;301:7–14.

111. French JA. The role of drug-resistance proteins in medically refractory epilepsy. Epilepsy Curr 2002;2:166–7.

112. Fetell MR, Grossman SA, Fisher JD, et al. Preirradiation paclitaxel in glioblastoma multiforme: efficacy, pharmacology, and drug interactions. New Approaches to Brain Tumor Therapy Central Nervous System Consortium. J Clin Oncol 1997;15:3121–8.

113. Grossman SA, Hochberg F, Fisher J, et al. Increased 9-aminocamptothecin dose requirements in patients on anticonvulsants. NABTT CNS Consortium. The New Approaches to Brain Tumor Therapy. Cancer Chemother Pharmacol 1998;42:118–26.

114. Mason WP, MacNeil M, Kavan P, et al. A phase I study of temozolomide and everolimus (RAD001) in patients with newly diagnosed and progressive glioblastoma either receiving or not receiving enzyme-inducing anticonvulsants: an NCIC CTG study. Invest New Drugs 2012;30:2344–51.

115. Loghin ME, Prados MD, Wen P, et al. Phase I study of temozolomide and irinotecan for recurrent malignant gliomas in patients receiving enzyme-inducing antiepileptic drugs: a North American Brain Tumor Consortium study. Clin Cancer Res 2007;13:7133–8.

116. Chalk JB, Ridgeway K, Brophy T, et al. Phenytoin impairs the bioavailability of dexamethasone in neurological and neurosurgical patients. J Neurol Neurosurg Psychiatry 1984;47:1087–90.

117. Haque N, Thrasher K, Werk EE, et al. Studies on dexamethasone metabolism in man: effect of diphenylhydantoin. J Clin Endocrinol Metab 1972;34:44–50.

118. Rüegg S. Dexamethasone/phenytoin interactions: neurooncological concerns. Swiss Med Wkly 2002;132:425–6.

119. Penry JK, Newmark ME. The use of antiepileptic drugs. Ann Intern Med 1979;90:207–18.

120. Wen PY, Schiff D, Kesari S, et al. Medical management of patients with brain tumors. J Neurooncol 2006;80:313–32.

121. Moots PL, Maciunas RJ, Eisert DR, et al. The course of seizure disorders in patients with malignant gliomas. Arch Neurol 1995;52:717–24.

122. Bosma I, Vos MJ, Heimans JJ, et al. The course of neurocognitive functioning in high-grade glioma patients. Neuro Oncol 2007;9:53–62.

123. Taphoorn MJB, Klein M. Cognitive deficits in adult patients with brain tumours. Lancet Neurol 2004;3:159–68.

124. Klein M, Engelberts NH, van der Ploeg HM, et al. Epilepsy in low-grade gliomas: the impact on cognitive function and quality of life. Ann Neurol 2003;54:514–20.

125. Vecht CJ, Wagner GL, Wilms EB. Interactions between antiepileptic and chemotherapeutic drugs. Lancet Neurol 2003;2:404–9.

126. Macdonald DR, Cascino TL, Schold SC, et al. Response criteria for phase II studies of supratentorial malignant glioma. J Clin Oncol 1990;8:1277–80.

127. Wen PY, Macdonald DR, Reardon DA, et al. Updated response assessment criteria for high-grade gliomas: response assessment in neuro-oncology working group. J Clin Oncol 2010;28:1963–72.

128. de Wit MCY, de Bruin HG, Eijkenboom W, et al. Immediate post-radiotherapy changes in malignant glioma can mimic tumor progression. Neurology 2004;63:535–7.

129. Brandsma D, Stalpers L, Taal W, et al. Clinical features, mechanisms, and management of pseudoprogression in malignant gliomas. Lancet Oncol 2008;9:453–61.

130. Chamberlain MC, Glantz MJ, Chalmers L, et al. Early necrosis following concurrent Temodar and radiotherapy in patients with glioblastoma. J Neurooncol 2007;82:81–3.

131. Taal W, Brandsma D, de Bruin HG, et al. Incidence of early pseudo-progression in a cohort of malignant glioma patients treated with chemoirradiation with temozolomide. Cancer 2008;113:405–10.

132. Shah AH, Snelling B, Bregy A, et al. Discriminating radiation necrosis from tumor progression in gliomas: a systematic review what is the best imaging modality? J Neurooncol 2013;112:141–52.

133. Vredenburgh JJ, Desjardins A, Herndon JE 2nd, et al. Bevacizumab plus irinotecan in recurrent glioblastoma multiforme. J Clin Oncol 2007;25:4722–9.

134. Xu T, Chen J, Lu Y, et al. Effects of bevacizumab plus irinotecan on response and survival in patients with recurrent malignant glioma: a systematic review and survival-gain analysis. BMC Cancer 2010;10:252.

135. Keunen O, Johansson M, Oudin A, et al. Anti-VEGF treatment reduces blood supply and increases tumor cell invasion in glioblastoma. Proc Natl Acad Sci U S A 2011;108:3749–54.

136. Villano JL, Williams LE, Watson KS, et al. Delayed response and survival from NovoTTF-100A in recurrent GBM. Med Oncol 2013;30:338.

137. Huang RY, Neagu MR, Reardon DA, et al. Pitfalls in the neuroimaging of glioblastoma in the era of antiangiogenic and immuno/targeted therapy – detecting illusive disease, defining response. Front Neurol 2015;6:33.

138. Motl S, Zhuang Y, Waters CM, et al. Pharmacokinetic considerations in the treatment of CNS tumours. Clin Pharmacokinet 2006;45:871–903.

139. Neuwelt EA. Mechanisms of disease: the blood-brain barrier. Neurosurgery 2004;54:131–40 [discussion: 141–2].

140. de Lange ECM, Danhof M. Considerations in the use of cerebrospinal fluid pharmacokinetics to predict brain target concentrations in the clinical setting: implications of the barriers between blood and brain. Clin Pharmacokinet 2002;41:691–703.

141. Ungerstedt U. Microdialysis–principles and applications for studies in animals and man. J Intern Med 1991;230:365–73.

142. Zhou Q, Gallo JM. In vivo microdialysis for PK and PD studies of anticancer drugs. AAPS J 2005;7:E659–67.

143. Dabrosin C. Variability of vascular endothelial growth factor in normal human breast tissue in vivo during the menstrual cycle. J Clin Endocrinol Metab 2003;88(6):2695–8. Available at: http://www.ncbi.nlm.nih.gov/pubmed/12788875. Accessed March 29, 2016.

144. Poca MA, Sahuquillo J, Vilalta A, et al. Percutaneous implantation of cerebral microdialysis catheters by twist-drill craniostomy in neurocritical patients: description of the technique and results of a feasibility study in 97 patients. J Neurotrauma 2006;23:1510–7.

145. During MJ, Spencer DD. Extracellular hippocampal glutamate and spontaneous seizure in the conscious human brain. Lancet 1993;341(8861):1607–10. Available at: http://www.ncbi.nlm.nih.gov/pubmed/8099987. Accessed March 29, 2016.

146. Salci K, Nilsson P, Howells T, et al. Intracerebral microdialysis and intracranial compliance monitoring of patients with traumatic brain injury. J Clin Monit Comput 2006;20:25–31.

147. Mindermann T, Zimmerli W, Gratzl O. Rifampin concentrations in various compartments of the human brain: a novel method for determining drug levels in the cerebral extracellular space. Antimicrob Agents Chemother 1998;42:2626–9.

148. Blakeley JO, Olson J, Grossman SA, et al. Effect of blood brain barrier permeability in recurrent high grade gliomas on the intratumoral pharmacokinetics of methotrexate: a microdialysis study. J Neurooncol 2009;91:51–8.

149. Portnow J, Badie B, Chen M, et al. The neuropharmacokinetics of temozolomide in patients with resectable brain tumors: potential implications for the current approach to chemoradiation. Clin Cancer Res 2009;15:7092–8.

150. Dhodapkar M, Rubin J, Reid JM, et al. Phase I trial of temozolomide (NSC 362856) in patients with advanced cancer. Clin Cancer Res 1997;3:1093–100.

Index

Note: Page numbers of article titles are in **boldface** type.

A

Adoptive cellular therapy (ACT)
  clinical application of, 242f
  in melanomas, 241
  T cell receptor-engineered T cells in, 241–242
  tumor-infiltrating lymphocytes in, 241
Adult diffuse gliomas
  astrocytomas
    ATRX mutation in, 34, 39f, 40f
    IDH-mutated, 34, 39f, 40f
  molecular classification model, 33–34, 39f
  oligodendrogliomas, 34, 39f, 40
    loss of 1p/19q in, 40, 41f
    types of, 40
Adult glioblastomas, 41–43. *See also*
  Astrocytomas
  CDK4/6-p16^{ink4-a}-RB1-E2F pathway in, 43–44
  genomic copy number alterations in, 42–43f
  IDH-mutant, 41–42
  IDH-wild-type, 41–41
  molecular classification of, 41
  mutations in
    MET, 45
    MYC, 45
    NOTCH1 gene, 45
  O6-methylguanine-DNA methyltransferase
    (MGMT) in, 45–46
  p14^{ARF}-MDM2-MDM4-p53 pathway in, 44
  RTK-RAS-P13K pathway in, 44–45
    in *EGRF* gene, 44
    MET in, 45
    MYC family and, 45
    in *PDGFRA* gene, 44
    phosphatase and tensin *(PTEN)* homolog
      and, 44–45
Afatinib, for recurrent glioblastoma, 154, 160f
5-Aminolevulinic acid as tumor marker
  in fluorescence-guided surgery, 171–172, 190,
    191–192f
  lessons learned, 280
  in spectroscopic MRI, 190
Angiopoietins, as angiogenic factor, 57
Antiangiogenic therapy, **143–149**
  acquired resistance
    compensatory activation of pathways in, 58
    hypoxia-induced resistance, 58–59
    pericyte-mediated vessel protection in, 58
  angiogenic factors in, 56–57
    angiopoietins, 57

    basic fibroblast growth factor, 56
    hepatocyte growth factor, 57
    platelet-derived growth factor, 57
    vascular endothelial growth factor, 56
  antivascular agents in, 57
  early research in angiogenesis
    growth and blood supply, 143–144
    transparent chambers, 143
  lessons learned, 281–282
  molecular basis for use, 143–144
    proangiogenic tumor secreted factors
      in, 144
  new directions in
    endothelial metabolism and, 59
    vascular detransformation and, 59
  plus targeted molecular therapy, 65
  potential therapeutic barriers
    acquired resistance, 58–59
    primary resistance, 57–58
  primary resistance
    angiogenic pathway redundancy in, 57–58
    microenvironment-dependent protection
      in, 58
    vascular transformation in, 58
  therapeutic targets and treatment efficacy,
    55–57, 56f
  translation from other oncologic fields to
    glioblastoma, 144–145
  tumor secreted factors
    tumor angiogenesis, 144
    tumor vascular permeability, 144
Antiepileptic drugs (AEDs), health-related quality
  of life and, 256
Astrocytomas. *See also* Adult glioblastomas
  adult and pediatric
    BRF and H3K27M expression in, 46–47, 47f
    molecular classification model of, 46f
    pilocytic astrocytoma, 46
    pleomorphic xanthoastrocytoma, 46
  ATRX mutation in, 34, 39f, 40f
  IDH-mutated, 34, 39f, 40f
Awake craniotomy, **177–186**
  anesthesia complications
    airway, 179
    hemodynamic instability, 180
    intraoperative seizure, 179–180
  anesthetic considerations
    asleep-awake-asleep technique, 178
    dexmedetomidine, 179

Awake (*continued*)
    local anesthetics, 178
    monitored care, 179
    premedication, 178
    propofol and propofol-opiod combination, 179
indications for, 177
and intraoperative brain mapping, 169–170
patient outcomes, 182–183
    with complete tumor resections, 183
    Karnofsky performance status in, 183
    recollection, total to partial, 183
patient selection for, 177–178
    ideal patient, 178
technique
    cortical motor mapping, 181
    language mapping, 181, 182*f*
    positioning and pinning, 180
    subcortical motor mapping, 181
    surgical incision and draping, 180–181

B

Bailey, Percival, 2, 4*f*
Basic fibroblast growth factor, as angiogenic factor, 56
BCNU, for recurrent glioblastoma, as single and in combination therapy, 154, 155*f*
O-benzylguanine, for recurrent glioblastoma, 154, 156*f*
Bevacizumab (BEV)
    cost and cost-per-life year gained, 273
    lessons learned, 281–282
    for recurrence, 154
    for recurrent glioblastoma
        as single and in combination therapy, 154, 156*f*, 157*f*, 158*f*, 159*f*
Bevacizumab (BEV) clinical trials
    becacizumab in addition to Stupp protocol, 146–147
    in newly diagnosed glioblastoma
        Avastin trial, 146
        with temozolomide and radiation, 146
    for recurrent glioblastoma
        in irinotecan combination, 145
        with lomustine, 146
        as monotherapy, 145
        in sorafenib combination, 145–146
    resistance to, variations in imaging of, 147, 147*f*
Bevacizumab with temozolomide-radiotherapy (Stupp protocol), 146
Biomarkers
    chromosomal, 35*f*
    circulating tumor cell detection, 250
    in clinical practice, **33–53**
    definition and types of, 33, 34

epigenetic, 37–38*f*
extracellular macromolecule detection and
    circulating DNA and, 248
    glial fibrillary acidic protein and, 249
    metabolomics and, 249
    microRNA profiles and, 248–249
extracellular vesicle detection and, 249–250
    mRNA expression in, 249–250
    proteins with, 250
genetic, 35–38*f*
overview of chromosomal, genetic, epigenetic, and phenotypic alterations as, 35–38*f*
phenotypic, 38*f*
Brachytherapy, interstitial, 6, 6*f*, 105–106
Brain-blood barrier, drug penetration of, microdialysis measurement of, 285–286
Brain plasticity and glioma resection
    anatomofunctional subcortical connectivity subserving neural functions, 231–232
    central nervous system reshaping
        time course of disease and, 226–227
    implications of, 232–233
        for direct electriostimulation mapping, 232
        for multistage surgical approach, 232–233
    intraoperative
        acute functional remapping, 228–230
        direct electrostimulation mapping, 227, 228*f*, 229*f*
        task selection for cognitive mapping, 227–228
    neuroplasticity
        compensatory phenomena and, 225–226
        definition and mechanisms of, 226
        eloquent and noneloquent regions and, 225
        equipotentiality and, 225
    oncofunctional balance concept and, 233
    preoperative functional reallocation, 227, 228*f*
    probabilistic atlases of postsurgical residue and of functional plasticity, 230–231
    subcortical connectivity and minimal common brain and, 230–231
    white matter tract as limit of, 230–232
Brain plasticity and reorganization, **225–236**

C

Carbon ion therapy, 123, 124
Carboplatin, for recurrent glioblastoma, 154, 156*f*
Carmustine wafer (Gliadel), 208–209
    advantages of, 280–281
    benefits of, 280
    with chemoradiation, safety and efficacy of, 280
    complications with, 209–210
    cost and cost-per-life year gained, 273
    implantation of, 209, 210*f*

maximum tolerated dose, 281
  with radiation, survival in, 209, 209f
  for recurrent glioblastoma, 154, 157f, 209
Cediranib, for recurrent glioblastoma, 154, 157f
Cetuximab, for recurrent glioblastoma, 154, 157f
Chemotherapeutics, **133–141**
  current gold standard
    acquired resistance from mutations in DNA
      mismatch repair enzymes, 136
    attempts to improve, 136–137
    BCNU plus radiotherapy, 133–134
    chemotherapy with radiotherapy, 134
    dose-dense dosing strategy, 136–137
    intrinsic resistance from *MGMT* promoter
      methylation, 136
    irinotecan, 134
    nitrosoureas, 134
    resistance mechanisms and, 136
    temozolomide-based chemoradiotherapy,
      135–136
  lessons learned
    angiogensis inhibitors, 281–282
    bevacizumab, 281–282
    dose-dense temozolomide, 283
    epidermal growth factor receptor
      inhibitors, 283–284
  modalities beyond the current gold standard,
    137–138
    alternating tumor-treating electric fields,
      137–138
    antiangiogenic therapy, 137
    bevacizumab with irinotecan combination,
      137
    cilengitide, 137
  representative targeted therapies, 28t
  temozolomide-based chemoradiotherapy
    overall survival with, 133, 134t
    in recurrent glioblastoma, 138–139
  traditional therapy, 133
Chimeric antigen receptor-T therapy (CART)
  limitations of, 242
  trials of, 242–243
Cilengitide, for recurrent glioblastoma, 154,
  156f, 158f
Cognitive decline, from radiation treatment,
  126
Convection-enhanced drug delivery
  blood-brain barrier bypass, 208
  clinical applications of, 208
  improved diffusion and distribution of drug
    with, 207–208, 208f
Cortical motor mapping, in awake craniotomy,
  181
Cortical stimulation, intraoperative, 170, 171f
CTC (circulating tumor cells), 250
ctDNA (circulating DNA), 248
Cushing, Harvey Williams, 2, 4f, 6

Cushing, Harvey Williams and Percival Bailey
  classification of presumed cell of origin, 1, 2, 3f

D
Dendritic cell vaccines
  clinical applications of, 241f
  polyvalent, 241
  targeting EGFRvlll, 240–241
Diffusion tensor imaging (DTI), intraoperative,
  188–189, 189f
Direct electrostimulation mapping (DEM),
  intrasurgical, 227, 228f, 229f
ctDNA, 248
Drug delivery, through blood-brain barrier, 65
Drug-eluting wafers. *See also* Carmustine wafer
  (Gliadel)
  BCNU, 208–209

E
Early detection, **247–252**. *See also* Biomarkers
  benefits of, 247
  biomarkers in, 247, 248–250
  surface markers and mutations in, 247–248
EGFRvlll (epidermal growth factor receptor vlll), in
  peptide targeting, 238–239, 238f
Elderly patient
  chemoradiation and adjuvant TMZ in, 111
  comparison of hypofractionated RT and
    standard RT in, 113
    RT alone *versus* supportive care alone, 113
  comparison of RT alone with TMZ alone for
    efficacy in, 113–114
  hypofractionated radiation with concurrent
    and adjuvant TMZ in, 111
  prognosis for
    recursive positioning analysis classification
      in, 114, 114t
  radiation therapy alone, 111, 113
  stereotactic radiosurgery in, 114, 115–117t,
    118
    survival rates with, 114, 115–117t, 118
Epidermal growth factor receptor vlll (EGFRvlll), in
  peptide targeting, 238–239, 238f
Erlotinib, for recurrent glioblastoma, as single and
  in combination therapy, 154, 156f, 157f
Etirinotecan, for recurrent glioblastoma, 154, 160f
Etoposide, for recurrent glioblastoma, 154, 156f
Everolimus, for recurrent glioblastoma, 154, 156f

F
Fluid-attenuated inversion recovery (FLAIR)-
  weighted imaging
  preoperative, intraoperative, and
    postoperative in diffuse glioma surgery,
    228f, 229f

Fluorescence-guided surgery
    5-aminolevulinic acid enhancement in,
        171–172, 190, 191–192f
    fluorescein *versus* 5-aminolevulinic acid in,
        192–193
Folkman, Judah, 4
Functional neuro-oncology, 6

G
Gefitinib, for recurrent glioblastoma, 154, 155f,
    156f
GFAP (glial fibrillary acidic protein), 249
Gliadel wafer (carmustine wafer)
    for recurrent glioblastoma, 154, 157f
Glial fibrillary acidic protein (GFAP), 249
Glioblastoma
    diagnosis of
        advanced imaging in, 2
        MR imaging in, 2
    historical perspectives on
        advanced imaging, 5–6
        agiogenesis concept of, 4
        biopsy locations indicated on stereotaxic
            CT slice, 5f
        brachytherapy, 6, 6f
        concurrent chemoradiotherapy with TMZ, 7
        diagnosis of, 2–4, 3f, 4f
        functional neuro-oncology, 6
        management of, 4–7
        microsurgical instruments and techniques
            and, 4–5, 6f
        stereotactic method, 6
    historical perspectives on the diagnosis, 2–4
    history and modern correlates, **1–9**
    history from trephination to World Health
        Organization classification, 1–2, 2f
    molecular and genetic alterations leading
        to, 25f
    molecular subclassifications, 25t
    O(6)-methylguanine-DNA-methyltransferase,
        promoter methylation of, 17–18
    overall survival rate, 237
    pediatric
        ACVR1 gene mutations in, 48
        FGFR1 and *FGFR3* gene mutations in,
            48–49
        H3.3-ATRX-DAXX chromatin remodeling
            pathway in, 47–48, 47f
        H3F3A gene mutation, 48
        SEDTD2 protein in, 48
    predictive biomarkers in, 49
    prognostic and predictive molecular features
        of, 16t
    risk factors for, 265
        CMV infection, 265
        neurocysticercosis and, 265

signaling pathways in, 26f
subtypes and survival, 15–16
    DNA methylation changes and, 17–18
    epigenetic alterations, 17–18
    gene expression, 16t, 17, 23f
    prognostic and predictive molecular
        features of, 16t
    somatic mutations in, 16–17
Glioma
    classification of, 21
    distribution by histology subtypes, 21, 22f
    histology of, characteristic findings in, 21,
        22f, 23f
    incidence of
        sex, race, ethnicity, and age and, 11, 12f
        time trends in, 11
    risk factors for
        environmental, 15
        genomic variants, 15
        heritable genetic, 15
    subtypes
        primary and secondary, 22–23, 25f
        proneuronal, survival and, 22, 24f

H
Health-related quality of life (HRQOL)
    cognitive deficits and
        assessment in research studies, 257, 257t
        instruments in evaluation and monitoring
            of, 256
        motivation to improve and, 258
        neuropsychological assessment in, 256–257
        prevalence variations in differing patient
            populations, 258
        psychoeducation for patients and families,
            258–259
        psychostimulants for, 259
        rehabilitation for, 258, 259
        treatment of, 258–259
    disease-specific symptoms affecting, 253
    neurocognitive functioning association with,
        254, 254f
        cognitive functioning integral to HRQOL,
            254f, 255
    neurocognitive issues and
        chemotherapy and, 255–256
        evaluation and treatment of, 256–258, 257t
        radiotherapy and, 255
        symptom management medications, 256
    treatment impact on
        age-bias in studies of, 254
        antiangiogenic agent in, 254
        radiotherapy and chemotherapy, 254
        surgery, 253–254
Health-related quality of life (HRQOL),
    253–264

Heat shock proteins (HSPs), in peptide targeting, 239

Hepatocyte growth factor (HGF), as angiogenic factor, 57

Hodotopy, white matter tracts as limit of neural plasticity, 230–232

HRQOL. *See* Health-related quality of life (HRQOL)

I

Imaging, advanced, **81–103**

Imatinib, for recurrent glioblastoma, as single and in combination therapy, 154, 155*f*, 156*f*

Immunotherapy, **237–246**
  adoptive cellular therapy, 242–243
  background
    infection-remission coincidence in, 237–238
  chimeric antigen receptor cells and, 242–243
  classification by mechanisms, 238
  defined, 238
  dendritic cell vaccines, 240–241, 241*f*
  limitations and challenges of
    with chimeric antigen receptor T cells, 243
    in clinical trial design, 243–244
    with epidermal growth factor receptor variant (VIII), 243
    immunologic escapes, 243
    targeting immunosuppressive pathways, 243
  peptide targeting, 238–239, 238*f*
  plus targeted molecular therapy, 65
  for recurrence, 154, 161*t*, 162

Intraoperative imaging, **187–195**
  diffusion tensor imaging, 188–189, 189*f*
    advantage and disadvantage of, 189
  intraoperative MRI, 189–190, 190*t*, 279–280
  MRI neuronavigation, 187–188, 188*f*
    advantages and limitations of, 187–188
    devices for, 187, 188*f*
  spectroscopic MRI, whole-brain, 190

K

Karnofsky performance status, in awake craniotomy, 183

L

Language mapping, in awake craniotomy, 181, 182*f*

Laser interstitial thermal therapy (LITT), **197–206**
  biological basis for, 197–198
  for brain tumors and CNS disorders, 197
  versus chemotherapeutic options, 199
  histologic changes during, 198
  historical context and evolution of

    with CT stereotactic technique, 199
    use of hyperthermia for tumors in, 198–199
  indications for, 199
  for maximal tumor cytoreduction, 200
  versus microsurgical resection, 199
  MRI thermography, 198
  newly diagnosed glioblastoma studies, 201
  physical effects of, 197–198
  for radiation necrosis, 125–126
  recurrent glioblastoma studies, 200–201
  versus surgical options, 199–200
  systems available for, 201–202
  technical nuances in, 201–202

Lessons learned, **279–291**
  assessing treatment efficacy and effectiveness, challenges in, 284–285
  chemotherapy, 281–284
  drug penetration at specific site, 285–286
  intraoperative techniques, 279–281
  radiation therapy, 281
  seizures and antiepileptic agents, 284
  surgery, 279

LITT. *See* Laser interstitial thermal therapy (LITT)

Local drug delivery, **207–211**
  blood-brain barrier and, 207
  cellular infiltrative nature of the disease, 207
  convection-enhanced, 207–208, 208l*f*
  drug-eluting wafers, 208–210, 209*f*, 210*f*
  limitations to drug-eluting biomaterials, 207
  recent advances
    hydrogels, 210
    thermal gel depots, 210–211

Lomustine, for recurrent glioblastoma, 154, 159*f*

M

MacDonald criteria
  for radiograpic imaging in recurrent glioma, 98–99
  for treatment efficacy and effectiveness, 284–285

Magnetic resonance imaging (MRI)
  intraoperative, 279–280
  in neuronavigation, 187–188, 188*f*
  T1-weighted
    preoperative, intraoperative, and postoperative in diffuse glioma surgery, 228*f*, 229*f*

Magnetic resonance spectroscopy (MRS), 90, 91*f*

Medicare and Medicaid patients, radiation treatment and, 266–267

Minimally invasive target therapy, **197–206**

miRNA (microRNA), 248–249

Molcular pathogenesis
  glioma stem cell hypothesis, 27–29
    neurospheres in, 29
    signaling pathways in, 29

Molcular (*continued*)
  MGMT promoter methylation, 27
  targeted therapies and, 28t
Molecular diagnostic testing
  FISH, 49
  immunohistochemical complex techniques, 49
  next generation sequencing, 49
  single nucleotide variants, 49
Molecular pathogenesis, **21–31**
  classification and histology and, 21–22, 22f, 24f
  EGFR gene in, 24–25, 28t
  isocitrate dehydrogenase in, 26–27
  loss of heterogeneity
    on chromosome 10 and *PTEN* gene, 24
  MDM2 gene in, 23–24
  in primary and secondary, 22–23, 25f
  TP53 gene in, 23–24
Molecular targeting
  for recurrence, 161t, 162
Multimodality targeting of cells, **56–72**. *See also*
  Antiangiogenic therapy; Targeted molecular
  therapy
  in antiangiogenic therapy, 55–59
  in targeted molecular therapy, 59–64

N

National and global economic impact,
  271–278
  economic background and, 271, 272t
  income disparity effect on standard of care for
    treatment and follow-up, 274–275
    advanced disease in lower SES patients,
      275
    care in private *versus* public hospitals,
      274–275
    effect on prognosis and otcomes, 275
    insurance quality and treatment decisions,
      275
  national and international perspectives on
    economics
    aggressive stance toward expensive
      treatment, 275
    willingness-to-pay threshold per
      quality-adjusted life year, 276
  treatment costs
    of approved chemotherapy agents,
      273–274
    of bevacizumab, 273
    of carmustine wafer, 273
    direct medical and nonmedical, 271–272,
      272t
    incremental cost-effectiveness ratios and,
      271, 272t
    indirect, 271, 272t, 274
    of recommended treatment, 272–273
    of temozolomide, 273

Neurocognitive functioning after treatment,
  253–264
Neuronavigation
  intraoperative, 168–169, 169f
  MRI, 187–188, 188f
Nitrosoureas, for recurrence, 154

P

Peptide targeting
  EGFRvlll targeting with cdx-110, 238f, 239
  with heat shock proteins, 239
Pioglitazone, 154, 157f
Platelet-derived growth factor (PDGF/PDGFR), as
  angiogenic factor, 57
Proton radiation
  as boost with concomitant x-ray therapy,
    122–123
  cost/access for, 124
  plus targeted molecular therapy, 65
Pulsed reduced-dose-rate (PRDR) radiation
  therapy, for recurrence, 118, 122

R

Radiation necrosis
  cause of, 125
  laser interstitial thermal therapy for, 125–126
  treatment of, 125
Radiation standard of care. *See also* Reirradiation
  for current gliomas
  current
    chemoradiation after maximal surgical
      resection, 106
    dose-volume histogram in, 109, 110f
    immobilization in, 106–107, 107f
    intensity modulated, 109
    management of elderly patients, 111,
      113–114
    organs at risk for fractionated, 109, 109f
    prognosis with, 109, 111, 113t
    recursive partitioning analysis classification
      and prognosis in, 111, 113t
    recursive partitioning analysis classification
      in, 111, 112t
    survival data 111, 113t
    target volumes in, 107–109, 107t, 108f
    temozolomide with, 106
    treatment planning and delivery, 109,
      110–111f
    volume modulated, 109
  historical context
    as adjuvant therapy, 105
    Eastern Cooperative Oncology Group/
      Radiation Therapy Oncology Group
      study, 105
    interstitial brachytherapy, 105–106
    three-dimensional conformal RT, 106

Radiation treatment, **105–132**
  cost/access in
    of carbon ion therapy, 124
    of proton therapy, 124
  follow-up imaging
    diffusion tensor imaging, 124
    diffusion-weighted MRI, 124
    dynamic contrast-enhanced MRI, 124–125
    imaging findings to differentiate tumor
      recurrence from radiation necrosis, 125t
    magnetic resonance spectroscopy, 125
    MRI findings to differentiate recurrence
      from pseudoprogression, 126t
    PET, 125
  follow-up/imaging
    MRI brain sequences, 124
    pseudoprogression on MRI, 124
  lessons learned, 281
    stereotactic radiosurgery added to
      radiation for brain metastases, 281
  for recurrence, 162
  side effects of
    cognitive decline, 126
    radiation necrosis, 125–126
    radiation somnolence symptoms, 126
  standard management techniques, 281
Radiographic detection, **81–103**
Radiographic imaging
  advanced
    dynamic contrast-enhancement, 89–90, 89f
    dynamic perfusion and permeability
      imaging, 87, 89–90, 89f
    dynamic susceptibility contrast-enhanced,
      89–90, 89f
    gliomatosis cerebri in, 91, 93f
    magnetic resonance spectroscopy, 90, 91f
    response assessment in, 88t
  conventional features of, 81, 83t
    on computed tomography, 82, 84–85,
      84f, 85f
    on contrast-enhanced MRI, 85–86, 85f
    with contrast enhancement, 87, 88f
    on diffusion-weighted images, 86–87
    on fluid-attenuated inversion recovery
      imaging, 86, 88f
    nonenhancing components and, 86–87
    with pathologic and radiologic correlates,
      81, 82t
    on T-1 and T-2 weighted MR images,
      85–86, 85f, 88f
    typical patterns, 81, 82f
  future directions in, 99–100
    nanoparticle agents, 100
    nuclear medicine techniques, 100
  glioblastoma mimics in, 91–92, 94f
    abscess, 96
    arterial infarct, 96

    lymphoma, 93–94
    metastases, 92–93
    other primary glial neoplasms, 94–96
    tumefactive demyelination, 96
  in multicentric and multifocal glioblastoma,
    90–91, 92f
  in other primary glial neoplasms, 94–96
  in recurrent disease *versus* treatment effects
    of chemoradiation, 97
    complication of anti-vascular endothelial
      growth factor monoclonal antibody
      (bevacizumab), 97, 99f
    guidelines for reponse to therapy and,
      98–99
    immediate postoperative period, 96–97
    MacDonald criteria, 98–99
    new enhancing lesions and, 97
    pseudoprogression radiation necrosis, 97,
      98f, 99f
    of radiation, 97, 98f
    Response Assessment in Neuro-Oncology
      criteria, 98–99
Recurrence
  chemotherapy for
    alternative delivery methods in, 162t
    bevacizumab, 154
    immunotherapy, 154, 161t, 162
    molecular targeting, 161t, 162
    nitrosoureas, 154
    novel agents, 154, 155–160t
    temozolomide, 154
    vaccine therapies, 161t
  definition of, 151–153
    MacDonald criteria, 151, 152t
    Response Assessment in Neuro-Oncology
      criteria for, 151, 152t
  radiotherapy for, 162
  surgical intervention in
    carmustine wafer implantation and,
      153–154
    gross total resection, 153
    subtotal resection, 153, 153f
  tumor-treating electric fields *versus* best
    physician's choice in, 218–219, 219f
    dexamethasone effect on survival,
      219, 220f
Recurrent glioblastoma, **151–165**
Reirradiation for recurrence, 118–122
  future directions
    carbon ion therapy, 123, 124
    proton therapy, 122–123, 124
    pulsed reduced-dose-rate radiation therapy,
      118, 122
    stereotactic radiosurgery, 118, 119–121t
Response Assessment in Neuro-oncology criteria
  for radiograpic imaging in recurrent glioma,
    98–99

Response (*continued*)
　for treatment efficacy and effectiveness,
　　284–285
microRNA, 248–249

S
Sagopilone, for recurrent glioblastoma, 154, 158*f*
Scherer, Hans Joachim, concept of primary *versus*
　secondary glioblastoma, 2
Seizures and brain tumor-related epilepsy,
　antiepileptic drugs for, 284
Socioeconomics and survival, **265–269**
Socioeconomic status
　and access to care, 268
　Australian patients, 267
　in Brazil, 268
　Canadian farmers, 267
　and diagnosis, 265–266
　　early *versus* late hospice enrollment, 267
　　gender and, 266
　　higher SES and increased survival, 267
　　high SES and higher risk, 266
　　Medicaid patient, 265–266
　Greek patients, 267–286
　radiation treatment in Medicare and Medicaid
　　patients and, 266–267
　and treatment and follow-up, 266–267
　UK National Health Service, 267
Sorafenib, for recurrent glioblastoma, 154, 158*f*
Spectroscopic MRI (sMRI)
　5-aminolevulinic acid enhancement in, 190
　intraoperative, 190
Standards of care, **73–80**
　for chemotherapy and radiation
　　in elderly patients, 77
　　specific patient subgroups, 77
　　survival with radiotherapy plus
　　　temozolomide *versus* radiotherapy
　　　alone, 76–77, 76*f*
　　temozolomide in, 75–76, 76*f*
　for newer treatment strategies
　　bevacizumab, 77–78
　　tumor-treating fields plus temozolomide,
　　　78*f*, 79
　for radiation. See Radiation standard of care
　for surgical intervention, 73–75
　　correlation between residual tumor volume
　　　and median overall survival, 74, 75*f*
　　survival based on extent of resection, 74*f*
　　survival with carmustine wafer adjuvant
　　　therapy, 75
Stem cell hypothesis, 27–29
　factors involved in stem cell renewal, 29*f*
　neurospheres in, 29
　signaling pathways in, 29
Stereotactic radiosurgery (SRS)

in elderly patient, 114, 115–117*t*, 118
　for recurrent gliobastoma, 118, 119–121*t*
Stupp protocol (bevacizumab with
　temozolomide-radiotherapy), 146
Subcortial motor mapping, in awake craniotomy,
　181
Subcortical connectivity
　anatomofunctional subserving neural
　　functions, 231–232
　and minimal common brain, 230–231
Sulfasalazine, for recurrent glioblastoma,
　154, 156*f*
Sunitinib, for recurrent glioblastoma, 154,
　158*f*, 159*f*
Surgical treatment, **167–176**
　intraoperative standards of resection, 168–172
　　awake craniotomy and intraoperative brain
　　　mapping, 169–170
　　cortical stimulation in, 170, 171*f*
　　fluorescence-guided with 5-aminolevulinic
　　　acid, 171–172
　　intraoperative MRI, 170–171
　　neuronavigation, 168–169, 169*f*
　lessons learned, 279
　outcome
　　extent of resection and, 172
　preoperative evaluation for
　　brain MRI with and without enhancement
　　　in, 167
　　corticosteroids in, 167
　　history and physical examination in, 167
　preoperative planning for
　　functional MRI in, 167–168, 168*f*
　　structural MRI in, 167–168, 168*f*
　tenets of, 172
Survival
　after diagnosis, 1-year, 2-year, 3-year, 4-year,
　　and 5-year, 11–12, 13*f*, 14
　long-term, 14–15
　subtypes and
　　mutations in *IDH1/1DH2* mutations a
　　　marker, 15
　　primary glioblastoma, 15
　　secondary, 15–16
　time trends in 1-year and 5-year, 14
　trends in, **11–19**

T
Tamoxifen, for recurrent glioblastoma, 154, 155*t*
Targeted molecular therapy, 59–64
　new directions
　　antiangiogenesis plus targeted molecular
　　　therapy, 65
　　combinations of multiple therapeutic
　　　modalities, 65
　　combined targeted molecular therapies, 64

immunotherapy plus targeted molecular therapy, 65
improvement in drug delivery through the blood-brain barrier, 65
multiple agent combinations, 64–65
new molecular targets, 64
proton radiation plus targeted molecular therapy, 65
single agents, 64
potential therapeutic barriers
blood-brain barrier, 64
intratumoral heterogeneity, 63–64
signaling pathway redundancy, 64
treatment-resistant glioma stem cells, 63
targets and treatment efficacy
hedgehog pathway, 62
histone deaceylase, 63
isocitrate dehydrogenase 1/2, 63
Janus kinase/signal transducer and activator of transcription pathway, 62
notch pathway, 62
phosphatidylinositol 3-kinase/Akt-mammalian target of rapamycin pathway, 61–62
proteasome inhibition, 63
rat sarcoma/rapidly activated fibrosarcoma/mitogen-activated erk kinase/extracellular signal-regulated kinase pathway, 62
receptor tyrosine kinases, 59, 61
transforming growth factor-beta pathway, 62
WNT/beta-catein pathway, 62–63
Temozolomide (TMZ)
adjuvant with chemoradiation, 111
adjuvant with chemoradiation in elderly patient, 111
cost and cost-per-life year gained, 273
with current chemoradiation, 106
dose-dense, lessons learned, 283
for recurrence, 154
for recurrent glioblastoma
as single and in combination therapy, 154, 155t, 158t, 159f, 160f
Temozolomide (TMZ)-based chemoradiation, 135–136
Temsirolimus, for recurrent glioblastoma, 154, 155f
Thalidomide, and derivatives, as antivascular agents, 57
TMZ. See Temozolomide (TMZ)
Treatment efficacy and effectiveness
MacDonald criteria for, 284–285
pseudoprogression, treatment-induced, 285
Response Assessment in Neuro-oncology criteria for, 285
Tumor-treating (electric) fields (TTFs), **213–224**
biological basis for, 213–214
cell biology effects during mitosis, 214, 214f
in clinical practice, 219, 221
electromagnetic spectrum in treatment of brain tumors, 214f
first-in-human trial of, 218
historical context of, 213, 214f
increased overall and progression-free survival compared with adjuvant temozolomide, 284
at interface of cerebrospinal fluid and brain tissue, 215, 217–218
intracranial distribution of, 215, 216f
for newly-diagnosed glioblastoma, efficacy of, 221
Patient Registry Data Set for, 221
physical properties of, 215–218
physical science supporting, 214, 214lf
physics of, 215
in recurrent glioblastoma, 218–219
sensitivity analysis of distribution, 215, 216f
with TMZ versus TMZ alone, 137–138
transducer array delivery of, 215, 216f
variation in electric properites of gliomas, 218

V

Vaccine therapies, for recurrence, 161t
Vascular endothelial growth factor (VEGF)
as angiogenic factor, 56
and tumor vascularity, 143
Vascular endothelial growth factor inhibitor, 146
Viral vaccines, 239
oncolytic
adenoviruses, 239
herpes simplex virus, 239
polioviruses, 239
timeline of development for glioblastomas, 240f
Vorinostat, for recurrent glioblastoma, 154, 156f, 158f

W

World Health Organization (WHO) classification, 2, 21

Y

Yasargil, M. Gazi, microsurgical instruments and techniques, 4–5, 6f

Printed and bound by CPI Group (UK) Ltd, Croydon, CR0 4YY

08/05/2025

01864757-0001